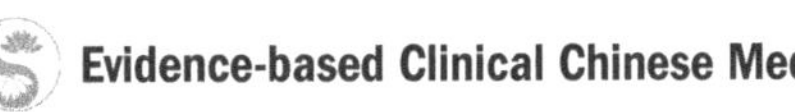 **Evidence-based Clinical Chinese Medicine**

Volume 17
Colorectal Cancer

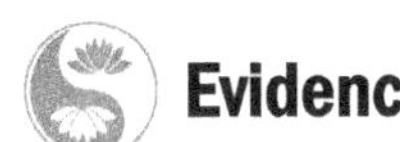

Evidence-based Clinical Chinese Medicine

Co Editors-in-Chief

Charlie Changli Xue
RMIT University, Australia

Chuanjian Lu
Guangdong Provincial Hospital of Chinese Medicine, China

Volume 17
Colorectal Cancer

Lead Authors

Brian H May
RMIT University, Australia

Yihong Liu
Guangdong Provincial Hospital of Chinese Medicine, China

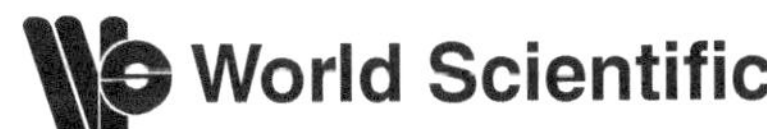

World Scientific

NEW JERSEY · LONDON · SINGAPORE · BEIJING · SHANGHAI · HONG KONG · TAIPEI · CHENNAI · TOKYO

Published by

World Scientific Publishing Co. Pte. Ltd.

5 Toh Tuck Link, Singapore 596224

USA office: 27 Warren Street, Suite 401-402, Hackensack, NJ 07601

UK office: 57 Shelton Street, Covent Garden, London WC2H 9HE

Library of Congress Cataloging-in-Publication Data
Names: Xue, Charlie Changli, author. | Lu, Chuan-jian, 1964–   author.
Title: Evidence-based clinical Chinese medicine / Charlie Changli Xue, Chuanjian Lu.
Description: New Jersey : World Scientific, 2016. | Includes bibliographical references and index.
Identifiers: LCCN 2015030389| ISBN 9789814723084 (v. 1 : hardcover : alk. paper) |
    ISBN 9789814723091 (v. 1 : paperback : alk. paper) |
    ISBN 9789814723121 (v. 2 : hardcover : alk. paper) |
    ISBN 9789814723138 (v. 2 : paperback : alk. paper) |
    ISBN 9789814759045 (v. 3 : hardcover : alk. paper) |
    ISBN 9789814759052 (v. 3 : paperback : alk. paper)
Subjects: | MESH: Medicine, Chinese Traditional--methods. | Clinical Medicine--methods. |
    Evidence-Based Medicine--methods. | Psoriasis. | Pulmonary Disease, Chronic Obstructive.
Classification: LCC RC81 | NLM WB 55.C4 | DDC 616--dc23
LC record available at http://lccn.loc.gov/2015030389

Volume 17: Colorectal Cancer
ISBN 978-981-121-418-9 (hardcover)
ISBN 978-981-123-542-9 (paperback
ISBN 978-981-121-419-6 (ebook for institutions)
ISBN 978-981-121-420-2 (ebook for individuals)

First published 2020
Reprinted 2021

British Library Cataloguing-in-Publication Data
A catalogue record for this book is available from the British Library.

For any available supplementary material, please visit
https://www.worldscientific.com/worldscibooks/10.1142/11661#t=suppl

Disclaimer

The information in this book is based on systematic analyses of the best available evidence for Chinese medicine interventions both historical and contemporary. Every effort has been made to ensure accuracy and completeness of the data herein. This book is intended for clinicians, researchers and educators. The practice of evidence-based medicine consists of consideration of the best available evidence, practitioners' clinical experience and judgment, and patients' preference. Not all interventions are acceptable in all countries. It is important to note that some of the substances mentioned in this book may no longer be in use, may be toxic, or may be prohibited or restricted under the provisions of the Convention on International Trade in Endangered Species of Wild Fauna and Flora (CITES). Practitioners, researchers and educators are advised to comply with the relevant regulations in their country and with the restrictions on the trade in species included in CITES appendices I, II and III. This book is not intended as a guide for self-medication. Patients should seek professional advice from qualified Chinese medicine practitioners.

Foreword

Since the late 20th century, Chinese medicine, including acupuncture and herbal medicine, has been increasingly used throughout the world. The parallel development and spread of evidence-based medicine has provided challenges and opportunities for Chinese medicine. The opportunities have been evidence-based medicine's emphasis on the effective use of the best available clinical evidence, incorporating the clinicians' clinical experience, subject to patients' preference. Such practices have a patient focus which reflects the historical nature of Chinese medicine practice. However, the challenges are also significant due to the fact that, despite the long-term development and very rich literature accumulated over 2,000 years, there is an overall lack of high-level clinical evidence for many of the interventions used in Chinese medicine.

To address this knowledge gap, we need to generate clinical evidence through high-quality clinical studies and to evaluate evidence to enable effective use of the available evidence to promote evidence-based Chinese medicine practice.

Modern Chinese medicine is rooted in its classical literature and the legacies of ancient doctors, grounded in the practice of expert clinicians and increasingly informed by clinical and experimental research efforts. In recognition of the unique features of Chinese medicine, for each of the conditions in this series a 'whole-evidence' approach is used to provide a synthesis of different types and levels of evidence to enable practitioners to make clinical decisions informed by the current best evidence.

There are four main components of this 'whole-evidence' approach. In the first component, we present the current approaches to the diagnosis, differentiation and treatment in each condition based on expert consensus expressed in textbooks and clinical guidelines. This provides an overview of how the condition is currently managed. The second component provides an analysis of the condition in historical context based on systematic searches of the *Zhong Hua Yi Dian* which includes the full texts of more than 1,000 classical medical books. These analyses provide objective views on how the condition has been treated over two millennia, reveal continuities and discontinuities between traditional and modern practice, and suggest avenues for future research.

The third component is the assessment of evidence derived from modern clinical studies of Chinese medicine interventions. The methods established by the *Cochrane Collaboration* are used for conducting systematic reviews and undertaking meta-analyses of outcome data for randomised controlled trials (RCTs). In addition, the clinical relevance of meta-analysis data is enhanced by examining the herbal formulas, individual herbs and acupuncture treatments that were assessed in the RCTs, and the evidence base is broadened by the inclusion of data from controlled clinical trials and non-controlled studies. The fourth component is to determine how the herbal medicine interventions may achieve the effects indicated by the clinical trials. Thus for each of the most frequently used herbs we provide reviews of their effects in pre-clinical models and their likely mechanisms of action.

For each condition, this 'whole-evidence' approach links clinical expertise, historical precedent, clinical research data and experimental research to provide the reader with assessments of the current state of the evidence for the efficacy, effectiveness and safety of Chinese medicine interventions using herbal medicines, acupuncture and moxibustion, and other health care practices such as *tai chi*.

Since these books are available in Chinese and English, they can benefit patients, practitioners and educators internationally and enable practitioners to make clinical decisions informed by the current best evidence.

These publications represent a major milestone in the development of Chinese medicine and make a significant contribution to the development of evidence-based Chinese medicine globally.

Co-Editors-in-Chief

Distinguished Professor Charlie Changli Xue, RMIT University, Australia

Professor Chuanjian Lu, Guangdong Provincial Hospital of Chinese Medicine, China

Purpose of this Book

This book is intended for clinicians, researchers and educators. It can be used to inform tertiary education and clinical practice by providing systematic, multidimensional assessments of the best available evidence for using Chinese medicine to manage each common clinical condition.

How to Use this Book

Some Definitions

A glossary is included, containing terms and definitions which frequently appear in the book. It also describes the definitions of statistical tests, methodological terms, evaluation tools and interventions. For example, in this book, integrative medicine refers to the combined use of a Chinese medicine treatment with conventional medical management, and combination therapies refer to two or more Chinese medicines from different therapy groups (e.g. Chinese herbal medicine, acupuncture or other Chinese medicine therapies) administered together. Terminology used throughout the book is based on the World Health Organisation's *Standard Terminologies on Traditional Medicine in the Western Pacific Region* (2007) where possible or from the cited reference.

Data Analysis and Interpretation of Results

In order to synthesise the clinical evidence, a range of statistical analysis approaches are used. In general, the effect size for dichotomous data is reported as a risk ratio (RR) with 95% confidence interval (CI), and for continuous data, they are reported as mean difference (MD) with 95% CI. Statistically significant effects are indicated with an asterisk*. Readers should note that statistical significance does not necessarily correspond with a clinically important effect. Interpretation of results should take into consideration the clinical significance, quality of studies (expressed as high, low or unclear risk of bias in this book) and heterogeneity amongst the studies. Tests for heterogeneity are conducted using the I^2 statistic. An I^2 score greater than 50% was considered to indicate substantial or considerable heterogeneity.

Use of Evidence in Practice

The Grading of Recommendations Assessment, Development and Evaluation (GRADE) approach was used to summarise the results and the certainty of the evidence for critical and important comparisons and outcomes. Due to the diverse nature of Chinese medicine practice, treatment recommendations are not included with the summary of findings tables. Therefore readers will need to interpret the evidence with reference to the local practice environment.

Limitations

Readers should note some of the methodological limitations of the classical literature and the clinical evidence.

- Search terms used to search the *Zhong Hua Yi Dian* database may not include all terms that have been used for the condition, which may alter the findings.
- Chinese language has changed over time. Citations have been interpreted for analysis, and such interpretations may be subject to disagreement.
- Chinese medicine theory has evolved over time. As such, concepts described in classical Chinese medical literature may no longer be found in contemporary works.

- Symptoms described in citations may be common to many conditions, and a judgment was required to determine the likelihood of the citation being related to the condition. This may have introduced some bias due to the subjective nature of the judgment.
- The vast majority of the clinical evidence for Chinese medicine treatments has come from China. The applicability of the findings to other populations and other countries requires further assessment.
- Many studies included participants with varying disease severity. Where possible, subgroup analyses were undertaken to examine the effects in different subpopulations. As this was not always possible, the findings may be limited to the population included, and not to subpopulations.
- The potential risk of bias found in many included studies suggested methodological limitations. The findings for GRADE assessments based on studies of very low to moderate quality evidence should be interpreted accordingly.
- Nine major English and Chinese language databases were searched to identify clinical studies, in addition to clinical trial registers. Other studies may exist which were not identified through searches, and which may alter the findings.
- The calculation of frequency of herbal formula use was based on formula names. It is possible that studies evaluated herbal treatments with the same or similar herb ingredients, but which were given different formula names. Due to the complexity of herbal formulas, it was considered not appropriate to make a judgment as to the similarity of formulas for analysis. As such, the frequency of formulas reported in Chapter 5 may be underestimated.
- The most frequently utilised herbs which may have contributed to the treatment effect have been described in Chapter 5. These herbs may provide leads for further exploration. Calculation of the herbs with potential effect is based on frequency of formulas reported in the studies, and does not take into consideration the clinical implications and functions of every herb in a formula.

Authors and Contributors

Co-editors-in-Chief
Dist. Prof. Charlie Changli Xue (*RMIT University, Australia*)
Prof. Chuanjian Lu (*Guangdong Provincial Hospital of Chinese Medicine, China*)

Co-deputy Editors-in-Chief
Assoc. Prof. Anthony Lin Zhang (*RMIT University, Australia*)
Dr. Brian H May (*RMIT University, Australia*)
Prof. Xinfeng Guo (*Guangdong Provincial Hospital of Chinese Medicine, China*)
Prof. Zehuai Wen (*Guangdong Provincial Hospital of Chinese Medicine, China*)

Lead Authors
Dr. Brian H May (*RMIT University, Australia*)
Dr. Yihong Liu (*Guangdong Provincial Hospital of Chinese Medicine, China*)

Co-authors
RMIT University (Australia):
Assoc. Prof. Anthony Lin Zhang
Prof. Charlie Changli Xue

Guangdong Provincial Hospital of Chinese Medicine (China):
Prof. Chuanjian Lu
Dr. Haibo Zhang
Prof. Xinfeng Guo

Members of Advisory Committee and Panel

Assoc. Prof. Ying Guo (*Department of Palliative, Rehabilitation and Integrative Medicine, MD Anderson Cancer Center, Texas, United States*)

Assoc. Prof. Wen Li Liu (*Integrative Medicine Program, MD Anderson Cancer Center, Texas, United States*)

Professor Charlie Changli Xue

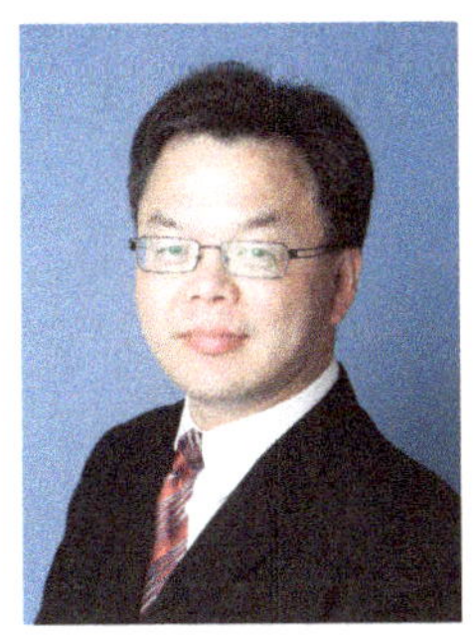

Distinguished Professor Charlie Changli Xue holds a Bachelor of Medicine (majoring in Chinese Medicine) from Guangzhou University of Chinese Medicine, China (1987) and a PhD from RMIT University, Australia (2000). He has been an academic, researcher, regulator and practitioner for almost three decades. Prof Xue has made significant contributions to evidence-based educational development, clinical research, regulatory framework and policy development, and provision of high-quality clinical care to the community. Professor Xue is recognised internationally as an expert in evidence-based traditional medicine and integrative health care.

Professor Xue is the Inaugural National Chair of the Chinese Medicine Board of Australia appointed by the Australian Health Workforce Ministerial Council (in 2011), and he was reappointed for a second term in 2014. Since 2007, he has been a Member of the World Health Organisation (WHO) Expert Advisory Panel for Traditional and Complementary Medicine, Geneva. Professor Xue is also Honorary Senior Principal Research Fellow at the Guangdong Provincial Academy of Chinese Medical Sciences, China.

At RMIT, Professor Xue is Executive Dean, School of Health and Biomedical Sciences. He is also Director of the WHO Collaborating Centre for Traditional Medicine.

Between 1995 and 2010, Professor Xue was Discipline Head of Chinese Medicine at RMIT University. He leads the development of five successful undergraduate and postgraduate degree programmes in Chinese Medicine at RMIT University which is now a global leader in Chinese medicine education and research.

Professor Xue's research has been supported by research grants of over AUD 15 million, including six project grants from the Australian Government's National Health and Medical Research Council (NHMRC) and two Australian Research Council (ARC) grants. He has contributed over 200 publications and has been frequently invited as keynote speaker for numerous national and international conferences. Professor Xue has contributed to over 300 media interviews on issues related to complementary medicine education, research, regulation and practice.

Professor Chuanjian Lu

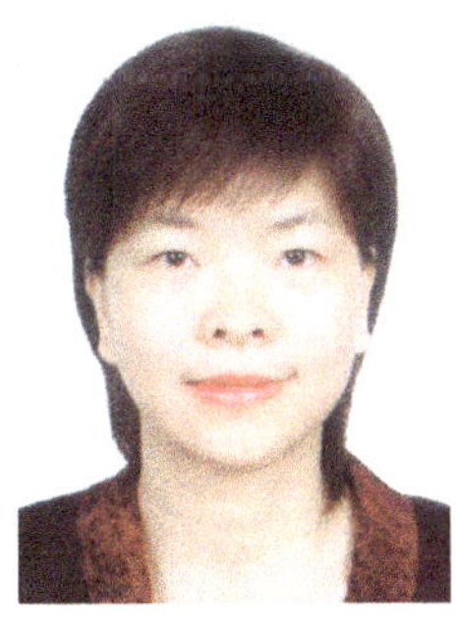

Professor Chuanjian Lu is the Vice-president of Guangdong Provincial Hospital of Chinese Medicine (Guangdong Provincial Academy of Chinese Medical Sciences, Second Clinical Medical College of Guangzhou University of Chinese Medicine). She also is the Chair of the Guangdong Traditional Chinese Medicine (TCM) Standardisation Technical Committee, and the Vice-chair of the Immunity Specialty Committee of the World Federation of Chinese Medicine Societies (WFCMS).

Professor Lu has engaged in scientific research into TCM, clinical practice and teaching for some 25 years. Her research has been devoted to integrating traditional and western medicine. She has edited and published 12 monographs and 120 academic research articles as first author and corresponding author with over 30 articles being included in SCI journals.

She has received widespread recognition for her achievements with awards for Excellent Teacher of South China, National Outstanding Women TCM Doctor and National Outstanding Young Doctor of TCM. She also received the Science and Technology Star of the Association of Chinese Medicine, the National Excellent Science and Technology Workers of China Award and the Five-continent Women's Scientific Awards of China Medical Women's Association.

Professor Lu has won the Award of Science and Technology Progress over ten times from Guangdong Provincial Government, China Association of Chinese Medicine and Chinese Hospital Association.

Acknowledgements

The authors and contributors would like to acknowledge the valuable contributions of the following people who assisted with database searches, data extraction, data screening, data assessment, translation of documents, editing, and/or administrative tasks: Su-yueh Chang, Dr Menghua Chen, Dr Meaghan Coyle, Dr Jhodie Duncan, Jiaming Fan, Shaonan Liu, Lihong Yang, Jing Chen, Yihan He, Qianqian Tian, Jinqiang Wei, Cuixian Huang, Yanhong Chen, Dr Claire Zhang, Dr Iris Zhou.

Contents

3. **Classical Chinese Medicine Literature**   **55**

Contents

List of Figures

List of Tables

1

Introduction to Colorectal Cancer

OVERVIEW

This chapter introduces colorectal cancer from the perspective of modern medicine. It outlines the pathological features of the disease, its epidemiology and risk factors, how the disease is diagnosed and how the stage is determined. The management of colorectal cancer in conventional medicine is described, including screening for early detection, adenoma management, surgery, chemotherapy, radiotherapy, chemo-radiotherapy, targeted therapies, post-therapy monitoring, survival rates and palliative care.

Definition of Colorectal Cancer

The term 'colorectal cancer' (CRC) includes tumours of the right colon (caecum, ascending colon), transverse colon, left colon from the splenic flexure downwards, and rectum to anus.[1] The *International Statistical Classification of Diseases* (ICD 10) specifies colorectal cancer under malignant neoplasms of the colon (C18), rectosigmoid junction (C19) and rectum (C20), with anal cancer as C21.[2]

More than 90% of tumours are classed as adenocarcinomas; however, there is variation in the characteristics of the disease and its treatment according to location.[1] In the United States about 72% of diagnoses were located in the colon and 28% in the rectum.[3] The majority of tumours of the colon are in the descending colon (left side).[4] Rectal cancer is located 15 cm or less from the anal margin and anal cancer is in the anal canal and/or anal margin.[1,5,6]

Clinical Presentation and Subtypes

In the early stages, CRC tends to be asymptomatic. Clinical indications of CRC include change in bowel habit, blood in the stool, bowel obstruction, abdominal pain, abdominal mass, tenesmus, unexplained constipation or diarrhoea, weight loss and/or unexplained anaemia. Such clinical indications are often indicative of more advanced cancer.[7] Rectal cancer can be detected by digital examination and endoscopy[5] and anal cancer by digital examination and/or observation.[6]

With the advent of screening programmes, diagnosis is often preceded by a positive result on a guaiac-based faecal occult blood test (gFOBT) which can detect about 50% of cancers, the more sensitive faecal immunochemical tests (FIT) and/or colonoscopy.[7] In people with higher risks of CRC, detection may be via barium enema, colonoscopy, flexible sigmoidoscopy or computed tomography (CT) colonography.[1,7,8]

Epidemiology

Based on the Global Cancer Incidence, Mortality and Prevalence (GLOBOCAN) survey in 2012, the age standardised rate (ASR) for incidence of CRC worldwide was estimated at 17.2 cases per 100,000 of the population. For males, the rate was 20.6 compared to 14.3 for females. The cumulative risk of developing CRC by the age of 75 was 2.0% overall and the cumulative risks were 2.4% and 1.6% for males and females respectively. Colorectal cancer was the third most common cancer in men and the second most common in women, with 1.36 million new cases and 694,000 deaths in 2012.[9]

In Europe, rectal cancer accounted for approximately 35% of CRC cases[5] and in China the estimated proportion was 60–75%.[10] Anal cancer is relatively rare with an incidence of 1–2 per 100,000.[6,11]

Australia and New Zealand had the highest estimated ASRs for CRC in 2012 (44.8 males; 32.2 females) compared to Europe (37.3 males; 23.6 females), Northern America (30.1 males; 22.7 females) and East Asia (22.4 males; 14.6 females).[9] In the United States, the average ASRs for 2009–2013 were 46.9 for men and 35.6 for women; however, the cumulative risks were similar (4.6% versus 4.2%), mainly due to the longer lifespan of women.[12]

In China, the ASR increased from 12.8 (14.1 males; 11.5 females) in 2003 to 16.8 per 100,000 (19.7 males; 14.0 females) in 2011 and overall mortality rose from 5.9 to 7.8 per 100,000.[13] In comparison, incidence and mortality rates in the United States declined over the period 1985 to 2013 in both men and women aged 50 years and over. However, there was a 13% increase in incidence in those aged 20–49 years from 2000 to 2013.[12] The ASR in Australia was fairly stable over this period and the mortality rate decreased.[14,15]

In general, the global incidence of CRC was higher in more developed regions, with ASRs of 36.3 for males and 23.6 for females, and lower in less developed regions (13.6 males; 9.8 females).[9] In China, ASRs were higher in urban populations (23.5 males; 16.8 females) than in rural areas (15.6 males; 11.0 females) and mortality was greater than 15 per 100,000 in the east coast provinces compared to less than 5 per 100,000 in Tibet.[13] In the United States, the incidence and mortality rates of colon and rectal cancers were higher for African Americans than white Americans.[12,16,17] In Australia, higher rates of CRC were associated with lower socio-economic status.[15]

Overall, CRC incidence tends to be positively associated with higher levels of economic development and socio-economic status but mortality appears to be declining in more developed regions. It is likely that the declines in mortality in some countries are at least partly associated with early diagnosis and screening programmes which have not been available to most people in China where most cases are symptomatic at diagnosis.[13]

Burden of Disease

Based on the Global Burden of Disease study, there were 1.7 million incident cases (95% uncertainty interval [UI], 1.6–1.8 million) of CRC in 2015.[18] The odds of developing CRC before 79 years of age were higher for men (1 in 28) than for women (1 in 43) but these odds were increased in countries with the highest socio-economic index

(1 in 14 men; 1 in 23 women). Colorectal cancer was the cause of 832,000 deaths (95% UI, 812,000–855,000) worldwide in 2015 and 17 million disability-adjusted life-years (DALYs)[18] (95% UI, 16.6–17.5 million).

Global survival rates for CRC have been estimated to be 83.4% at one year, 64.9% at five years and 58.3% at ten years post-diagnosis but these rates improved considerably when there was early diagnosis with 90% at five years. Survival rates were higher in countries with a higher socio-economic index.[19]

A review of studies of the economic burden of CRC found considerable variations in the methods used and costs included. Of the US studies, one estimated the mean cancer-related costs (based on 2004 dollars) in the 12 months following diagnosis at USD 29,609 for men and USD 29,930 for women, while another estimated the total costs at USD 41,134 (2003 dollars) per person.[20]

In terms of cost to the US health care system, it was estimated that in 2014 there were 1.6 million office visits for malignant neoplasm of the colon or rectum and 3,910 deaths in hospital, and that the aggregate charges were USD 9.86 billion.[21] In Australia in 2008–2009, CRC incurred the highest health system expenditure of any cancer at AUD 388 million for hospital inpatient services, AUD 18.25 million for out-of-hospital services, and AUD 21.2 million for prescription pharmaceuticals, while AUD 33 million was spent on screening programmes. Based on 14,624 new cases, the direct costs were AUD 29,229 per person, per year.[22]

Risk Factors

The risk of CRC tends to increase with age. In the United States, the median age at diagnosis was 68 years for males and 72 years for females in 2013, but rates are increasing in younger age groups.[23] In China, the median age at diagnosis was 56.8 years in 1980–1989 and 59.7 years in 1990–1999.[24] In 2009–2011, the incidence rates were highest in the age range 60–74 years for both males and females.[25]

Most cases of CRC are considered 'sporadic' and have no identifiable cause. In about 20% of cases, CRC occurs in familial clusters.[1]

Having a parent, sibling or child with CRC doubles the risk of the disease but a family history of small adenomas does not appear to increase the risk.[7] About 5% of CRC cases have been linked to genetic predisposition.[7] Of the inherited syndromes, Lynch syndrome appears the most common with 50% of affected people developing CRC or other cancers. In such cases, tumours tend to be right-sided, have distinctive histology (mucinous, signet ring) and microsatellite instability (MSI). Less common syndromes include familial adenomatous polyposis, Peutz-Jeghers syndrome and MUTYH-associated polyposis.[7]

Chronic inflammation plays an important role in the initiation and continuation of tumour growth; notably, ulcerative colitis and Crohn's disease are significant risk factors.[8,26] In sporadic CRC, diet plays an important role. Meta-analyses of cohort studies found increased risks for CRC associated with intake of red and processed meats and alcohol consumption. Conversely, risks decreased with increased intake of whole grains and dairy products, with weaker evidence for vegetables and fish.[27] A meta-analysis that focused on dietary patterns found that lower CRC risk was associated with high intake of fruits and vegetables, whole grains, nuts and legumes, fish and other seafood, and milk and other dairy products, while high intake of red meat, processed meat, sugar-sweetened beverages, refined grains, desserts and potatoes were linked to higher risks of developing CRC.[28] Obesity, weight gain, smoking and sedentary lifestyle have all been linked to increased CRC risk.[29–32] In addition to sporadic CRC, diet and lifestyle factors increase CRC risk in those with a familial history[33] and increased physical activity appears preventative in this subgroup.[34]

In contrast, anal cancer is associated with human papillomavirus (HPV) infection, anal intercourse and suppression of the immune system due to various causes, rather than to dietary factors.[6]

Pathological Processes and Histology

In the early stages of colon cancer, there is an outgrowth of an adenomatous polyp from the colonic mucosa or a flat dysplasia. There is also the presence of inflammation. Only a small proportion of such lesions progress to a carcinoma.[1,35] Tissue may be sampled by endoscopy and examined by histology. In cancerous lesions, the main histological type is adenocarcinoma with small proportions of mucinous adenocarcinomas, signet-ring tumours, squamous cell carcinomas, adenosquamous carcinomas and undifferentiated carcinomas.[1] Histopathological features associated with poor prognosis include deep infiltration of the bowel wall layers, poor differentiation of the cells, high levels of angiogenesis in the tumour and metastasis to numerous regional lymph nodes or to distant lymph nodes. A favourable prognostic feature is host response with intense inflammatory infiltrate.[1,35]

Colorectal cancer evolves through an accumulation of genetic and epigenetic alterations in the colonic mucosa, especially within pre-existing adenomas, which transform normal cells into invasive cancers. In sporadic CRC, the following three main molecular pathways have been identified:

1. The chromosomal instability (CIN) pathway (about 85% of cases) involves the gain or loss of chromosomal regions or whole chromosomes affecting more than 20 genes. Typical features are dysfunction in the Wnt pathway which regulates cell cycle progression, notably loss of function of the Adenomatous Polyposis Coli (APC) gene leading to inactivation of Wnt signalling, mutations of the proto-oncogene KRAS which is involved in cell proliferation and differentiation, and mutations in the transcription factor p53 (TP53) altering its tumour-suppressive actions.

2. The MSI pathway (about 15% of cases) involves dysfunction in the DNA mismatch repair (MMR) system. This repairs the base-pair mismatches that occur in microsatellites, which are short repeat nucleotide sequences, during DNA replication. Instability in two or more marker genes is defined as MSI-high; those with instability in one marker are MSI-low. Tumours with no apparent instability are defined as microsatellite stable (MSS). Microsatellite instability-high is associated with mutation in the oncogene BRAF in the RAS/MAPK pathway which is involved in cell differentiation, migration and apoptosis.

3. The CpG Island Methylator Phenotype (CIMP) pathway is related to the MSI pathway. It involves silencing of genes by DNA hypermethylation. Methylation of at least three markers is defined as CIMP-high (15–25% of cases).[36,37]

The majority of adenocarcinomas are well to moderately differentiated with intermediate sized glands lined with columnar epithelium and stratified columnar or rounded nuclei. Tumours with high MSI have variegated histology and include moderate to poorly differentiated adenocarcinomas, mucinous adenocarcinomas, tumours with cribriform or serrated architectures, signet-ring adenocarcinomas and undifferentiated adenocarcinomas. Tumours with more than 50% gland-forming component are classified as low grade while those with less are classified as high grade. High-grade neuroendocrine carcinomas are aggressive but relatively rare. These are classified into small cell and large cell types.[35] Immunohistochemistry is used to identify biomarkers in tumour samples that may help in the prediction of prognosis and/or the selection of therapies for CRC. These include MSI/MMR; deletions on chromosome 18q; DCC (deleted in colorectal cancer) gene mutation; p53 (TP53) status (wild type/mutant); mutations of oncogenes in the RAS family, notably KRAS and NRAS; mutations in BRAF; mutations of transforming growth factor beta receptor 2 (TGFBR2); and others.[26]

Anal cancer develops from the squamous epithelium rather than the columnar epithelium of the rectum. Anal intraepithelial neoplasia (AIN) is a precursor to anal cancer. Progression is slow in immunocompetent patients and there can be regression. Tumours of the anal margin tend to be well differentiated, whereas those in the anal canal tend to be poorly differentiated.[1,6,11]

Diagnosis

The main method of diagnosis of CRC, provided the patient is sufficiently fit, is by colonoscopy and biopsy to provide samples for histological evaluation. When histology is inconclusive, further biopsies may be required. An alternative to colonoscopy is CT pneumocolonography.[8] Anal tumours can be detected by digital examination followed by biopsy.[6,11] When malignancy is identified or suspected, high-resolution CT scanning is used to identify any spread. Further imaging using ultrasound, magnetic resonance imaging (MRI) or fluorodeoxyglucose (FDG)-positron emission tomography (PET) scanning may be required.[8]

Staging

A number of systems are used to classify the stage of the tumour. The older Dukes system involves four stages based on degree of invasion and metastasis. It has since been modified into several versions. Stage A indicates invasion of, but not through, the bowel wall; stage B involves penetration of the bowel wall into the muscle layer without lymph node involvement; stage C indicates involvement of lymph nodes and stage D indicates widespread metastases.[38]

Dukes staging was superseded by the American Joint Cancer Committee (AJCC)/Union for International Cancer Control (UICC) TNM classification system which has been in use since 1968 and was last updated in 2010.[26] 'T' is for tumour and denotes the extent of invasion of the intestinal wall; 'N' is for the number of lymphatic nodes invaded and the amount of lymphatic node involvement and 'M' is for distant metastasis. Within each of these categories are a number of subcategories which have been revised in various versions of the system. Within the 'T' there are five main stages: stage 0 refers to polyps without invasive characteristics; stage I indicates invasion of the submucosa only; while stage IV indicates the most advanced stage of the disease. Accurate staging requires proper examination of resection specimens, in conjunction with the clinical history, and can depend on whether the location of the tumour was in the rectum, sigmoid colon, transverse colon or caecum.[26,35]

Management

The management of CRC involves prevention and early detection at the population level, and at the individual level involves surgical resection, chemotherapy, targeted therapy, radiotherapy and/or palliative care depending on the stage and presentation of the disease, which can be complex. The main clinical guidelines used internationally are produced by the European Society for Medical Oncology (ESMO) and the National Comprehensive Cancer Network (NCCN). This chapter can only provide an overview of current CRC management (Table 1.1). Readers should consult the latest versions of these guidelines and other country-specific guidelines for more detailed information.

Prevention

In theory, CRC is preventable since disease progression is slow and early-stage disease is curable via the surgical removal of adenomas.[7] Early detection is possible by a combination of screening, genetic testing, endoscopy and other methods but universal screening is costly, may only be available to older people or to those with identified hereditary syndromes or inflammatory bowel disease, and there are the issues of patient uptake of screening and adherence to colonoscopy recommendations.[7,39]

Dietary modification appears a promising approach to risk reduction with studies showing benefits for higher fibre, calcium, milk, whole grains and possibly vitamin D, folate and non-starchy vegetables.[40] Exercise, physical activity and reduced central adiposity appear protective against the development of colon cancer and increase survival.[8,34,41]

A study of the relationship between adherence to the World Cancer Research Fund/American Institute for Cancer Research 2007 recommendations on cancer prevention in cohort studies of Italian adults found significant reductions in CRC risk with adherence to specific recommendations for body fatness, physical activity, foods and drinks that promote weight gain, eating mostly foods of plant origin, limiting red meat and processed meat, limiting alcohol, and limiting salt. This suggests that modification of lifestyle factors can translate into reduced risk.[42] Also, weight loss resulting from change in diet and lifestyle has been shown to reduce inflammation and biomarkers associated with CRC in colonic tissue.[43,44]

Table 1.1 Treatment Algorithm

Clinical Presentation	Finding		Primary Treatment*	Adjuvant Treatment*
Colon Cancer				
Appropriate for RE (non-metastatic)	Non-obstructing or obstruction		RE	Based on the result of pathologic stage, choose observation or chemo.
	Clinical T4b		Consider neoadjuvant chemo, and then RE.	
	Locally unresectable or medically inoperable		Systemic therapy, then RE ± RT or systemic therapy.	
Suspected or proven metastatic synchronous adenocarcinoma (Any T, and N, M1)	Synchronous liver only and/or lung only metastases	Resectable	RE and/or local therapy or neoadjuvant therapy followed by RE or RE followed by chemo.	Chemo
		Unresectable (potentially convertible or unconvertible)	Systemic therapy, consider RE only if imminent risk of obstruction, significant bleeding, perforation or other significant tumour-related symptoms.	Re-evaluate for conversion to resectability every two months if conversion to resectability is a reasonable goal.
	Synchronous abdominal/ peritoneal metastases	Non-obstructing	Systemic therapy	—
		Obstructed or imminent obstruction	RE or diverting ostomy or bypass of impending obstruction or stenting.	Systemic therapy
	Synchronous unresectable metastases of other sites		Systemic therapy	

Clinical Presentation	Finding		Primary Treatment*	Adjuvant Treatment*
Rectal Cancer				
Appropriate for RE	T1, N0		Transanal local excision, if appropriate	Based on the result of pathologic finding after RE, choose observation or chemo, RT or others.
	T1–2, N0		Transabdominal RE	
	T3, N any with CRM (by MRI); T1–2, N1–2		Neoadjuvant treatment (chemo and/ or RT), then primary treatment (RE/chemo/RT)	Based on the primary treatment, choose the adjuvant treatment.
	T3, N any with involved CRM (by MRI); T4, N and/or locally unresectable or medically inoperable			
Suspected or proven metastatic synchronous adenocarcinoma (T any, N any, M1)	Synchronous liver only and/or lung only metastases	Resectable	Chemo and/or RT	Restaging, staged or synchronous RE and/or local therapy for metastasis, and RE of rectal lesion.
		Unresectable or medically inoperable	Chemo ± targeted therapy	Reassess response to determine resectability, choose chemo, RT, RE, or others.
	Synchronous abdominal/ peritoneal metastases	Non-obstructing	Systemic therapy	
		Obstructed or imminent obstruction	RE, or diverting ostomy, or bypass of impending obstruction, or stenting.	Systemic therapy
	Synchronous unresectable metastases of other sites		Systemic therapy	

*See NCCN guidelines version 1, 2018 for more detail. Abbreviations: RE, resection; chemo, chemotherapy; RT, radiotherapy; CRM, clear circumferential margin; T, tumour. N, number of lymphatic nodes invaded; M, distant metastasis (see TNM staging).

Epidemiological studies have found that aspirin consumption reduces the incidence of CRC and there is some evidence of a similar effect for other non-steroidal anti-inflammatory drugs (NSAIDs).[8] However, NSAIDs are not without risk and a recent study of aspirin in the healthy elderly found increased CRC incidence in the aspirin group.[45]

Management of Adenomas

The effective management of adenomas (polyps) can reduce progression to CRC. Endoscopy can be used to characterise a lesion and differentiate neoplastic from non-neoplastic lesions based on the Paris classification of polyp morphology, the granularity of flat lesions and the surface architecture of excavated lesions. Depending on the characteristics of the lesion, resection can be performed using endoscopic mucosal resection, endoscopic diathermy knife and/or other endoscopic techniques.[8,46] The main complications of resection are bleeding (5–10%) and perforation (0.5–1.0%). Post-resection surveillance is important, especially when adenomas are greater than 1 cm in size and show histological features of a significant villous component, high-grade dysplasia or sessile serrated morphology.[46] When there is high-grade dysplasia there may be submucosal invasion and further biopsy may be required.[35] In cases where there are multiple polyps, this is suggestive of familial history which should be investigated.[46] In general, when a polyp has unfavourable histological features and the patient has average or lower operative risk, surgical resection is the recommended option.[26]

Surgical Resection of Primary Tumours

Surgical resection is the main treatment for tumours, provided that the patient is fit enough based on preoperative assessments that consider pre-existing medical conditions and assess the risk of complications. In patients with poor performance status, programmes of preoperative optimisation can be used to improve performance status. If these are ineffective, non-surgical interventions may need to be considered.[8]

Prior to admission for elective surgery, a multidisciplinary team is assembled and perioperative care commences. This involves preoperative patient education and nutritional supplements followed by postoperative pain control, thromboprophylaxis, enteral nutrition, early feeding and early mobilisation to reduce hospital stay.[8]

In colon cancer, radical surgery involves complete removal of the section of colon containing the tumour and about 5 cm of normal colon proximally and distally, together with the lymph nodes that drain the area. The two sections are then joined via an anastomosis. The surgical procedure varies according to the size and location of the lesion in the colon and the local arterial and lymphatic features.[8] Surgery may be open or use laparoscopic techniques where possible. Since it is less invasive, laparoscopic surgery is associated with earlier recovery, but due to the challenges of laparoscopic surgery, about 10% of cases require conversion to open surgery.[8] In rectal cancer, radical total mesorectal excision (TME) is the main procedure.[5]

Lymph node sampling is an important aspect of surgical resection in primary CRC. The AJCC recommends at least 10–14 lymph nodes be examined to determine the 'N' stage. In general, the higher the number of negative lymph nodes, the better the survival.[35]

In cases of colorectal metastases to the liver, lung, ovary or non-regional lymph nodes, surgical resection of the distant tumour is standard practice.[35] Where possible this surgery can be conducted at the same time as the resection of the primary tumour. Hepatic metastases that were previously considered unresectable, can be downstaged using neoadjuvant chemotherapy to enable subsequent resection.[8]

In anal cancer, surgery is not a primary treatment and is not recommended for AIN. Local excision may be used for tumours of the anal margin that are not poorly differentiated.[6,11] In locally advanced primary rectal cancer, pelvic exenteration may be required. When negative resection margins were attained, survival was enhanced with a three-year survival rate of 56.4%.[47]

Chemotherapy

The main cytotoxic drugs used in CRC are 5-fluorouracil (5-FU), capecitabine, irinotecan (IR), oxaliplatin (OX) and raltitrexed. These are used singly or in a range of combinations. Leucovorin (LV, LF) is often combined with 5-FU to increase its effect. Typical regimens include FOLFIRI (5-FU, LV, IR), FOLFOX (5-FU, LV, OX), XELOX/CapeOX (capecitabine, OX), S-1 (tegafur, gimeracil, oteracil potassium) and SOX (S-1, OX).[8,48,49]

All lymph node-positive (stages III–IV) primary CRC patients are recommended postoperative adjuvant chemotherapy. In stage II colon cancer perforations, at or proximal to, the tumour site are associated with higher risk of recurrence and are an indication for postoperative adjuvant chemotherapy.[35] Adjuvant chemotherapy reduces risk of death in stage III and stage II CRC patients.[26] In rectal cancer, adjuvant chemotherapy may be used in people with high risk of recurrence but the benefit appears smaller than for colon cancer.[5] In anal cancer, chemotherapy is the main treatment with 5-FU and mitomycin C being the main agents for stages I to III. Complete regression is achieved in 80–90% of these patients.[6]

Radiotherapy and Chemo-radiotherapy

In advanced rectal cancer when the tumour has spread to the pelvic wall and sacrum, preoperative radiotherapy or chemoradiotherapy may be used to shrink the cancer to enable resection. Postoperative chemoradiotherapy may be used in people with adverse histopathological findings.[5]

In colon cancer adjuvant radiotherapy is not a well-established practice. Adjuvant chemo-radiotherapy is mainly used in selected patients with advanced disease involving invasion of fixed structures. It may be used preoperatively to downstage advanced or difficult-to-resect tumours.[26] In people with liver metastasis, stereotactic body radiotherapy (SBRT) is a new method that can be focused on lesions while sparing normal tissue.[8]

Intraoperative radiation therapy (IORT) is a technique requiring specialised equipment that may be used in selected patients at the time of surgery when complete resection of the cancer is not feasible.[26] Brachytherapy is a related method in which the radiation source is placed close to the tumour.[8]

Chemoradiotherapy is a standard treatment in anal cancer, with the principal chemotherapeutic agents 5-FU and mitomycin C being combined with radiotherapy, ideally guided by CT or other 3D imaging to improve accuracy.[6]

Targeted Therapies

A number of new biological therapies are used in metastatic disease in selected patients based on characterisation of the molecular pathology of the tumour. These monoclonal antibodies include the vascular endothelial growth factor (VEGF) antibody bevacizumab, the epidermal growth factor receptor (EGFR) antibodies cetuximab and panitumumab, and the BRAF-mutant inhibitors dabrafenib, vemurafenib and encorafenib. These are used in conjunction with various chemotherapy regimens and are selected based on the results of biomarker testing including RAS and BRAF mutation status, testing for MSI or tumour MMR, and testing for biomarkers of chemotherapy sensitivity and toxicity. Clinical trials have indicated better outcomes for the use of these personalised approaches in metastatic disease but results have been inconclusive in the adjuvant setting.[8,50,51] Currently, targeted therapies are not available for rectal or anal cancers. In the case of distant metastases, therapy is the same as for colon cancer.[5]

Hyperthermic Intraperitoneal Chemotherapy

Hyperthermic intraperitoneal chemotherapy (HIPEC) involves the direct delivery of highly concentrated, warmed chemotherapy drugs to the abdominal cavity during surgery. It can be used in cases where there is peritoneal metastasis, usually in conjunction with cytoreductive surgery.[50]

Elderly Patients

In people aged over 75 years and those with poor performance status or cognitive impairment, surgery and adjuvant chemotherapy may not be considered appropriate. In such cases, the multidisciplinary team should formulate an individualised management plan in consultation with a geriatrician for elderly patients and inform the patient and their family of the risks, possible functional impairments and likely outcomes of planned treatments. Even in elderly patients, individualised chemotherapy and/or targeted therapies can extend life but clinical trial data is limited.[52]

Side-effects of Cancer Therapy

An important part of therapy is the management of the distressing side effects of various cancer therapies. These are too numerous for complete elaboration in this chapter. Criteria for their grading can be found in the World Health Organisation (WHO) guidelines[53] and Common Terminology Criteria for Adverse Events (CTCAE).[54]

Nausea and vomiting can accompany chemotherapy with over 70% of patients receiving oxaliplatin-based regimens experiencing symptoms.[55] To prevent acute and delayed nausea and vomiting following therapy current guidelines recommend the administration of combinations of anti-emetic drugs prior to chemotherapy, radiotherapy and chemo-radiotherapy. Although there have been advances in the control of emesis in recent years, nausea remains an issue.[49,56]

Chemotherapy-induced diarrhoea can be a serious adverse event. The frequency of grades 3–4 events in randomised clinical trials is in the range 5–47%, with 11–14% in studies of FOLFIRI, and acute diarrhoea can result from radiotherapy and chemo-radiotherapy. The diarrhoea may be associated with fat malabsorption, bile acid malabsorption, bacterial overgrowth, viral infection or other causes and can lead to fatigue, dehydration, pain, and physical and psychological distress. The first-line therapies are loperamide, codeine and octreotide, with antibiotics being used for bacterial overgrowth.[57]

Myelosuppression and neutropenia is an adverse reaction to chemotherapy for CRC, with incidence of grade 3/4 neutropenia ranging from 37% to 56% in different populations.[58] In small proportions of patients, the more severe condition of febrile neutropenia can arise. Granulocyte colony-stimulating factor (G-CSF), which initiates the proliferation of granulocyte precursor cells and their differentiation into mature granulocytes in bone marrow, is used as a primary prophylaxis for severe neutropenia and antimicrobials are used for febrile neutropenia.[59]

A side effect of long-term oxaliplatin-based chemotherapy regimens used in advanced CRC is neurotoxicity. This is related to the cumulative dose of oxaliplatin and can produce numbness, tingling, cold sensitivity, and/or pain in the extremities which adversely affect quality of life and can lead to cessation of therapy prior to disease progression.[50,60,61] Currently, treatment options are limited to duloxetine for neuropathic pain and discontinuous treatment with oxaliplatin.[49,50]

Post-therapy Follow-up and Monitoring

Even with optimal management, between 30% and 50% of CRC patients relapse, with most relapses in the three years following resection of the primary cancer. The follow-up measures recommended by ESMO for colon cancer include recording the history of the patient, physical examination, and testing of serum carcinoembryonic antigen (CEA) every three to six months for three years and every six to 12 months at Year 4 and Year 5 after surgery; and colonoscopy one year post-surgery and every three to five years after. In patients at higher risk, CT scans of the chest and abdomen every six to 12 months for the first three years should be considered. In addition, cancer survivors require a care plan to assist them with managing co-morbidities, stoma, rehabilitation, and maintenance of a healthy lifestyle and weight in order to reduce the risk of recurrence.[8,26]

Palliative Care

Advanced disease, advanced age, relapse, treatment refusal and treatment failure can all lead to the need for palliative care which focuses on the effective management of pain and suffering and supports the best possible quality of life for patients and their family. Collaboration between the multidisciplinary oncology team and the palliative care team enables development of a care plan that integrates physical and psycho-social aspects of care. The benefits and burden of anti-cancer treatment, relative to estimated life expectance, should be assessed and discussed with the patient. When the assessment indicates months to weeks, discontinuation of cancer treatment should be considered in favour of treatment of specific symptom complexes. These can include constipation, diarrhoea, bleeding, bowel obstruction, painful metastasis to bone, dyspnea, anorexia and cachexia, nausea and vomiting, insomnia and sedation, and delirium. Pain management may require opioids, and obstructive tumours and metastases can be relieved with radiotherapy or surgery depending on the case.[35,62]

Prognosis

In the United States, overall mortality rates for CRC have declined since 1975. The overall five-year survival rate for patients diagnosed from 2006 to 2012 was 65%.[3,12] In the United Kingdom, the five-year survival rate increased from 22% in 1971–1975 to 51% in 2001–2006.[8] In Australia, the five-year survival rates for CRC in 2017 were 68% for males and 69% for females for cancers diagnosed between 2009 and 2013. Notably, 39% of people aged 50–74 had taken part in the National Bowel Cancer Screening Programme.[15] In China, analysis of cancer registry data showed an increase from 2003 to 2015 for five-year survival rates for all cancers. For colorectal cancer, the age-standardised five-year relative survival for 2012–2015 was 56.9% (95% confidence interval, 56.2 to 57.5) with 56.3% for males and 57.7% for females.[63] For anal cancer, the five-year survival rate in the United States was 60% for men and 78% for women.[6]

Mortality rates vary according to the stage of the CRC at diagnosis, age of the patient, population group and other variables. In the United Kingdom for those diagnosed between 1996 and 2002, the five-year survival rate was 93.2% for stage I CRC, 77% for stage II, 47.7% for stage III and 6.6% for Stage IV.[8] Elective surgery for CRC had low mortality (1–4%) and relatively low morbidity (1–20%) based on multi-centre trials.[8] In the United States, the five-year survival rate was 90% for cancers diagnosed at the local stage, declining to 71% for those with regional disease and 14% for distant disease. Survival rates were higher in younger (<65 years = 69%) than in older (≥65 years = 62%) patients.[12]

References

1. International Agency for Research on Cancer. (2014) World cancer report 2014. WHO Press, Lyon.
2. World Health Organisation. (2004) ICD-10 international statistical classification of diseases and related health problems. World Health Organisation, Geneva.
3. Pande M, Frazier ML. (2014) Chapter 1: Epidemiology. In: Scholefield JS, Eng C (eds), *Colorectal Cancer: Diagnosis and Clinical Management*. Wiley-Blackwell, Chichester, pp. 1–26.
4. Kerr DJ, Haller DG, van de Velde CJH, Baumann M, eds. (2017) *Oxford Textbook of Oncology*, 3rd ed. Oxford University Press, UK.
5. Glynne-Jones R, Wyrwicz L, Tiret E, *et al.* (2017) Rectal cancer: ESMO clinical practice guidelines for diagnosis, treatment and follow-up. *Ann Oncol* **28(Suppl 4)**: iv22–iv40.
6. Glynne-Jones R, Nilsson PJ, Aschele C, *et al.* (2014) Anal cancer: ESMO-ESSO-ESTRO clinical practice guidelines for diagnosis, treatment and follow-up. *Ann Oncol* **25(Suppl 3)**: iii10–iii20.
7. Steele RJC, MacDonald P. (2014) Chapter 2: Screening for colorectal cancer. In: Scholefield JS, Eng C (eds), *Colorectal Cancer: Diagnosis and Clinical Management*. Wiley-Blackwell, Chichester, pp. 27–50.
8. Zalcberg J, Fox S, Heriot A, *et al.* (2016) Chapter 39: Colon cancer. In: Kerr DJ, Haller DG, van de Velde CJH, Baumann M (eds), *Oxford Textbook of Oncology*, 3rd ed. Oxford University Press, UK.
9. Ferlay J, Soerjomataram I, Dikshit R, *et al.* (2015) Cancer incidence and mortality worldwide: Sources, methods and major patterns in GLOBOCAN 2012. *Int J Cancer* **136(5):** E359–E386.
10. Chen RS. (2003) 陈锐深. 现代中医肿瘤学. 北京: 人民卫生出版社.
11. Roberts JR, Siekas LL, Kaz AM. (2017) Anal intraepithelial neoplasia: A review of diagnosis and management. *World J Gastrointest Oncol* **9(2):** 50–61.

12. Siegel RL, Miller KD, Fedewa SA, *et al.* (2017) Colorectal cancer statistics, 2017. *CA Cancer J Clin* **67(3):** 177–193.

13. Zhu J, Tan Z, Hollis-Hansen K, *et al.* (2017) Epidemiological trends in colorectal cancer in China: An ecological study. *Dig Dis Sci* **62(1):** 235–243.

14. Australian Institute of Health and Welfare and Australasian Association of Cancer Registries. (2012) Cancer in Australia: An overview, 2012. Cancer series no. 74. Cat. no. Can 70. Australian Institute of Health and Welfare, Canberra.

15. Australian Institute of Health and Welfare and Australasian Association of Cancer Registries. (2017) Cancer in Australia: In brief, 2017. Cancer series no. 102. Cat. no. Can 101. Australian Institute of Health and Welfare, Canberra.

16. White A, Joseph D, Rim SH, *et al.* (2017) Colon cancer survival in the United States by race and stage (2001–2009): Findings from the CONCORD-2 study. *Cancer* **123(Suppl 24):** 5014–5036.

17. Joseph DA, Johnson CJ, White A, *et al.* (2017) Rectal cancer survival in the United States by race and stage, 2001 to 2009: Findings from the CONCORD-2 study. *Cancer* **123(Suppl 24):** 5037–5058.

18. Global Burden of Disease Cancer Collaboration, Fitzmaurice C, Allen C, *et al.* (2017) Global, regional, and national cancer incidence, mortality, years of life lost, years lived with disability, and disability-adjusted life-years for 32 cancer groups, 1990 to 2015: A systematic analysis for the global burden of disease study. *JAMA Oncol* **3(4):** 524–548.

19. Favoriti P, Carbone G, Greco M, *et al.* (2016) Worldwide burden of colorectal cancer: A review. *Updates Surg* **68(1):** 7–11.

20. Yabroff KR, Borowski L, Lipscomb J. (2013) Economic studies in colorectal cancer: Challenges in measuring and comparing costs. *J Natl Cancer Inst Monogr* **2013(46):** 62–78.

21. Peery AF, Crockett SD, Murphy CC, *et al.* (2019) Burden and cost of gastrointestinal, liver, and pancreatic diseases in the United States: Update 2018. *Gastroenterology* **156(1):** 254–272.e11.

22. Australian Institute of Health and Welfare. (2013) Health system expenditure on cancer and other neoplasms in Australia 2008–09, cancer series 81. Cat. no. Can 78. Australian Institute of Health and Welfare, Canberra.

23. American Cancer Society. (2017) Colorectal cancer facts and figures 2017–2019. American Cancer Society, Atlanta.

24. Li M, Gu J. (2004) Changing patterns of colorectal cancer over the recent two decades in China. *Chin J Gastrointest Surg* **7(3):** 214–217.

25. Chen W, Zheng R, Baade PD, *et al.* (2016) Cancer statistics in China, 2015. *CA Cancer J Clin* **66(2):** 115–132.

26. Labianca R, Nordlinger B, Beretta GD, *et al.* (2013) Early colon cancer: ESMO clinical practice guidelines for diagnosis, treatment and follow-up. *Ann Oncol* **24(Suppl 6):** vi64–vi72.

27. Vieira AR, Abar L, Chan DSM, *et al.* (2017) Foods and beverages and colorectal cancer risk: A systematic review and meta-analysis of cohort studies, an update of the evidence of the WCRF-AICR continuous update project. *Ann Oncol* **28(8):** 1788–1802.

28. Tabung FK, Brown LS, Fung TT. (2017) Dietary patterns and colorectal cancer risk: A review of 17 years of evidence (2000–2016). *Curr Colorectal Cancer Rep* **13(6):** 440–454.

29. Lynch BM. (2010) Sedentary behavior and cancer: A systematic review of the literature and proposed biological mechanisms. *Cancer Epidemiol Biomarkers Prev* **19(11):** 2691–2709.

30. Karahalios A, English DR, Simpson JA. (2015) Weight change and risk of colorectal cancer: A systematic review and meta-analysis. *Am J Epidemiol* **181(11):** 832–845.

31. Grace MS, Lynch BM, Dillon F, *et al.* (2017) Joint associations of smoking and television viewing time on cancer and cardiovascular disease mortality. *Int J Cancer* **140(7):** 1538–1544.

32. Dong Y, Zhou J, Zhu Y, *et al.* (2017) Abdominal obesity and colorectal cancer risk: Systematic review and meta-analysis of prospective studies. *Biosci Rep* **37(6).**

33. Fardet A, Druesne-Pecollo N, Touvier M, Latino-Martel P. (2017) Do alcoholic beverages, obesity and other nutritional factors modify the risk of familial colorectal cancer? A systematic review. *Crit Rev Oncol Hematol* **119:** 94–112.

34. Shaw E, Farris MS, Stone CR, *et al.* (2018) Effects of physical activity on colorectal cancer risk among family history and body mass index subgroups: A systematic review and meta-analysis. *BMC Cancer* **18(1):** 71.

35. Maru DM. (2014) Chapter 4: How histopathology affects the management of the multidisciplinary team. In: Scholefield JS, Eng C (eds), *Colorectal Cancer: Diagnosis and Clinical Management.* Wiley-Blackwell, Chichester, pp. 67–83.

36. Bosman FT, Hamilton SR, Lambert R. (2014) 5.5. Colorectal cancer. In: Stewart BW, Wild C (eds), *World Cancer Report 2014*. International Agency for Research on Cancer, Lyon, pp. 392–402.

37. Al-Sohaily S, Biankin A, Leong R, *et al.* (2012) Molecular pathways in colorectal cancer. *J Gastroenterol Hepatol* **27(9):** 1423–1431.

38. Astler VB, Coller FA. (1954) The prognostic significance of direct extension of carcinoma of the colon and rectum. *Ann Surg* **139(6):** 846–852.

39. Connell LC, Mota JM, Braghiroli MI, Hoff PM. (2017) The rising incidence of younger patients with colorectal cancer: Questions about screening, biology, and treatment. *Curr Treat Options Oncol* **18(4):** 23.

40. Song M, Garrett WS, Chan AT. (2015) Nutrients, foods, and colorectal cancer prevention. *Gastroenterology* **148(6):** 1244–1260 e16.

41. Haydon AMM, Macinnis RJ, English DR, Giles GG. (2006) Effect of physical activity and body size on survival after diagnosis with colorectal cancer. *Gut* **55(1):** 62–67.

42. Turati F, Bravi F, Di Maso M, *et al.* (2017) Adherence to the World Cancer Research Fund/American Institute for Cancer Research recommendations and colorectal cancer risk. *Eur J Cancer* **85:** 86–94.

43. Beeken RJ, Croker H, Heinrich M, *et al.* (2017) The impact of diet-induced weight loss on biomarkers for colorectal cancer: An exploratory study (INTERCEPT). *Obesity* **25:** S95–S101.

44. Pendyala S, Neff LM, Suarez-Farinas M, Holt PR. (2011) Diet-induced weight loss reduces colorectal inflammation: Implications for colorectal carcinogenesis. *Am J Clin Nutr* **93(2):** 234–242.

45. McNeil JJ, Nelson MR, Woods RL, *et al.* (2018) Effect of aspirin on all-cause mortality in the healthy elderly. *N Engl J Med* **379(16):** 1519–1528.

46. Dolwani S, Singh R, Uedo N, Ragunath K. (2014) Chapter 3: Management of adenomas. In: Scholefield JS, Eng C (eds). *Colorectal Cancer: Diagnosis and Clinical Management*. Wiley-Blackwell, Chichester, pp. 51–65.

47. PelvEx Collaborative, Kelly ME, Glynn R, *et al.* (2019) Surgical and survival outcomes following pelvic exenteration for locally advanced primary rectal cancer: Results from an international collaboration. *Ann Surg* **269(2):** 315–321.

48. Watanabe T, Muro K, Ajioka Y, *et al.* (2018) Japanese Society for Cancer of the Colon and Rectum (JSCCR) guidelines 2016 for the treatment of colorectal cancer. *Int J Clin Oncol* **23(1):** 1–34.

49. National Comprehensive Cancer Network. (2017) Clinical practice guidelines in oncology: Colon cancer, version 2.2017. Available from: https://www.nccn.org.

50. Van Cutsem E, Cervantes A, Adam R, *et al.* (2016) ESMO consensus guidelines for the management of patients with metastatic colorectal cancer. *Ann Oncol* **27(8):** 1386–1422.

51. Yoshino T, Arnold D, Taniguchi H, *et al.* (2018) Pan-asian adapted ESMO consensus guidelines for the management of patients with metastatic colorectal cancer: A JSMO-ESMO initiative endorsed by CSCO, KACO, MOS, SSO and TOS. *Ann Oncol* **29(1):** 44–70.

52. Papamichael D, Audisio RA, Glimelius B, *et al.* (2015) Treatment of colo-rectal cancer in older patients: International society of geriatric oncology (SIOG) consensus recommendations 2013. *Ann Oncol* **26(3):** 463–476.

53. Miller AB, Hoogstraten B, Staquet M, Winkler A. (1981) Reporting results of cancer treatment. *Cancer* **47(1):** 207–214.

54. National Institutes of Health and National Cancer Institute. (2008) Common terminology criteria for adverse events (CTCAE), version 4. In: U.S. Department of Health and Human Services, National Institutes of Health, Bethesda, MD.

55. Navari RM. (2009) Pharmacological management of chemotherapy-induced nausea and vomiting: Focus on recent developments. *Drugs* **69(5):** 515–533.

56. Roila F, Molassiotis A, Herrstedt J, *et al.* (2016) 2016 MASCC and ESMO guideline update for the prevention of chemotherapy- and radiotherapy-induced nausea and vomiting and of nausea and vomiting in advanced cancer patients. *Ann Oncol* **27(Suppl 5):** v119–v133.

57. Andreyev J, Ross P, Donnellan C, *et al.* (2014) Guidance on the man-agement of diarrhoea during cancer chemotherapy. *Lancet Oncol* **15(10):** E447–E460.

58. Sugihara K, Ohtsu A, Shimada Y, *et al.* (2012) Safety analysis of FOLFOX4 treatment in colorectal cancer patients: A comparison between two Asian studies and four western studies. *Clin Colorectal Cancer* **11(2):** 127–137.

59. Klastersky J, de Naurois J, Rolston K, *et al.* (2016) Management of febrile neutropaenia: ESMO clinical practice guidelines. *Ann Oncol* **27(Suppl 5):** v111–v118.

60. Padman S, Lee J, Kumar R, *et al.* (2015) Late effects of oxaliplatin-induced peripheral neuropathy (LEON): Cross-sectional cohort study of

patients with colorectal cancer surviving at least 2 years. *Support Care Cancer* **23(3):** 861–869.

61. Beijers AJ, Mols F, Tjan-Heijnen VC, *et al.* (2015) Peripheral neuropathy in colorectal cancer survivors: The influence of oxaliplatin administration. Results from the population-based profiles registry. *Acta Oncol* **54(4):** 463–469.

62. National Comprehensive Cancer Network. (2017) Clinical practice guidelines in oncology: Palliative care, version 2.2017. Available from: https://www.nccn.org.

63. Zeng HM, Chen WQ, Zheng RS, *et al.* (2018) Changing cancer survival in China during 2003–15: A pooled analysis of 17 population-based cancer registries. *Lancet Glob Health* **6(5):** E555–E567.

2

Colorectal Cancer in Chinese Medicine

OVERVIEW

This chapter introduces the main aetiology, pathogenesis and syndromes of colorectal cancer in contemporary Chinese medicine based on guidelines and major textbooks. For each syndrome a guiding herbal formula is provided based on an authoritative clinical guideline, and additional formulas from major textbooks are provided in a table. Treatments with external herbal preparations and acupuncture/moxibustion, as well as management with other Chinese medicine therapies, cancer prevention, nursing and dietary therapy are included based on major textbooks.

Introduction

In Chinese, the term *da chang ai* 大肠癌 includes cancers of the large intestine and rectum and is equivalent to the English term colorectal cancer (CRC). In pre-modern and ancient times, the term *da chang ai* 大肠癌 was not used and CRC was included under other disorders including *ji ju* 积聚, *zheng jia* 癥瘕, *zang du* 脏毒, *chang feng* 肠风, *xia li* 下痢 and *suo gang zhi* 锁肛痔. [1-12]

Aetiology and Pathogenesis

The large intestine is one of the six hollow (*fu* 腑) organs, whose functions involve transportation. In Chinese medicine (CM), the aetiology of CRC involves internal and external factors. The internal factors include internal damage due to disorder of the seven emotions, deficiency of the healthy *qi* (*zheng qi* 正气) and *yin-yang* disharmony.

The external factors include external contraction of the six excesses, dietary irregularities and irregular lifestyle. The key feature in the pathogenesis is the loss of the transporting function of the large intestine which leads to accumulation of dampness and heat (*shi re* 湿热) and/or toxins and stasis (*yu du* 瘀毒) which produce obstruction and blockage of passage through the intestine. Over a long time, the obstructions undergo pathological transformation into cancer.[7]

In CM, CRC is located in the large intestine and is considered to have a close relationship with the Spleen, Stomach, Liver and Kidney. Its aetiology has deficiency as its root and excess as its branch. As the root, deficiency of Spleen and Kidney *yang*, deficiency of *qi* and blood, and/or deficiency of Liver and Kidney *yin* are often seen. As the branch, the common pathogenic factors are *qi* stagnation, Blood stasis, dampness and toxic heat which can combine together, and gradually clump and accrete to form blockages in the intestine. In the early stages of the disease, the pathogenic factors (*xie* 邪) are abundant and the healthy *qi* is not too deficient, so the principal syndromes relate to *qi* stagnation, Blood stasis, dampness and toxic heat. In the middle and late stages of the disease the *qi* and Blood, and *yin* and *yang* all become deficient. As the pathogenic factors become more abundant, the healthy *qi* becomes more and more deficient, so the disease becomes more complex and serious.[2,4–8,10]

Syndrome Differentiation and Treatments

There is no national standard for syndrome differentiation in CRC since syndromes can vary considerably from patient to patient and according to the clinical symptoms and the stage of the disease.[4,6] We consulted textbooks and other books on CRC and obtained expert advice to select the *Guideline of Diagnosis and Treatment of Tumours in Traditional Chinese Medicine* 肿瘤中医诊疗指南 which was produced in 2008 by the China Association of Chinese Medicine 中华中医药学会 as the basis for syndrome differentiation and treatment (Table 2.1).[1] Syndromes and treatments from major textbooks are presented in Table 2.2.

Table 2.1   Summary of Chinese Herbal Medicines for Colorectal Cancer

Syndrome Differentiation	Treatment Principle	Oral Formula
Spleen deficiency with qi stagnation 脾虚气滞	Fortify Spleen and regulate *qi* 健脾理气	*Xiang sha liu jun zi tang* with modifications 香砂六君子汤加减
Dampness-heat agglomeration 湿热蕴结	Clear heat, drain dampness and resolve toxins 清热利湿解毒	*Bai tou weng tang* plus *Huai jiao wan* with modifications 白头翁汤合槐角丸加减
Stasis of Blood and toxins block the interior 瘀毒内阻	Move *qi* to activate Blood, and resolve stasis and toxins 行气活血, 化瘀解毒	*Ge xia zhu yu tang* with modifications 膈下逐瘀汤加减
Spleen and Kidney yang deficiency 脾肾阳虚	Warm and tonify Spleen and Kidney 温补脾肾	*Li zhong wan* plus *Si shen wan* with modifications 理中丸合四神丸加减
Liver-Kidney *yin* deficiency 肝肾阴虚	Enrich and nourish Liver and Kidney, clear heat and resolve toxins 滋养肝肾,清热解毒	*Zhi bai di huang wan* with modifications 知柏地黄丸加减
Dual deficiency of *qi* and Blood 气血两虚	Tonify *qi* and replenish Blood 补益气血	*Bu zhong yi qi tang* plus *Si wu tang* with modifications 补中益气汤合四物汤加减

See reference 1 in the References list at the end of this chapter.

Treatment Based on Syndrome Differentiation

Six syndromes are described, each with typical symptoms and signs, a principle of treatment and an oral herbal formula.

1. Spleen deficiency with *qi* stagnation (*pi xu qi zhi* 脾虚气滞)
Clinical manifestations: Abdominal distension with borborygmus, pain in the abdomen that moves around, no appetite, lack of mental and physical strength, dull yellowish complexion, loose stool, pale red tongue body, thin slimy tongue coat and soggy-slippery (*ru hua* 濡滑) pulse.

Treatment principle: Fortify the Spleen and regulate *qi* (*jian pi li qi* 健脾理气).

Oral formula: *Xiang sha liu jun zi tang* with modifications 香砂六君子汤加减.

Herbs: *Mu xiang* 木香, *sha ren* 砂仁, *dang shen* 党参, *ban xia* 半夏, *chao bai zhu* 炒白术, *fu ling* 茯苓, *chen pi* 陈皮, *ba yue zha* 八月札, *zhi ke* 枳壳, *wu yao* 乌药, *lv e mei* 绿萼梅, *ye pu tao teng* 野葡萄藤 and *she mei* 蛇莓.

Main actions of herbs: *Mu xiang* 木香 fortifies the Spleen, moves *qi* and relieves pain; *sha ren* 砂仁 resolves dampness and enlivens the Spleen, and moves *qi* and harmonises the Stomach; *dang shen* 党参 replenishes *qi* and fortifies the Spleen; *ban xia* 半夏, *chao bai zhu* 炒白术 and *fu ling* 茯苓 fortify the Spleen and resolve dampness; *chen pi* 陈皮 and *zhi ke* 枳壳 regulate *qi* and harmonise the middle, move stagnation and reduce distension; *ba yue zha* 八月札 regulates *qi* and activates the Blood to relieve pain, and disperses nodules; *wu yao* 乌药 moves *qi* and relieves pain; *lv e mei* 绿萼梅 harmonises the Spleen and Stomach, and soothes and regulates *qi* and the Blood; *ye pu tao teng* 野葡萄藤 and *she mei* 蛇莓 drain dampness, resolve toxins and resist cancer.

2. Dampness-heat agglomeration (*shi re yun jie* 湿热蕴结)

Clinical manifestations: Abdominal distension and pain, rectal tenesmus, burning sensation in the anus, sticky malodorous stool or stool with mucus and blood, thirst and poor appetite, red tongue body, yellow slimy tongue coat and slippery rapid pulse.

Treatment principle: Clear heat, drain dampness and resolve toxins (*qing re li shi jie du* 清热利湿解毒).

Oral formula: *Bai tou weng tang* 白头翁汤 plus *Huai jiao wan* with modifications 槐角丸加减.

Herbs: *Huai hua* 槐花, *di yu* 地榆, *bai tou weng* 白头翁, *bai jiang cao* 败酱草, *hong teng* 红藤, *ma chi xian* 马齿苋, *huang bai* 黄柏, *ku shen* 苦参, *sheng yi ren* 生苡仁, *huang qin* 黄芩 and *chi shao* 赤芍.

Main actions of herbs: *Huai hua* 槐花 and *di yu* 地榆 purge fire and clean the intestines, cool the Blood and stop bleeding; *bai tou weng*

白头翁 clears heat, resolves toxins and cools the Blood; *bai jiang cao* 败酱草 and *sheng yi ren* 生苡仁 clear heat, resolve toxins and expel pus; *hong teng* 红藤 clears heat, resolves toxins and disperses nodules; *ma chi xian* 马齿苋, *ku shen* 苦参, *huang bai* 黄柏 and *huang qin* 黄芩 clear heat, resolve toxins and dispel dampness; *chi shao* 赤芍 clears heat, cools the Blood and relieves pain.

3. Stasis of the Blood and toxins block the interior (*yu du nei zu* 瘀毒内阻)

Clinical manifestations: Abdominal distension with pain that is exacerbated by pressure, palpable mass in the abdomen, rectal tenesmus, stool with profuse pus and blood, purple tongue body with petechiae, thin yellow tongue coat, and string-like or rough pulse.

Treatment principle: Move *qi* to activate Blood, resolve stasis and resolve toxins (*xing qi huo xue* 行气活血, *hua yu jie du* 化瘀解毒).

Oral formula: *Ge xia zhu yu tang* with modifications 膈下逐瘀汤加减.

Herbs: *Dang gui* 当归, *hong hua* 红花, *tao ren* 桃仁, *chi shao* 赤芍, *dan shen* 丹参, *sheng di* 生地, *chuan xiong* 川芎, *sheng yi ren* 生苡仁, *ban zhi lian* 半枝莲, *teng li gen* 藤梨根, *bai jiang cao* 败酱草, *hong teng* 红藤 and *bai hua she she cao* 白花蛇舌草.

Main actions of herbs: *Dang gui* 当归 and *chi shao* 赤芍 nourish and activate the Blood; *hong hua* 红花 and *tao ren* 桃仁 break the Blood and expel stasis, and disperse nodules; *dan shen* 丹参 activates the Blood, dispels stasis and relieves pain; *sheng di* 生地 cools the Blood to stop bleeding; *chuan xiong* 川芎 moves *qi* to activate the Blood and frees the collateral vessels to relieve pain; *sheng yi ren* 生苡仁 and *bai jiang cao* 败酱草 clear heat, resolve toxins and expel pus; *ban zhi lian* 半枝莲, *teng li gen* 藤梨根, *hong teng* 红藤 and *bai hua she she cao* 白花蛇舌草 clear heat, resolve toxins, resist cancer and disperse nodules.

4. Spleen and Kidney yang deficiency (*pi shen yang xu* 脾肾阳虚)

Clinical manifestations: Abdominal pain that does not stop and is relieved by warmth and pressure; emaciation and fatigue; dullish complexion; fear of cold; cold hands and feet; poor appetite; thin sloppy stool; frequent defecations or 'fifth watch diarrhea'; pale tongue body; thin white tongue coat and sunken fine pulse.

Treatment principle: Warm and tonify the Spleen and Kidney (*wen bu pi shen* 温补脾肾).

Oral formula: *Li zhong wan* 理中丸 plus *Si shen wan* with modifications 四神丸加减.

Herbs: *Zhi fu zi* 制附子, *dang shen* 党参, *bai zhu* 白术, *fu ling* 茯苓, *sheng yi ren* 生苡仁, *bu gu zhi* 补骨脂, *he zi* 诃子, *rou dou kou* 肉豆蔻, *wu zhu yu* 吴茱萸, *gan jiang* 干姜, *chen pi* 陈皮 and *wu wei zi* 五味子.

Main actions of herbs: *Zhi fu zi* 制附子 tonifies fire and assists *yang*, dissipates cold and relieves pain; *dang shen* 党参 replenishes *qi* and fortifies the Spleen; *bai zhu* 白术, *fu ling* 茯苓 and *sheng yi ren* 生苡仁 fortify the Spleen and dispel dampness; *bu gu zhi* 补骨脂 warms the Kidney, assists *yang* and checks diarrhoea; *he zi* 诃子 astringes the intestines and checks diarrhoea; *rou dou kou* 肉豆蔻 warms the Spleen and Kidney, and checks diarrhoea; *wu zhu yu* 吴茱萸 and *gan jiang* 干姜 warm the middle to restore *yang*, dissipate cold, eliminate dampness and relieve pain; *chen pi* 陈皮 regulates *qi* and fortifies the Spleen, and prevents the supplementing herbs from causing stagnation; *wu wei zi* 五味子 secures the Kidney and astringes the Essence, promotes contraction and checks diarrhoea.

5. Liver-Kidney yin deficiency (*gan shen yin xu* 肝肾阴虚)
Clinical manifestations: Vexing heat in the chest, palms and soles, dizziness and blurred vision, low-grade fever and night sweating, bitter taste in the mouth and dry throat, aching low back and tired legs, constipation, red tongue body with scanty coat or no coat, and fine, string-like pulse or fine rapid pulse.

Treatment principle: Enrich and nourish the Liver and Kidney (*zhi yang gan shen* 滋养肝肾), clear heat and resolve toxins (*qing re jie du* 清热解毒).

Oral formula: *Zhi bai di huang wan* with modifications 知柏地黄丸加减.

Herbs: *Sheng di* 生地, *shu di* 熟地, *zhi mu* 知母, *huang bai* 黄柏, *bai shao* 白芍, *dan pi* 丹皮, *shan zhu yu* 山茱萸, *wu wei zi* 五味子, *mai dong* 麦冬, *ze xie* 泽泻, *sha shen* 沙参, *gou qi zi* 枸杞子, *ye pu tao teng* 野葡萄藤 and *ban zhi lian* 半枝莲.

Main actions of herbs: *Sheng di* 生地, *zhi mu* 知母 and *sha shen* 沙参 clear heat and nourish *yin*, engender fluid and allay thirst; *shu di* 熟地 nourishes *yin* and tonifies the Kidney, replenishes the Essence and nourishes the Marrow; *huang bai* 黄柏 clears heat and resolves toxins; *bai shao* 白芍 nourishes the Blood and emolliates the Liver, constrains *yin* and restrains sweat; *shan zhu yu* 山茱萸 warms and tonifies the Liver and Kidney, and restrains the essential *qi*; *dan pi* 丹皮 clears and purges Liver fire, and counters the warm astringing property of *shan zhu yu* 山茱萸; *ze xie* 泽泻 clears and purges Kidney fire, and counters the moist sticky properties of *shu di* 熟地; *wu wei zi* 五味子 and *mai dong* 麦冬 replenish *qi*, nourish *yin* and engender fluid; *gou qi zi* 枸杞子 enriches and tonifies the Liver and Kidney; *ye pu tao teng* 野葡萄藤 and *ban zhi lian* 半枝莲 clear heat, resolve toxins, resist cancer and disperse nodules.

6. Dual deficiency of qi and Blood (*qi xue liang xu* 气血两虚)

Clinical manifestations: Lack of mental and physical strength, pale complexion, dizziness and blurred vision, pale lips and nails, lack of appetite, repeated instances of blood in the stool, prolapse of the anus, loose stool, pale tongue body, thin coat and fine weak pulse.

Treatment principle: Tonify *qi* and replenish the Blood (*bu yi qi xue* 补益气血).

Oral formula: *Bu zhong yi qi tang* 补中益气汤 plus *Si wu tang* with modifications 四物汤加减.

Herbs: *Dang shen* 党参, *dang gui* 当归, *fu ling* 茯苓, *huang qi* 黄芪, *shu di* 熟地, *bai shao* 白芍, *chuan xiong* 川芎, *sheng ma* 升麻, *bai zhu* 白术, *dan shen* 丹参, *chen pi* 陈皮, *ba yue zha* 八月札, *da zao* 大枣, *gan cao* 甘草, *hong teng* 红藤, *ye pu tao teng* 野葡萄藤 and *teng li gen* 藤梨根.

Main actions of herbs: *Dang shen* 党参, *bai zhu* 白术 and *gan cao* 甘草 tonify *qi* and fortify the Spleen; *dang gui* 当归, *bai shao* 白芍 and *dan shen* 丹参 nourish the Blood and harmonise the nutrient aspect (*ying* 营); *fu ling* 茯苓 fortifies the Spleen and dispels dampness; *huang qi* 黄芪 tonifies the middle and replenishes *qi*, upraises the *yang* and secures the exterior; *shu di* 熟地 nourishes the Blood and enriches *yin*; *chuan xiong* 川芎 moves *qi* to activate the Blood and open stagnation; *sheng ma* 升麻 upraises the *yang* and lifts prolapse; *chen pi* 陈皮 regulates *qi* and harmonises the Stomach, and prevents the supplementing herbs from causing stagnation; *ba yue zha* 八月札 regulates *qi*, activates the Blood and disperses nodules; *da zao* 大枣 harmonises the middle and fortifies the Spleen; *hong teng* 红藤, *ye pu tao teng* 野葡萄藤 and *teng li gen* 藤梨根 clear heat, resolve toxins, resist cancer and disperse nodules.

Additional Sources for Treatment Based on Syndrome Differentiation

Since there is no single national standard for the CM differential diagnosis and management of CRC, a summary is provided in Table 2.2 of the syndromes, principles of treatment and guiding oral formulas from five additional authoritative monographs and textbooks.[3–8] These books list between three and five syndromes and their associated formulas.

Manufactured Medicines

A number of orally administered manufactured medicines (*zhong cheng yao* 中成药) are available for use in cancers including CRC.

1. *Zhong jie feng pian* 肿节风片
Actions: Clear heat and resolve toxins, dispel masses and disperse nodules. Can be used to assist in the treatment of cancers.

Dose: Three tablets, three times per day.[1,3,11]

2. *Ping xiao pian* 平消片
Actions: Activate the Blood and resolve stasis, disperse nodules and dispel masses, and resolve toxins and relieve pain. Can be used by cancer patients whose condition is characterised by toxins and stasis binding internally (*du yu nei jie* 毒瘀内结) in order to alleviate symptoms, reduce

Table 2.2 Summary of Chinese Herbal Medicines for Colorectal Cancer in Additional Monographs and Textbooks

Book Name	Syndrome Differentiation	Treatment Principle	Oral Formula
Shi Yong Zhong Yi Zhong Liu Shou Ce 1996 实用中医肿瘤手册[3]	Dampness-heat agglomeration 湿热蕴结	Clear heat and resolve dampness 清热化湿	*Bai tou weng tang* with modifications 白头翁汤加减
	Stasis of Blood and toxins block the interior 瘀毒内阻	Move *qi* to activate Blood, resolve stasis and toxins 行气活血, 化瘀解毒	*Ge xia zhu yu tang* with modifications 膈下逐瘀汤加减
	Spleen deficiency with *qi* stagnation 脾虚气滞	Fortify Spleen and regulate *qi* 健脾理气	*Xiang sha liu jun zi tang* with modifications 香砂六君子汤加减
	Spleen and Kidney *yang* deficiency 脾肾阳虚	Warm and tonify Spleen and Kidney 温补脾肾	*Li zhong tang* with modifications 理中汤加减
	Liver-Kidney *yin* deficiency 肝肾阴虚	Enrich and nourish Liver and Kidney, clear heat and resolve toxins 滋养肝肾, 清热解毒	*Liu wei di huang wan* with modifications 六味地黄汤加减
Zhong Liu Ke Zhuan Bing Zhong Yi Lin Chuang Zhen, 3rd ed. 2013 肿瘤科专病中医临床诊治 (第3版)[4]	Dampness-heat agglomeration 湿热蕴结	Clear heat, drain dampness and resolve toxins 清热利湿解毒	*Huai jiao di yu tang* with modifications 槐角地榆汤加减
	Qi stagnation with Blood stasis 气滞血瘀	Move *qi* to resolve stasis, resolve toxins and eliminate masses 行气化瘀, 解毒消癥	*Tao hong si wu tang* with modifications 桃红四物汤加减
	Spleen and Kidney *yang* deficiency 脾肾阳虚	Warm and tonify Spleen and Kidney 温补脾肾	*Shen ling bai zhu san* with modifications 参苓白术散

(Continued)

Table 2.2   (Continued)

Book Name	Syndrome Differentiation	Treatment Principle	Oral Formula
	Liver-Kidney *yin* deficiency 肝肾阴虚	Enrich and nourish Liver and Kidney 滋养肝肾	*Zhi bai di huang tang* with modifications 知柏地黄汤加减
	Dual deficiency of *qi* and Blood 气血两虚	Tonify *qi* and nourish Blood 补气养血	*Bu zhong yi qi tang* plus *Si wu tang* with modifications 补中益气汤合四物汤加减
Zhong Yi Lin Chuang Zhi Liao Te Se Yu You Shi Zhi Nan 2007 中医临床治疗特色与优势指南[5]	Dampness-heat agglomeration 湿热蕴结	Clear heat, drain dampness and resolve toxins 清热利湿解毒	*Huai jiao di yu tang* with modifications 槐角地榆汤加减
	Qi stagnation with Blood stasis 气滞血瘀	Move *qi* to resolve stasis, resolve toxins and eliminate masses 行气化瘀, 解毒消癥	*Tao hong si wu tang* with modifications 桃红四物汤加减
	Spleen and Kidney *yang* deficiency 脾肾阳虚	Warm and tonify Spleen and Kidney 温补脾肾	*Fu zi li zhong wan* with modifications 附子理中丸加减
	Liver-Kidney *yin* deficiency 肝肾阴虚	Enrich and nourish Liver and Kidney 滋养肝肾	*Zhi bai di huang tang* with modifications 知柏地黄汤加减
	Dual deficiency of *qi* and Blood 气血两虚	Tonify *qi* and nourish Blood 补气养血	*Bu zhong yi qi tang* plus *Si wu tang* with modifications 补中益气汤合四物汤加减

(*Continued*)

Table 2.2   (*Continued*)

Book Name	Syndrome Differentiation	Treatment Principle	Oral Formula
Xian Dai Zhong Yi Zhong Liu Xue 2005 现代中医肿瘤学[7]	Dampness-heat agglomeration in the interior 湿热内蕴	Clear heat and drain dampness, resolve toxins and resist cancer 清热利湿,解毒抗癌	*Huai jiao di yu tang* with modifications 槐角地榆汤加减
	Stasis of Blood and toxins block the interior 瘀毒内阻	Move *qi* to eliminate stasis, resolve toxins and resist cancer 行气消瘀,解毒抗癌	*Tao hong si wu tang* plus *si xiao san* with modifications 桃红四物汤和失笑散
	Spleen and Kidney *yang* deficiency 脾肾阳虚	Warm and tonify Spleen and Kidney, resolve toxins and resist cancer 温补脾肾,解毒抗癌	*Shen ling bai zhu san* plus *si shen wan* with modifications 参苓白术散合四神丸化裁
	Liver-Kidney *yin* deficiency 肝肾阴虚	Enrich and nourish Liver and Kidney, resolve toxins and resist cancer 滋养肝肾,解毒抗癌	*Zhi bai di huang tang* with modifications 知柏地黄汤加减
	Deficiency of both *qi* and Blood 气血双亏	Supplement *qi* and nourish Blood, resolve toxins and resist cancer 益气养血,解毒抗癌	*Shi quan da bu tang* with modifications 十全大补汤加减
Xian Dai Zhong Yi Zhong Liu Xue 2003 现代中医肿瘤学[8]	Dampness-heat agglomeration 湿热蕴结	Clear heat and drain dampness, resolve toxins and disperse nodules 清热利湿,解毒散结	*Bai tou weng tang* with modifications 白头翁汤加减
	Stasis of Blood and toxins block the interior 瘀毒内阻	Clear heat and resolve toxins, dispel stasis and disperse nodules 清热解毒,祛瘀散结	*Huai hua san* with modifications 槐花散加减

(*Continued*)

Table 2.2 (*Continued*)

Book Name	Syndrome Differentiation	Treatment Principle	Oral Formula
	Deficiency of Spleen and Kidney 脾肾亏虚	Fortify Spleen and tonify Kidney, supplement *qi* and activate Blood 健脾补肾,益气活血	*Si jun zi tang* with modifications 四君子汤加减

See references 3, 4, 5, 7 and 8 in the References list at the end of this chapter.

the size of the tumour, improve immunity, strengthen the body and prolong survival time.

Dose: Four to eight tablets, three times per day.[1,3]

3. *Yi shen jian pi chong ji* 益肾健脾冲剂

Actions: Fortify the Spleen and replenish the Kidney. Used to reduce the adverse effects of surgery, chemotherapy and radiotherapy, improve immunity and strengthen the body. Also used for other symptoms due to Spleen and Kidney weakness (*pi shen xu ruo* 脾肾虚弱).

Dose: One packet, twice a day.[1,6]

4. *Ping xiao jiao nang* 平消胶囊

Actions: Activate Blood and resolve stasis, disperse nodules and dispel masses, resolve toxins and relieve pain. For cancer patients whose condition involves toxins and stasis binding internally (*du yu nei jie* 毒瘀内结), this medicine can alleviate symptoms, reduce tumour volume, strengthen the immune system and the body, and prolong survival.

Dose: Four to eight tablets, three times per day.[4–6,8]

5. *Xi huang wan* 西黄丸

Actions: Clear heat and resolve toxins, dispel masses and disperse nodules. Used for toxic boils, ulcers and carbuncles, scrophula, deep abscesses and tumours.

Dose: Three grams, twice per day.[4]

6. *Huai er ke li* 槐耳颗粒

Actions: Used in combination with standard chemotherapy drugs to alleviate symptoms including lack of mental and physical strength, weak *qi* and no energy to speak, stomach and abdominal pain and/or distension, distressed rapid breathing, poor appetite, dry stool or loose stool, cough, excessive phlegm, pale complexion, chest pain, phlegm containing blood, and/or discomfort in the chest and rib area, to improve the patient's quality of life.

Dose: One packet, three times per day.[5]

7. *Fu fang ban mao jiao nang* 复方斑蝥胶囊

Actions: Break Blood and eliminate stasis, counteract toxins and drain sores.

Dose: Three tablets, twice per day.[6,8]

8. *Zhen qi fu zheng jiao nang* 贞芪扶正胶囊

Actions: Tonify *qi* and nourish *yin*, used in patients who have been sick for a long time and have insufficiency of *qi* and *yin* (*qi yin bu zu* 气阴不足). When combined with surgery, radiotherapy or chemotherapy, it can promote recovery.

Dose: Six tablets, twice per day.[6]

9. *Hua chan su pian* 华蟾素片

Actions: Resolve toxins, dispel masses and relieve pain. Used in the middle and later stages of cancer.

Dose: Three to four tablets, three or four times per day.[6]

External Chinese Herbal Medicine Treatment

External herbal medicine is an important component of CM treatment. It can have effects that are similar to those of oral Chinese herbal medicine (CHM) and can be used in cases where oral CHM cannot be applied. External CHM therapies used in CRC include enemas (*guan chang* 灌肠), suppositories (*yao shuan* 药栓), sitz baths (*zuo yu* 坐浴), topical applications (*wai fu* 外敷), and hand and foot baths (*pao xi* 泡洗).

Herbal Enemas

1. *Bao liu guang chang fang* 保留灌肠方: *Huang bai* 黄柏, *huang qin* 黄芩, *zi cao* 紫草, *ku shen* 苦参, *hu zhang* 虎杖, *teng li gen* 藤梨根 and *wu mei* 乌梅. Boil until 500 ml of water remains. Use 30–50 ml before sleep as a retention enema. Use once a day for rectal cancer.[1,5,9]

2. *Ya dan zi* 鸦胆子 (15 seeds), *bai ji* 白芨 (15 g), *ku shen* 苦参, *bai tou weng* 白头翁, *xu chang qing* 徐长卿, *ru xiang* 乳香 and *mo yao* 没药 (30g each). Use 1,000 ml of water and boil until 300–500 ml remains. When the temperature has reduced to 37°C, use as a retention enema. Use once every two days.[5,9]

3. *Huai hua* 槐花, *ya dan zi* 鸦胆子 (15 g each), *zao jiao ci* 皂角刺, *xue xie* 血竭 (10 g each), *bai hua she she cao* 白花蛇舌草, *sheng da huang* 生大黄 and *bai jiang cao* 败酱草 (40 g each). Boil until 200 ml of water remains. Use as a retention enema for 1–2 hours for rectal cancer.[5,9,10]

4. *Sheng da huang* 生大黄, *di yu tan* 地榆炭 (15 g each), *san qi* 三七, *wu bei zi* 五倍子 (10 g each), *bai hua she she cao* 白花蛇舌草 and *teng li gen* 藤梨根 (30 g each). Boil until 100 ml of water remains. Use before sleep as a retention enema every night for 10 days as a cycle. Then take 3–5 days' break. Used to restrain and stop bleeding.[6]

5. *Sheng da huang* 生大黄 (10 g, decoct later 后下), *mang xiao* 芒硝 (9 g, dissolve in solution after boiling), *zhi shi* 枳实 (12 g), *hou pu* 厚朴 (15 g), *bai hua she she cao* 白花蛇舌草 (30 g) and *ban zhi lian* 半枝莲 (30 g). Boil twice. Use 100–150 ml per time as a retention enema for more than one hour, twice per day. Used to discharge heat, free bowel movement and resolve toxins. Used for cancer-related intestinal obstruction.[6]

6. *Bai hua she she cao* 白花蛇舌草 (30 g), *ban zhi lian* 半枝莲, *hu zhang* 虎杖, *chao di yu* 炒地榆 (20 g each), *shan ci gu* 山慈菇 (15 g),

chao da huang 炒大黄 (6 g) and *yan hu suo* 延胡索 (10 g). Reduce to 50–100ml, use twice per day. Combine with chemotherapy to reduce adverse effects.[6]

7. *Da suan* 大蒜. Soak in water for a long time. Add 5% of the solution to water. Use as a retention enema for CRC.[9]

8. *Huang yao zi* 黄药子 (15 g) and *gan cao* 甘草 (4.5 g). Boil, then cool to a warm temperature for use as an enema for colon cancer with bleeding that does not stop.[9]

Suppositories

1. *Kang ai shuan* 抗癌栓: *Nao sha* 硇砂, *ya dan zi* 鸦胆子, *wu mei rou* 乌梅肉, *bing pian* 冰片 and excipients. Make into a suppository and insert one into the anus once or twice per day. Used for rectal cancer with intestinal stenosis, or difficult defecation. This medicine has an erosive action so be careful of bleeding.[1,9,10]

2. *Kang ai shuan* No 4 抗癌栓4号: *Chan chu* 蟾蜍, *xiong huang* 雄黄, *bai ji fen* 白芨粉, *dian qie jin gao* 颠茄浸膏, *gan you ming jiao* 甘油明胶 and *gan you* 甘油. Make into a suppository. Insert about 10 cm inside the anus with the patient lying prone for half an hour. Use twice per day for 30 days as one cycle.[1,9]

Sitz Baths

1. *Zuo yu fang* 坐浴方: *ku shen* 苦参, *wu bei zi* 五倍子, *long kui* 龙葵, *ma chi xian* 马齿苋, *bai jiang cao* 败酱草, *huang bai* 黄柏, *tu fu ling* 土茯苓, *shan dou gen* 山豆根, *huang yao zi* 黄药子, *ku fan* 枯矾, *bing pian* 冰片 and *lou lu* 漏芦. Boil, then cool to a temperature suitable for a sitz bath for the anus. Used for late stage anal cancer with cauliflower tumour or suppuration.[1,2]

2. *Huang bai* 黄柏 (60 g), *ku shen* 苦参 (30 g), *zi hua di ding* 紫花地丁 (60 g), *pu gong ying* 蒲公英 (60 g), *zhi ru xiang* 制乳香 (30 g), *zhi mo yao* 制没药 (30 g), *wu bei zi* 五倍子 (15 g), *lian fang* 莲房 (30 g), *huai hua* 槐花 (15 g), *di yu* 地榆 (15 g), *da huang* 大黄 (25 g), *she chuang zi* 蛇床子 (15 g) and *fang feng* 防风 (15 g). Boil in

2,000 ml of water, use 1,000 ml per time, at 37°C, twice per day, for 30 minutes per time, for ten days as a cycle. Used to clear heat and stop ulcers, for anastomotic inflammation after surgery for low rectal cancer.[6]

Topical Applications

Topical therapies include pastes, powders, sprays and the application of CHMs onto acupuncture points.

1. *Jiu hua gao* 九华膏, *huang lian gao* 黄连膏 or *si huang gao* 四黄膏 can be used for anal cancer with suppuration.[4]
2. *Ren shen* 人参 (15 g), *bu gu zhi* 补骨脂 (10 g), *dang gui* 当归 (10 g), *hong hua* 红花 (10 g), *shu fu zi* 熟附子 (6 g), *gan jiang* 干姜 (6 g) and *xue xie* 血蝎 (6 g). Make into a power and add saline water to form a paste. Apply bilaterally to BL20 *Pishu* 脾俞, BL21 *Weishu* 胃俞, BL23 *Shenshu* 肾俞 and other points for leukopenia.[5]
3. *Jiang ni zhi tu gao* 降逆止吐膏: *ban xia* 半夏, *fu ling* 茯苓, *ze xie* 泽泻, *bai dou kou* 白豆蔻 powder in equal proportions. Mix with ginger juice and honey to make a paste. During chemotherapy, apply to CV8 *Shenque* 神阙 and ST36 *Zusanli* 足三里 to prevent and treat chemotherapy-related vomiting.[6]
4. *Xing qi tong fu gao* 行气通腑膏: *sheng da huang fen* 生大黄粉 (100 g), *hou pu fen* 厚朴粉 (100 g), *bing pian fen* 冰片研粉 (20 g). Mix the powder with vinegar to form a paste. Apply to CV8 *Shenque* 神阙 and KI1 *Yongquan* 涌泉 bilaterally to prevent and treat chemotherapy-related constipation and opioid-induced constipation (OIC).[6]
5. *Qu tong pen wu ding* 祛痛喷雾酊: Soak *yuan hu* 元胡, *wu yao* 乌药, *di bie chong* 地鳖虫, *dan shen* 丹参 and *hong hua* 红花 in 2,000 ml of 75% alcohol for one week. Drain the liquid and add *xue xie* 血蝎 and *bing pian* 冰片 until dissolved. Use the liquid as a spray. Spray on painful areas three times a day. Used to relieve pain, reduce inflammation and dispel swelling.[7]
6. *Ma qian zi* 马钱子 powder mixed with vinegar can be applied to the anus for anal cancer.[9]

7. *Qing dai* 青黛 (15 g), *chan yi* 蝉衣 (30 g), and *bing pian* 冰片 (3 g). Make into a fine powder. Put on a tissue and apply to the anus for rectal and anal cancer with pus, pain and itch.[9,10]
8. *Nao sha ruan gao* 硇砂软膏: *zi nao sha* 紫硇砂 (30–50 g). Make into a powder and mix with 100 g petroleum jelly. Use for rectal cancer.[9]
9. Dry *qu gen* 瞿根 in the sun and make into a powder, and sprinkle onto the surface of the tumour for rectal and anal cancer.[9]

Hand and Foot Bath

The hands and feet can be soaked in a bath containing CHMs to relieve symptoms.

1. *Huang qi* 黄芪 (60 g), *di long* 地龙 (15 g), *tu bie chong* 土鳖虫 (10 g), *quan xie* 全蝎 (10 g), *chuan wu* 川乌 (15 g), *shui zhi* 水蛭 (10 g), *hong hua* 红花 (30 g) and *fu zi* 附子 (40 g). Boil in 2,000 ml of water and cool to 45°C. Soak the hands and feet once a day for 40 minutes, five days per week. Used to promote circulation and prevent and relieve neurotoxicity due to oxaliplatin.[6]

Acupuncture/Moxibustion Therapies

Therapies include manual acupuncture, electroacupuncture, moxibustion and ear acupressure. These treatments are used to alleviate symptoms (Table 2.3).

1. Abdominal distension and pain: Needle ST36 *Zusanli* 足三里, ST25 *Tianshu* 天枢, GB25 *Jingmen* 京门, BL20 *Pishu* 脾俞 and BL25 *Dachangshu* 大肠俞. For patients with deficiency add moxibustion on ST36 *Zusanli* 足三里, CV8 *Shenque* 神阙, CV4 *Guanyuan* 关元, SP6 *Sanyinjiao* 三阴交.[1]
2. Diarrhoea: Needle BL20 *Pishu* 脾俞, BL25 *Dachangshu* 大肠俞, and ST36 *Zusanli* 足三里. For rectal tenesmus add BL29 *Zhonglushu* 中膂俞; for patients with deficiency add moxibustion

on ST36 *Zusanli* 足三里, GV4 *Mingmen* 命门, CV4 *Guanyuan* 关元 and GV20 *Baihui* 百会.[1]

3. Blood in the stool: Needle SP6 *Sanyinjiao* 三阴交, BL57 *Chengshan* 承山, SP3 *Taibai* 太白, ST36 *Zusanli* 足三里, LI10 *Shousanli* 手三里 and add moxibustion on GV20 *Baihui* 百会.[1]

4. Nausea and vomiting: Needle PC6 *Neiguan* 内关, ST36 *Zusanli* 足三里, SP4 *Gongsun* 公孙, LR3 *Taichong* 太冲, BL21 *Weishu* 胃俞, CV14 *Juque* 巨阙 and BL17 *Geshu* 膈俞.[1]

5. Low blood cell counts and low immune function: Needle or moxibustion on ST36 *Zusanli* 足三里, CV4 *Guanyuan* 关元, GV20 *Baihui* 百会, BL20 *Pishu* 脾俞, BL23 *Shenshu* 肾俞, SP6 *Sanyinjiao* 三阴交 and CV6 *Qihai* 气海.[1]

6. Urinary retention after CRC surgery: Needle SP6 *Sanyinjiao* 三阴交, BL28 *Pangguangshu* 膀胱俞, KI3 *Taixi* 太溪 and SP9 *Yinlingquan* 阴陵泉 once a day for three days.[4,5]

7. Intestinal obstruction after CRC surgery: Needle PC6 *Neiguan* 内关, ST36 *Zusanli* 足三里, ST25 *Tianshu* 天枢, CV13 *Shangwan* 上脘, CV12 *Zhongwan* 中脘 and CV10 *Xiawan* 下脘, once a day for three days.[4]

8. Myelosuppression after chemotherapy or radiotherapy for CRC: Needle ST36 *Zusanli* 足三里, SP6 *Sanyinjiao* 三阴交, SP10 *Xuehai* 血海, BL17 *Geshu* 膈俞, LR3 *Taichong* 太冲 and KI3 *Taixi* 太溪, every day or every other day, six times as one cycle, for 1–3 cycles. Add warm needling (*wen zhen* 温针) on ST36 *Zusanli* 足三里 and SP6 *Sanyinjiao* 三阴交.[4,5]

9. Prevention and treatment of gastrointestinal reactions due to chemotherapy or radiotherapy for CRC: Needle PC6 *Neiguan* 内关, LI11 *Quchi* 曲池 and ST36 *Zusanli* 足三里, once every other day before and during therapy.[4,5]

10. Rectal and bladder reactions due to chemotherapy or radiotherapy for CRC: Needle LI4 *Hegu* 合谷, ST25 *Tianshu* 天枢, ST37 *Shangjuxu* 上巨虚 and ST36 *Zusanli* 足三里. For rectal tenesmus add CV6 *Qihai* 气海; for mucus in the stool add GB34 *Yanglingquan* 阳陵泉 and SP6 *Sanyinjiao* 三阴交; for blood in the stool add ST39 *Xiajuxu* 下巨虚. Treat once per day for one to two weeks.[4,5]

11. Late-stage CRC with intestinal obstruction: Needle ST36 *Zusanli* 足三里, CV6 *Qihai* 气海, ST37 *Shangjuxu* 上巨虚, ST25 *Tianshu* 天枢, CV4 *Guanyuan* 关元 and ST39 *Xiajuxu* 下巨虚.[4]

12. Leukopenia: Use moxa on a slice of ginger on BL20 *Pishu* 脾俞, BL23 *Shenshu* 肾俞, BL21 *Weishu* 胃俞 and BL17 *Geshu* 膈俞.[5]

13. Cancer pain: Needle ST36 *Zusanli* 足三里 bilaterally, once a day for 15 days.[4]

14. Electro-acupuncture for gastrointestinal reactions due to chemotherapy: Use LI11 *Quchi* 曲池, LI4 *Hegu* 合谷, ST36 *Zusanli* 足三里, SP6 *Sanyinjiao* 三阴交, PC6 *Neiguan* 内关, CV12 *Zhongwan* 中脘, BL20 *Pishu* 脾俞 and BL21 *Weishu* 胃俞.[5]

15. Ear acupressure for gastrointestinal reactions due to chemotherapy: For nausea and vomiting use CO18 *Neifenmi* 内分泌 and CO4 *Wei* 胃; for poor appetite use CO4 *Wei* 胃, CO18 *Neifenmi* 内分泌 and AH6a *Jiaogan* 交感; for hiccups 呃逆 use CO2 *Shidao* 食道 and CO3 *Benmen* 贲门. For all gastrointestinal reactions you can add CO10 *Shen* 肾, CO3 *Benmen* 贲门, CO2 *Shidao* 食道, CO13 *Pi* 脾 and CO4 *Wei* 胃. Apply Vaccaria seeds to points and press 3–4 times per day. Use for seven days.[4,5]

Table 2.3   Summary of Acupuncture Therapies for Colorectal Cancer

Symptoms	Acupuncture Points	Treatment Frequency
Acupuncture and/or Moxibustion[1,4,5]		
Abdominal distension and pain	Needle ST36 *Zusanli* 足三里, ST25 *Tianshu* 天枢, GB25 *Jingmen* 京门, BL20 *Pishu* 脾俞, BL25 *Dachangshu* 大肠俞. For patients with deficiency add moxibustion on ST36 *Zusanli* 足三里, CV8 *Shenque* 神阙, CV4 *Guanyuan* 关元 and SP6 *Sanyinjiao* 三阴交.	Not mentioned

(Continued)

Table 2.3   (*Continued*)

Symptoms	Acupuncture Points	Treatment Frequency
Diarrhoea	Needle BL20 *Pishu* 脾俞, BL25 *Dachangshu* 大肠俞 and ST36 *Zusanli* 足三里. For rectal tenesmus add BL29 *Zhonglushu* 中膂俞; for patients with deficiency add moxibustion on ST36 *Zusanli* 足三里, GV4 *Mingmen* 命门, CV4 *Guanyuan* 关元, and GV20 *Baihui* 百会.	Not mentioned
Blood in the stool	Needle SP6 *Sanyinjiao* 三阴交, BL57 *Chengshan* 承山, SP3 *Taibai* 太白, ST36 *Zusanli* 足三里, LI10 *Shousanli* 手三里 and add moxibustion on GV20 *Baihui* 百会.	Not mentioned
Nausea and vomiting	Needle PC6 *Neiguan* 内关, ST36 *Zusanli* 足三里, SP4 *Gongsun* 公孙, LR3 *Taichong* 太冲, BL21 *Weishu* 胃俞, RN14 *Juque* 巨阙 and BL17 *Geshu* 膈俞.	Not mentioned
Low blood cell counts and low immune function	Needle or moxibustion on ST36 *Zusanli* 足三里, CV4 *Guanyuan* 关元, GV20 *Baihui* 百会, BL20 *Pishu* 脾俞, BL23 *Shenshu* 肾俞, SP6 *Sanyinjiao* 三阴交 and CV6 *Qihai* 气海.	Not mentioned
Urinary retention after CRC surgery	Needle SP6 *Sanyinjiao* 三阴交, BL28 *Pangguangshu* 膀胱俞, KI3 *Taixi* 太溪 and SP9 *Yinlingquan* 阴陵泉.	Once a day for three days
Intestinal obstruction after CRC surgery	Needle PC6 *Neiguan* 内关, ST36 *Zusanli* 足三里, ST25 *Tianshu* 天枢, CV13 *Shangwan* 上脘, CV12 *Zhongwan* 中脘 and CV10 *Xiawan* 下脘.	Once a day for three days
Myelosuppression after chemotherapy or radiotherapy for CRC	Needle ST36 *Zusanli* 足三里, SP6 *Sanyinjiao* 三阴交, SP10 *Xuehai* 血海, BL17 *Geshu* 膈俞, LR3 *Taichong* 太冲 and KI3 *Taixi* 太溪. Add warm needling on ST36 *Zusanli* 足三里 and SP6 *Sanyinjiao* 三阴交.	Every day or every other day, six times as one cycle, for 1–3 cycles

(Continued)

Table 2.3 (*Continued*)

Symptoms	Acupuncture Points	Treatment Frequency
Prevention and treatment of gastrointestinal reactions due to chemotherapy or radiotherapy for CRC	Needle PC6 *Neiguan* 内关, LI11 *Quchi* 曲池 and ST36 *Zusanli* 足三里.	Once every other day before and during therapy
Rectal and bladder reactions due to chemotherapy or radiotherapy for CRC	Needle LI4 *Hegu* 合谷, ST25 *Tianshu* 天枢, ST37 *Shangjuxu* 上巨虚 and ST36 *Zusanli* 足三里. For rectal tenesmus add CV6 *Qihai* 气海; for mucus in the stool add GB34 *Yanglingquan* 阳陵泉 and SP6 *Sanyinjiao* 三阴交; for blood in the stool add ST39 *Xiajuxu* 下巨虚.	Once per day for one to two weeks
Late-stage CRC with intestinal obstruction	Needle ST36 *Zusanli* 足三里, CV6 *Qihai* 气海, ST37 *Shangjuxu* 上巨虚, ST25 *Tianshu* 天枢, CV4 *Guanyuan* 关元 and ST39 *Xiajuxu* 下巨虚.	Not mentioned
Cancer pain	Needle ST36 *Zusanli* 足三里 bilaterally.	Once a day for 15 days
Electroacupuncture[5]		
Gastrointestinal reactions due to chemotherapy	LI11 *Quchi* 曲池, LI4 *Hegu* 合谷, ST36 *Zusanli* 足三里, SP6 *Sanyinjiao* 三阴交, PC6 *Neiguan* 内关, CV12 *Zhongwan* 中脘, BL20 *Pishu* 脾俞 and BL21 *Weishu* 胃俞.	Not mentioned
Ear Acupressure[4,5]		
Gastrointestinal reactions due to chemotherapy	For nausea and vomiting use CO18 *Neifenmi* 内分泌 and CO4 *Wei* 胃; for poor appetite use CO4 *Wei* 胃, CO18 *Neifenmi* 内分泌 and AH6a *Jiaogan* 交感; for hiccups 呃逆 use CO2 *Shidao* 食道 and CO3 *Benmen* 贲门. For all gastrointestinal reactions you can add CO10 *Shen* 肾, CO3 *Benmen* 贲门, CO2 *Shidao* 食道, CO13 *Pi* 脾 and CO4 *Wei* 胃.	Apply Vaccaria seeds to points and press 3–4 times per day. Use for seven days.

See references 1–5 in the References list at the end of this chapter.

Other Chinese Medicine Therapies

These include *qi gong* 气功 therapies, *tui na* 推拿 and dietary therapy.

Qi gong Therapies

Qi gong 气功 therapies include *guo lin qi gong* 郭林气功, *tai ji quan* 太极拳, *zhou tian gong* 周天功, *yuan ji gong* 元极功 and *xiang gong* 香功. These aim to soothe and free the channels and connecting vessels, promote the flow of *qi* and the Blood, strengthen the constitution, regulate mood and emotions, build physique and improve health, prevent and treat cancer, reduce the adverse effects of chemotherapy and radiotherapy, and delay progression of the disease. Different people have different capacities for exercise, so it is important to avoid over-exercise and excessive fatigue.[9,13]

Tui na Therapy

Use the points LI4 *Hegu* 合谷, CV4 *Guanyuan* 关元, PC6 *Neiguan* 内关, ST36 *Zusanli* 足三里, and SP6 *Sanyinjiao* 三阴交. Manipulation methods include scrubbing (*ca* 擦), grasping (*na* 拿), rotating (*zhuan* 转) and rocking (*yao* 摇). To fortify the Spleen and harmonise the Stomach, recover the Stomach and Intestine function, and improve health.[9]

Dietary Therapy

In CM, medicine and food share the same source, and some foods are considered to have beneficial effects for the prevention and treatment of cancers by improving immune function, promoting recovery after surgery, reducing the adverse effects of chemotherapy and radiotherapy, and preventing tumor recurrence and metastasis.[11] The following are examples of dietary recipes.

1. *Ma chi xian lv dou tang* 马齿苋绿豆汤
Ingredients: *Ma chi xian* 马齿苋 (20 g) and *lv dou* 绿豆 (10 g).

Preparation method: Put into a pot with 1,000 ml of water. Boil on high heat for five mins, then simmer for 30 mins. Pour off the liquid and separate into portions for drinking.

Applications: To clear dampness and heat. Can use for damp-heat flowing downward type CRC with symptoms that include abdominal pain, rectal tenesmus, burning sensation in the anus, nausea and vomiting. It cannot be used in patients with Spleen-deficient damp diarrhoea (*pi xu shi xie* 脾虚湿泻).[4,13]

2. *Chi xiao dou yi mi zhou* 赤小豆薏米粥

Ingredients: *Chi xiao dou* 赤小豆 (50 g), *jing mi* 粳米 (50 g) and *sheng yi yi ren* 生薏苡仁 (30 g).

Preparation method: Soak the azuki beans (*chi xiao dou* 赤小豆) and Job's tears (*sheng yi yi ren*生薏苡仁) in water, then boil until all the beans burst. Add glutinous rice (*jing mi* 粳米) and cook until you have a congee. Add sugar and eat.

Applications: To clear heat and induce diuresis, disperse Blood stasis and resolve toxins. *Chi xiao dou* 赤小豆 is sweet, sour and mild in flavor; it moves water, clears heat and resolves toxins, disperses Blood stasis and dispels masses; *sheng yi yi ren* 生薏苡仁 is sweet and bland (*gan dan* 甘淡) in flavor and slightly cold in nature (*wei han* 微寒). It fortifies the Spleen and excretes dampness, clears heat and expels pus, dispels wind and eliminates dampness. *Jing mi* 粳米 tonifies the Spleen and harmonises the Stomach. Used for dampness-heat agglomeration (s*hi re yun jie* 湿热蕴结) type CRC. Can consume often.[4,13]

3. *Fo shou gan zhou* 佛手柑粥

Ingredients: *Fo shou gan* 佛手柑, water, *jing mi* 粳米 and *bing tang* 冰糖 (rock sugar).

Preparation method: Use *fo shou gan* 佛手柑 (10–15 g), add 200 ml water and boil until 100 ml remains. Add 50 g of *jing mi* 粳米 to the 100 ml of liquid, add *bing tang* 冰糖 and an extra 400 ml of water, and cook until you have a congee. Eat twice per day.

Applications: This congee first appeared in the book *Huan You Ri Li* 宦游日礼 in which it was used to move *qi* to relieve pain, fortify the Spleen and increase appetite. Used for CRC with abdominal distension.[4,13]

4. *Tao hua zhou* 桃花粥

Ingredients: Use 4 g of fresh peach flower petals *xian tao hua ban* 鲜桃花瓣 (or use 2 g dried petals) and *jing mi* 粳米 (100 g).

Preparation method: Cook the *jing mi* 粳米 to a congee. Then add the peach flower petals and boil.

Applications: To dispel swelling and distension, descend malign *qi*, drain retained fluids, dispel phlegm-fluid and stagnation, and alleviate difficult defaecation. During the *Tang* dynasty, *tao hua zhou* 桃花粥 was used as a food before and after the *Han shi jie* 寒食节 festival (no fire was used during the festival so only cold food was eaten). The custom was also present in the later *Ming* dynasty. *Tao hua* 桃花 is slightly cold, so stop eating after the difficulty in defaecation has been alleviated. Do not consume long term.[4,13]

5. *He tao lian rou gao* 核桃莲肉糕

Ingredients: *He tao ren* 核桃仁 (100 g), *lian rou* 莲肉 (after removing the embryo — called *lian zi xin* 莲子芯) (300 g), *qian shi fen* 芡实粉 (60 g) and *nuo mi* 糯米 (500 g).

Preparation method: Cook *he tao* 核桃 and *lian rou* 莲肉 in water until they burst. Mash into a puree. Soak *nuo mi* 糯米 in water for two hours. Add all ingredients into a pot and steam. Cool and solidify. Divide into portions, add a little sugar and eat morning and evening for 10–15 days.

Applications: To warm the Kidney and fortify the Spleen, nourish the intestine and check diarrhoea. *He tao* 核桃 is sweet and warm in nature and tonifies the Kidney. *Lian rou* 莲肉 is sweet and astringent, and mild in nature. It fortifies the Spleen and astringes the intestine, and promotes interaction between the Heart and Kidney. *Qian shi* 芡实 is sweet and warm, and mild in nature. It fortifies the Spleen and checks diarrhoea, nourishes the Kidney and secures the Essence. When all ingredients are combined into a solid cake (*gao* 糕), they nourish the stomach and intestine and disperse cold and dampness.[4,13]

6. *Zhen qi zhu gan* 贞杞猪肝

Ingredients: *Nv zhen zi* 女贞子 (30 g), *gou qi zi* 枸杞子 (35 g), pig liver (250 g), ginger, shallots, vegetable oil, sugar and yellow wine (*huang jiu* 黄酒).

Preparation method: Put *nv zhen zi* 女贞子 and *gou qi zi* 枸杞子 in a cloth bag and boil in water for 30 minutes, then discard. Clean the pig liver. Make a lot of small holes in the liver with a bamboo skewer. Add the liver to the liquid and boil for one hour. Remove and cut into pieces. Fry the liver pieces in vegetable oil with ginger and shallots, yellow wine, soy sauce, sugar and the herb liquid. Thicken the liquid with cornstarch (*dian fen* 淀粉).

Applications: To nourish the Liver and supplement Kidney, enrich *yin* and supplement deficiency. Used for CRC patients with deficiency of Liver and Kidney *yin*.[4,13]

7. *Huang qi hou tou tang* 黄芪猴头汤

Ingredients: *Hou tou gu* 猴头菇 (250 g), *huang qi* 黄芪 (50 g), chicken meat (500 g), pepper, sliced ginger, shallot, wine 料酒, salt and monosodium glutamate (MSG).

Preparation method: Soak the dried *hou tou gu* 猴头菇 mushroom in warm water until soft. Remove the mushroom and slice. Keep the water for cooking. Slice the chicken meat and *huang qi* 黄芪. Add the chicken, *huang qi* 黄芪, sliced ginger, shallot, wine and the mushroom water to a clear soup stock (*qing tang* 清汤) and boil for 90 minutes. Then add the mushroom slices and boil for a further 45 minutes. Add salt, MSG and pepper to taste.

Applications: To tonify the middle and supplement *qi*, nourish the Blood and generate fluids. Used for CRC patients with dual deficiency of *qi* and Blood (*qi xue liang xu* 气血两虚).[4,13]

8. *Huang qi shen zao zhou* 黄芪参枣粥
Ingredients: *Sheng huang qi* 生黄芪 (300 g), *dang shen* 党参 (30 g), *gan cao* 甘草 (15 g), *jing mi* 粳米 (100 g) and *da zao* 大枣 (10 dates).

Preparation method: Put *sheng huang qi* 生黄芪, *dang shen* 党参 and *gan cao* 甘草 in a cloth bag and boil in water, then discard. Add the *jing mi* 粳米 and *da zao* 大枣 and more water. Cook until it forms a congee.

Applications: To tonify the middle and supplement *qi*, fortify the Spleen and nourish the Blood. For patients with insufficiency of *qi* and Blood (*qi xue bu zu* 气血不足).[4,13]

9. *Ma chi xian zhou* 马齿苋粥
Ingredients: Fresh *ma chi xian* 马齿苋 (100 g) and *jing mi* 粳米 (60 g).

Preparation method: Finely cut the *ma chi xian* 马齿苋. Cook *jing mi* 粳米 in water to make a congee. Add the *ma chi xian* 马齿苋 and boil. Add seasoning and eat.

Applications: To clear heat and resolve toxins, fortify the Spleen and astringe intestines. For CRC patients with diarrhoea with pus and blood, who are thirsty but do not want to drink.[7,8,12]

10. *Mu er fu zhu men tu rou* 木耳腐竹焖兔肉
Ingredients: *Mu er* 木耳 (15 g), *fu zhu* 腐竹 (one piece), rabbit meat (250 g) and sliced ginger (two pieces).

Preparation method: Place all ingredients in a pot and cook. Add oil, salt and seasoning.

Applications: To activate the Blood, dispel stasis and resolve toxins. Used for CRC with stasis of Blood and toxins blocking the interior (*yu du nei zu* 瘀毒内阻).[7,8]

11. *Chi xiao dou bou ji* 赤小豆煲鸡
Ingredients: *Chi xiao dou* 赤小豆 (60 g) and one small whole hen (about 500 g).

Preparation method: Clean the hen, put the *chi xiao dou* 赤小豆 (azuki beans) inside the hen. Put in a pot with water and cook. Add seasoning and eat.

Applications: To activate the Blood, dispel stasis and resolve toxins. Used for CRC with stasis of Blood and toxins blocking the interior.[7,8]

12. *Lu dou nuo mi dun zhu chang* 绿豆糯米炖猪肠
Ingredients: Pig intestine (about 40 cm), *lv dou* 绿豆 (mung bean), *nuo mi* 糯米 (ratio *lv dou* versus *nuo mi* = 2:1), and *dong gu* 冬菇 (2–3 mushrooms).

Preparation method: Put all the ingredients in water and cook for two hours. After cooking, cut up the pig intestine, add seasoning and eat.

Applications: To fortify the Spleen and tonify the Kidney. For CRC patients with deficiency of Spleen and Kidney (*pi shen liang xu* 脾肾亏虚).[7,8]

13. *Tai zi shen, wu hua guo dun tu rou* 太子参, 无花果炖兔肉
Ingredients: Rabbit meat (150 g), *tai zi shen* 太子参 (30 g) and *wu hua guo* 无花果 (60 g).

Preparation method: Put all the ingredients in water and cook for two hours. Add seasoning and eat the meat and drink the soup.

Applications: To fortify the Spleen and tonify the Kidney. For CRC patients with deficiency of Spleen and Kidney (*pi shen kui xu* 脾肾亏虚).[7,8]

Principles for Combining Chinese and Western Medicine for Colorectal Cancer

At present, the combination of Western and Chinese treatment is widely used by CRC patients. The combination of the two approaches to treatment can take advantage of the strengths and counter the weaknesses of both therapies. Chinese herbal medicine treatment is applied at all stages in the treatment of CRC. The advantages of CHM are as follows: it extends life in patients with tumour burden, improves the patient's quality of life, prolongs survival time, speeds up recovery after surgery, prevents recurrence and/or metastasis, reduces the adverse effects and improves the effects of chemotherapy and/or radiotherapy.

In the early stages of CRC the main treatment is radical surgery. After surgery, CHMs for supporting health and eliminating pathogens (*fu zheng qu xie* 扶正祛邪) are used to improve recovery time, prevent recurrence of the tumour and prevent metastasis. In the middle and later stages of CRC, if there are no contraindications, the main treatments are surgery, chemotherapy or radiotherapy, combined with CHM to alleviate adverse effects, improve treatment effects and enhance recovery. For CRC patients who cannot receive surgery, chemotherapy or radiotherapy, the main treatment is CHM in order to relieve symptoms, improve quality of life and prolong survival.[2,5]

Prevention

To prevent pre-cancerous lesions, people should reduce their intakes of certain foods such as high-fat, fried, mouldy and very spicy foods, and reduce meat intake. People should consume more fresh vegetables, fresh fruits and foods high in fibre and vitamins to maintain daily defaecation. Patients who have symptoms of weight loss, blood in the stool, mucus in the stool, change in bowel habit or change in the form of the stool, should have an examination to determine the diagnosis and receive treatment as soon as possible. Early-stage patients who have received surgery and/or radiotherapy should receive regular check-ups.[3,4,7–9,11]

Nursing and Care of the Patient

Lifestyle

Patients should undertake appropriate physical exercise to enhance immunity, have a regular lifestyle and meals, and get enough sleep to promote health and resist disease. Adjust lifestyle according to the season to avoid cold and prevent seasonal diseases.[4,11]

Psychology

Colorectal cancer patients often experience psychological problems following diagnosis, including depression and anxiety. Doctors and nurses should talk to patients, provide scientific information on CRC and its treatment, and provide psychological treatment to dispel fear, despair and other negative emotions in order to maintain peace of mind and support the patient's courage to face the cancer and follow the treatment plan. The doctors and patient's family should be optimistic, improve the patient's mood, assist the patient to relax and encourage resilience.[4,7]

Prognosis

The prognosis depends on early detection of lesions, early diagnosis and early treatment, as well as the biological characteristics and pathological type of the tumour, and other factors. The use of CHM treatment in a timely manner that is in accordance with the stage of the disease and that uses correct syndrome differentiation and treatment can affect the prognosis.[2,4,8]

References

1. 中华中医药学会. (2008) 肿瘤中医诊疗指南. 北京: 中国中医药出版社.
2. 郁仁存. (1983) 中医肿瘤学. 北京: 科学出版社.
3. 刘嘉湘. (1996) 实用中医肿瘤手册. 上海: 上海科技教育出版社.
4. 吴万垠, 刘伟胜. (2013) 肿瘤科专病中医临床诊治 (第3版). 北京: 人民卫生出版社.
5. 罗云坚. (2007) 中医临床治疗特色与优势指南. 北京: 人民卫生出版社.
6. 林洪生. (2014) 恶性肿瘤中医诊疗指南. 北京: 人民卫生出版社.
7. 何裕民. (2005) 现代中医肿瘤学 (普通高等教育"十五"国家级规划教材面向21世纪课程教材). 北京: 中国协和医科大学出版社.
8. 陈锐深. (2003) 现代中医肿瘤学. 北京: 人民卫生出版社.
9. 李家庚, 屈松柏. (2001) 实用中医肿瘤学. 北京: 科学技术文献出版社.
10. 汪悦. (2002) 中医内科学. 上海: 上海中医药大学出版社.
11. 张蓓, 周志伟. (2004) 实用中西医结合肿瘤学. 广州: 广东人民出版社.
12. 周岱翰, 林丽珠. (2012) 中医肿瘤食疗学. 贵阳: 贵州科技出版社.
13. 徐振晔. (2013) 常见肿瘤的中医预防和护养. 上海: 复旦大学出版社.

3

Classical Chinese Medicine Literature

OVERVIEW

Classical Chinese medicine literature is a valuable source of information on intestinal and abdominal disorders that have symptoms and signs which are consistent with colorectal cancer. Besides descriptions of the disorders, the classical medical books suggest approaches to their management using Chinese herbal medicine, acupuncture, moxibustion and other therapies. This chapter reports the results of a search of *Zhong Hua Yi Dian* 中华医典, one of the largest collections of classical Chinese medicine texts. Six terms of relevance to colorectal cancer were searched and these identified 468 citations of which 409 referred to a treatment using Chinese herbal medicine, 54 referred to the use of acupuncture points and five referred to other methods. In general, the citations referred to conditions characterised by presence of a mass and those characterised by gastrointestinal bleeding. The symptoms, aetiology and treatments of these two categories of conditions are analysed separately and their relevance to colorectal cancer is discussed.

Introduction

Written records of the professional practice of Chinese medicine (CM) date back to the Spring and Autumn (770–476 BC) and Warring states (474–221 BC) periods. In these passages, concepts such as *yin* and *yang* are evident and therapeutic methods included the use of mugwort (*ai* 艾) for moxibustion, herbal decoctions and acupuncture.[1]

In order to obtain a sample of the classical and pre-modern medical literature, we conducted electronic searches of the *Zhong Hua Yi Dian* 中华医典 (ZHYD) 5th edition, a database of more than

1,150 medical books.[2] This collection is the largest currently available and is representative of other large collections of the classical and pre-modern CM literature.[3,4]

Search Terms

In CM, a number of disease and symptom names are of potential relevance to colorectal cancer (CRC). To select terms, 30 books and guidelines[5–34] were consulted and a list of 21 potential terms was compiled. Each term was searched in the ZHYD and a sample of citations for each term was read to determine the proportion of citations that were potentially relevant to CRC. In addition, ten clinical experts and consultant physicians provided their rankings of these terms regarding their relevance to CRC. Based on test searches, terms which had high frequencies but low specificity for CRC, for example *chang pi* 肠澼 (dysentery), *chang feng* 肠风 (intestinal bleeding), *bian xue* 便血 (blood in the stool) and *xia xue* 下血 (gastrointestinal bleeding), were excluded. Terms directly relating to masses (also called aggregation-accumulations) included *ji ju* 积聚 and *zheng jia* 癥瘕 (also written as 症瘕). In the case of *ji ju* 积聚, due to its relatively low specificity, it was combined with *chang* 肠 (intestine). Similarly, the terms *zheng jia* 症瘕 and *zheng* 癥 were combined with *chang* 肠 to improve the specificity of the search. The term *zang du* 脏毒 was included since experts agreed that this was relevant to CRC and the searches showed high specificity. *Suo gang zhi* 锁肛痔 was included since the experts agreed this was relevant to anal cancer.

Procedures for Search, Data Coding and Data Analysis

Each term was entered into the ZHYD database and the search results were downloaded to spreadsheets (Fig. 3.1).

A 'citation' was defined as a distinct passage of text referring to one or more of the search terms. Codes were allocated for the types of citations, books and the dynasties in which they were written

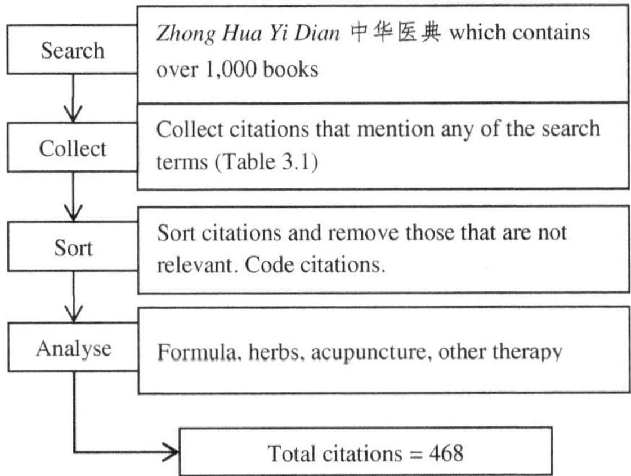

Fig. 3.1   Process for identifying classical literature citations.

according to the procedures described in May *et al.* (2014).[35] Books written after 1949 were excluded.

The number of hits identified by each search term was calculated by summing the results of the searches. The combination of the terms of *ji ju* 积聚, *zheng* 癥 and *zheng* 症 with *chang* 肠 (intestine) improved the specificity of these search results, but this did not limit all the results to disorders located in the intestine since the result was based on proximity to the term *chang* 肠 (within 100 characters) rather than any logical linkage between the two terms within a citation.

After removing duplicates, exclusion criteria were then applied to remove citations which were considered not related to CRC. The following exclusion criteria were applied to identify citations that were unlikely to refer to CRC: masses that disappear spontaneously, disorders of children, masses related to gynaecological disorders, conditions due to parasites, abscesses and carbuncles, haemorrhoids and other physical disorders unlike CRC.

Citations were scored by location in the intestine, abdomen, anus or rectum, and by symptoms and signs suggestive of CRC including a mass located in the intestine, rectum or anus; blood in the stool (*bian xue* 便血 and related terms); intestinal obstruction (*chang geng zu* 肠梗阻 and related terms); abdominal pain (*fu tong* 腹痛 and related terms); abdominal distension (*fu zhang* 腹胀 and related terms); emaciation (*xiao shou* 消瘦 and related terms) and change in bowel habit (*pai ben xi guan gai bian* 排便习惯改变 and related terms).

Citations were reviewed to identify any detailed descriptions relevant to CRC and its aetiology or pathogenesis. Citations that included a treatment were included in the further analyses. Data are presented below for the frequencies of identified formulas, herbs and acupuncture points.

The final data set included citations considered to potentially refer to CRC and which described CM treatments including Chinese herbal medicine (CHM), acupuncture and related therapies, or other CM therapies. When a citation referred to multiple treatments, each treatment was considered as a separate citation for calculating the frequency of formulas, herbs or acupuncture points. In the case of herbal formulas, those with the same or similar name and the same ingredients were considered to be the same formula, whereas those with the same name and different ingredients were considered different formulas, and these were distinguished with a number. Herbal treatments comprising two or more ingredients that had no name were all scored together as 'unnamed formula' in the formula frequencies. In the case of single-ingredient treatments, when these had a specific 'formula-like' name (such as names ending in *tang* 汤, *san* 散 or *wan* 丸), they were scored with the multi-ingredient formulas. When the treatment was a single herb with no special name, it was not included as a formula. These citations were scored separately and presented in the tables of herb frequencies, together with the frequencies of herbs in the formulas. In a number of citations, the treatment comprised a combination of formula names, with or without additional ingredients. In these cases, each named formula was scored separately.

In the case of acupuncture, citations tend to fall into two types: (1) lists of the uses of a specific point which may include a variety of symptoms that may, or may not, be all related to CRC; and (2) disorders or symptoms related to CRC and the points used to treat them.

Both types of citations were included, and these were distinguished in the analyses.

Included citations were grouped according to the CM intervention for further analysis. An additional screening process was performed to identify citations considered 'most likely' to be CRC based on the absence of the exclusion criteria and presence of key clinical symptoms including location in the intestine, blood in the stool and chronic nature. Data are presented for the frequencies of identified formulas, herbs and acupuncture points for the main sub-groups of citations and for those 'most likely' to have been CRC.

Search Results

Six terms, or combinations of terms, were used in the comprehensive searches. These identified 15,695 potential passages ('hits') in the database (Table 3.1). Following removal of duplicates, irrelevant or unclear hits, and citations that did not include a treatment, 468 citations were included in the data set. The most frequent search term was the combination of *ji ju* 积聚 and *chang* 肠 (within 100 characters) accounting for 46.9% of the hits and 17.9% of the included

Table 3.1   Hit Frequency by Search Term

Pinyin	Chinese Characters	Hit Frequency (%)[1]	Included Citations *n* (%)[2]
Ji ju + chang	积聚 + 肠	7,354 (46.9)	84 (17.9)
Zheng + chang	癥/症 + 肠	4,103 (26.1)	7 (1.5)
Zheng jia 1	癥瘕	1,751 (11.2)	8 (1.7)
Zheng jia 2	症瘕	1,562 (10.0)	2 (0.4)
Zang du	脏毒	922 (5.9)	380 (81.2)
Suo gang zhi	锁肛痔	3 (0.02)	0 (0)
Total		15,695	468*

*Some citations were located by two or more search terms.

[1]Before duplicate removal and screening.

[2]After duplicate removal and screening.

citations. In some books *zheng* 癥 was written, while in others it had been simplified to *zheng* 症 but had the same meaning. To reflect this difference, we use the term *zheng* 症/癥 in this chapter. *Zheng* 症/癥 plus *chang* 肠 found 26.1% of the hits but only 1.5% of the citations. The most productive search term was *zang du* 脏毒, with 5.9% of the hits and 81.2% of the citations. The term *suo gang zhi* 锁肛痔 was rare, with only three hits and zero included citations.

The included citations were derived from 143 different books written between 282 AD (*Zhen Jiu Jia Yi Jing* 针灸甲乙经) and 1938 (*Ben Cao Jian Yao Fang* 本草简要方). The most commonly cited book was *Pu Ji Fang* 普济方 (73 citations) followed by *Ben Cao Gang Mu* 本草纲目 (14 citations).

Citations Related to the Definitions of the Main Terms

Overall, the search results were derived from four main groups of terms: (1) *ji ju* 积聚; (2) *zheng* 癥/症 and/or *zheng jia* 癥瘕/症瘕; (3) *zang du* 脏毒; and (4) *suo gang zhi* 锁肛痔. The meanings of each of these terms are explored based on references from the Chinese classical literature.

Ji Ju and Related Terms

The characters *ji* 积 and *ju* 聚 appear in the ancient dictionaries *Shuo Wen Jie Zi* 说文解字 (c. 100 AD) and *Shi Ming* 释名 (c. 210). In the disease section of *Shi Ming* (*shi ji bing* 释疾病), *ji* 积 could refer to a breast abscess (*ru yong* 乳痈), while *ju* 聚 was used in the explanations of *zhong* 肿 (swellings) and *lu* 瘤 (lumps).

The composite term *ji ju* 积聚 appears in the ancient CM literature in the *Huang Di Nei Jing Ling Shu* 黄帝内经灵枢 (c. 100 BC), Chapter 46 *Wu bian* 五变. *Huang di* 黄帝 asked about the features of a disorder of the intestines called *ji ju* 积聚. The physician *Shao shu* 少俞 explained it as follows:

'When a person has thin skin and dull complexion (i.e. has poor nourishment), muscles that are weak and flaccid, and whose stomach and intestines are in poor condition, evil pathogenic *qi* (*e ze xie qi* 恶则邪气) can lodge in the interior, forming a mass (*ji ju* 积聚), which damages the Spleen and Stomach (*pi wei* 脾胃). When cold and warmth are disordered (*han wen bu ci* 寒温不次) in the Spleen and Stomach (*pi wei zhi jian* 脾胃之间), more pathogenic *qi* enters, accumulates and lodges. Firstly, large *ju* 聚 emerge.'

In this passage *ji ju* 积聚 is used as a composite term, with *ju* 聚 appearing to be early-stage masses. In a passage in Chapter 68 *Shang ge* 上膈, in a discussion on disorders associated with immoderate lifestyle, the term *ji ju* 积聚 is used to refer to an accumulation in the abdomen due to worms and cold (*chong han* 虫寒).[36]

In *Jin Gui Yao Lue* 金匮要略 (c. 206) Chapter 11 *Wu zang feng han ji ju bing mai zheng bing zhi* 五脏风寒积聚病脉证并治, the terms *ji* 积 and *ju* 聚 are distinguished as follows: *ji* 积 is a mass associated with the solid (*zang* 藏) organs which does not move; *ju* 聚 is a mass associated with the hollow organs (*fu* 府), which appears and disappears, can move location, and the pain moves. *Ju* 聚 can be treated.[37]

The *Nan Jing* 难经 (c. 220) contains a similar passage in Chapter 4 Difficulty 55, which aims to distinguish *ji* 积 and *ju* 聚. This passage says that *ji* 积 is related to *yin qi* 阴气, while *ju* 聚 is related to *yang qi* 阳气. *Yin* sinks and hides, *yang* floats and moves. In the case of *ji* 积, it does not move; the pain is always in the same place and you can feel the edges of the mass. In the case of *ju* 聚, it has no root, so it has no edges to feel, and the pain moves from place to place.[38]

Although the above books distinguish *ji* 积 and *ju* 聚, in later books these terms are more often used as the composite term *ji ju* 积聚. For example, *Zhen Jiu Jia Yi Jing* 针灸甲乙经 (c. 282) mentions *ji ju* 积聚 in the abdomen (*fu zhong ji ju* 腹中积聚) in Scroll 8 and Scroll 9. In *Zhou Hou Bei Ji Fang* 肘后备急方 (c. 363) the term *ji ju* 积聚 appears a number of times; however, there was little clinical information in most passages; for example, the formula *Lu su wan* 露宿丸 is simply for 'great cold *ji ju*' (*da han leng ji ju* 大寒冷积聚).

In the *Zhu Bing Yuan Hou Lun* 诸病源候论 (c. 610) section on *Ji ju hou* 积聚候, it explains that *ji* 积 is related to the *zang* 脏 organs and *yin qi* 阴气, while *ju* 聚 is related to the *fu* 腑 organs and *yang qi* 阳气. However, in the sections on specific disorders the composite term *ji ju* 积聚 is used and it is evident that this term can refer to various types of masses, with a number of references to *ji ju* 积聚 in a gynaecological context.

In *Bei Ji Qian Jin Yao Fang* 备急千金要方 (c. 652), the term *ji ju* 积聚 appears frequently. It is mainly a gynaecological disorder located in the abdomen, but it can also be associated with the upper abdomen, with the costal area and with malaria (*nue* 疟). In Scroll 37, the pill *Shen ming du ming yuan* 神明度命圆 is for 'long term *ji ju* 积聚 inside the abdomen which obstructs defaecation and urination, *qi* rising to oppress the heart area, middle abdominal distension and fullness, which harms eating and drinking.' In this citation, the disorder is chronic, and the symptoms appear to be mainly associated with intestinal blockage, so CRC seems a possibility.

The term 'five *ji* and six *ju*' (*wu ji liu ju* 五积六聚) appears in *San Yin Ji Yi Bing Zheng Fang Lun* 三因极一病证方论 (c. 1174) but it was not found in other major books from the Song dynasty or earlier. These types of masses were not distinguished and appear to be all due to the same process (see below). However, the *Ru Men Shi Qin* 儒门事亲 (c. 1228) says that the *wu ji* 五积 are located in the five *zang* organs and bitter cold (*ku han* 苦寒) medicines are used to treat them, while the *liu ju* 六聚 are located in the six *fu* organs and are treated with acrid warm (*xin wen* 辛温) medicines. The *wu ji* 五积 of each of the five *zang* organs are named using terms for existing disorders. Symptoms are given for each, but none show symptoms characteristic of CRC. In another section (Scroll 14) in the same book, there is a list of prognoses for many conditions including *ji ju* 积聚 of the abdomen which says that when the pulse is big (*mai da* 脉大), the abdomen is very distended and the four limbs are cold, the prognosis is death. If the abdomen is distended and full, there is blood in the stool and the pulse is big, whenever the gastrointestinal bleeding is extreme the prognosis is death. In this example, *ji ju* 积聚 is clearly associated with the intestine and with bleeding.

Zheng Jia and Related Terms

The character *zheng* 症 (also written as 癥) is not listed in the dictionary *Shuo Wen Jie Zi* 说文解字 (c. 100 AD) but the term *jia* 瘕 is defined as a women's disease. In the dictionary *Shi Ming* 释名 (c. 210), *zheng* 癥/症 does not appear as an entry.

The composite term *zheng jia* 症/癥瘕 does not appear in the *Huang Di Nei Jing* 黄帝内经, although there are separate mentions of *jia* 瘕 which do not appear relevant to cancer. In the *Jin Gui Yao Lue* 金匮要略 (c. 206) Chapter 87 *Nue bing mai zheng bing zhi* 疟病脉证并治, the term *zheng jia* 症/癥瘕 appears, but since the context is malaria (*nue bing* 疟病) this is possibly a reference to splenomegaly rather than to cancer.[37] In the *Zhou Hou Bei Ji Fang* 肘后备急方 Scroll 5, the term *zheng jia* 症/癥瘕 appears in a gynaecological context but the nature of the disease is unclear.

In the *Zhu Bing Yuan Hou Lun* 诸病源候论 (c. 610), Scroll 19 section on *Jia bing zhu hou* 瘕病诸候, the terms *zheng* 癥/症 and *jia* 瘕 are distinguished as follows:

'*Zheng* 癥/症 is due to disorder(s) of cold and warmth; leading to emptiness and weakness of the *qi* of the *zang* and *fu* organs 腑脏, so food and drink are not digested and accumulate (*ju jie* 聚结) inside; [this accumulation] gradually grows and extends. The mass (*kuai jia* 块叚) attaches and cannot move to another location. It is called *zheng* 症/癥. You can feel the shape and it is evident to everyone. If this *ji* 积 is there for a long time, the person will become emaciated, the abdomen will get big, the pulse will be string-like and hidden. If the *zheng* 癥/症 cannot be shifted, the person must die.

Jia 瘕 are all caused by dysregulation of cold and warmth. Food and drink are not transformed, and (these pathogenic factors) fight with the *zang qi* 脏气 to produce (this disease). When this disease does not move, it is called *zheng* 症/癥. If this disease produces a mass which can move, it is called *jia* 瘕. This *jia* 瘕 means '*jia* 假' (not true) and is called 'empty *jia*' (*xu jia* 虚假) since the mass can move.'

In *Bei Ji Qian Jin Yao Fang* 备急千金要方 (c. 652) the term *zheng jia* 症/癥瘕 appears separately as a gynaecological disorder, and in Scroll 37 it also appears together with *ji ju* 积聚 in the context of a formula for men and women for *jiu pi* 久癖 and *zheng ji ji ju* 症瘕积聚. However, it is not clear where these masses were located and there are no intestinal symptoms given.

In these books, the term *zheng jia* 症/癥瘕 could appear separately and combined with *ji ju* 积聚 as *zheng jia ji ju* 癥瘕积聚. Both referred to masses, but it is unclear whether these terms were used to refer to different types of conditions.

In the *Sheng Ji Zong Lu* 圣济总录 (c. 1117) section on *ji ju men* 积聚门, it says that *zheng jia* 症/癥瘕 and *jie pi* 结癖 are other names for *ji ju* 积聚. The symptoms are different, but the root is similar. Later in the same section there are formulas for treating *ji ju* 积聚 that are also used for *zheng jia* 症瘕, but there is insufficient information to determine the identity of the diseases or the differences between the symptoms of these two disorders.

In another passage, the *Sheng Ji Zong Lu* 圣济总录 distinguishes the terms *zheng* 症/癥, *jia* 瘕 and *pi* 癖 as follows: 'Zheng 症/癥 is hidden inside the lower abdomen, when you palpate it there is a shape that everyone can see; *jia* 瘕 is a *jia ju* 瘕聚 (false accumulation), when you push it, it moves around and is not fixed; *pi* 癖 is located on the side, in the rib area.'

Zang Du and Related Terms

The term *zang du* 脏毒 does not appear in the *Huang Di Nei Jing* 黄帝内经, *Shang Han Lun* 伤寒论, *Jing Gui Yao Lue* 金匮要略, *Zhou Hou Bei Ji Fang* 肘后备急方, *Zhu Bing Yuan Hou Lun* 诸病源候论, *Bei Ji Qian Jin Yao Fang* 备急千金要方 or other major pre-Song dynasty medical book.

It appears in the Song dynasty in the *Ben Cao Tu Jing* 本草图经 (c. 1061) which gives an unnamed two-herb formula (*di bai* 地柏 plus *huang qi* 黄芪) for *zang du* 脏毒 with gastrointestinal bleeding (*xia xue* 下血). The *Tai Ping Hui Min He Ji Ju Fang* 太平惠民和剂局方 (c. 1107) gives the two-herb formula *Wu jing wan* 乌荆丸 (*pao chuan wu* 炮川乌 plus *jing jie sui* 荆芥穗) for the composite term *chang feng zang du* 肠风脏毒 with gastrointestinal bleeding that does not stop, but the formula was also used for multiple other conditions. *Chang feng* 肠风 was a term used in *Su Wen* 素问 Chapter 42 *Feng lun* 风论 and in *Zhen Jiu Jia Yi Jing* 针灸甲乙经 Scroll 10 where it was associated with diarrhoea.

In the *Sheng Ji Zong Lu* 圣济总录 (c. 1117) chapter on *chang feng xia xue* 肠风下血 (intestine wind with bleeding), there were two formulas that were also used for *zang du* 脏毒. Both were also for symptoms of gastrointestinal bleeding and a further four formulas that mentioned the term *zang du* 脏毒 were all for stopping bleeding. So, although there was no definition of the term, it is apparent that *zang du* 脏毒 referred to an intestinal disorder with gastrointestinal bleeding. Since haemorrhoids (*zhi* 痔) has been a common term since at least the *Huang Di Nei Jing* 黄帝内经 (100 BC), and was distinguished from *chang feng* 肠风 in *Sheng Ji Zong Lu* 圣济总录, it is unlikely that *zang du* 脏毒 also referred to palpable haemorrhoids.

The composite term *chang feng zang du* 肠风脏毒 was used in multiple citations from the Song, Jin and Yuan dynasties. In the *Yan Shi Ji Sheng Fang* 严氏济生方 (c. 1253) chapter *Chang feng zang du lun zhi* 肠风脏毒论治, it says that 'in *chang feng* 肠风 the blood is clear and fresh, but in *zang du* 脏毒 the blood is turbid and dark.'

In the Ming dynasty, the *Ben Cao Gang Mu* 本草纲目 (c. 1578) section on *xia xue* 下血 says: 'when the blood is clear it is *chang feng* 肠风, due to empty heat generating wind, or the combination of dampness and *qi*; when the blood is turbid, it is called *zang du* 脏毒, due to accumulation of heat, food, and toxins, combined with dampness and heat.' A similar passage is found in *Lei Zheng Pu Ji Ben Shi Fang Shi Yi* 类证普济本事方释义 (c. 1746).

Suo Gang Zhi and Related Terms

Finally, the term *suo gang zhi* 锁肛痔 was defined in *Wai Ke Da Cheng* 外科大成 (c. 1665) as follows: '*Suo gang zhi* 锁肛痔 is just inside or outside the anus and is tightly attached. The shape is like a jelly fish (*hai zhe* 海蜇). There is rectal tenesmus, the shape of the stool is thin and flat like a ribbon (*dai bian* 带匾), and there is smelly fluid. There is no way to treat this.'

Summary of the Meanings of the Main Terms

The above quotations indicate that the four groups of terms referred to three main groups of conditions. The terms *ji ju* 积聚 and *zheng jia* 症/癥瘕 both referred to conditions characterised by abdominal masses. Both *ji* 积 and *zheng* 症/癥 were terms for fixed, unmovable masses and both *ju* 聚 and *jia* 瘕 were terms for insubstantial and/or movable masses. However, the composite terms were used in the formula citations. Therefore, these terms form a distinct group. Within this group, most citations were in a gynaecological context, especially those for *zheng jia* 症/癥瘕, but there were certain citations that were suggestive of intestinal involvement which could have included CRC. In the case of *zang du* 脏毒, the key features were rectal bleeding with a chronic presentation, so this group was likely to include CRC. In addition, *suo gang zhi* 锁肛痔 was due to a mass obstructing the anus which is suggestive of anal cancer but the only citation that mentioned treatment said it could not be treated, so this term could not be included in the further analyses.

Citations Related to Aetiology and Syndromes

Syndrome differentiation of the type used in contemporary CM was not found in any of the citations. However, a number of citations mentioned aspects of aetiology from which the likely syndromes could be inferred. The following are representative examples.

Regarding *ji ju* 积聚, the previous passage from the *Huang Di Nei Jing Ling Shu* 黄帝内经灵枢 (100 BC) Chapter 46 indicated that *ji ju* 积聚 within the intestines was due to evil pathogenic *qi* (*e ze xie qi* 恶则邪气) lodging and accumulating.

In the *Bei Ji Qian Jin Yao Fang* 备急千金要方 (c. 652), *ji ju* 积聚 was listed as one of the disorders of the channels (*jing luo* 经络) that affect the stomach and intestines. It was due to cold causing blockage which produces a mass (*ji* 积). In the case of *ji* 积 within the intestine (*chang zhong ji* 肠中积), the above passage from *Ling Shu* 灵枢 Chapter 46 was quoted verbatim.

In the *San Yin Ji Yi Bing Zheng Fang Lun* 三因极一病证方论 (c. 1174) passage on *wu ji liu ju* 五积六聚, the condition was due to 'damp *qi* from food and drink, lodging hidden inside and not dispersing (*fu liu bu san* 伏留不散), producing stagnation in the interior tunnels (*sui dao jie zhi* 隧道節滯), leading to all the vessels becoming blocked.' However, no symptoms were given so the disease cannot be determined. In other sections, there are numerous mentions of *ji ju* 積聚, some of which show gastrointestinal symptoms, but none were characteristic of CRC. There was no mention of *zheng jia* 症瘕.

The *Ren Zhai Zhi Zhi Fang Lun* (*Fu Bu Yi*) 仁斋直指方论 (附补遗) (c. 1224) section on *Ji ju, zheng jia, pi kuai fang lun* 積聚, 症瘕, 痞块方论 said that 'damage to the *luo* 络 vessels of the stomach and intestines, leads to bleeding from the intestine. Cold fluids in the intestine combine with the bleeding, these coalesce and cannot disperse, and become *ji* 积.'

The *Dan Xi Xin Fa* 丹溪心法 (c. 1481) said: 'The five flavours (i.e. food and drink) enter through the mouth and go into the stomach, but when toxins lodge and do not disperse, *ji ju* 积聚 can form over the long-term, damaging the harmonious function (of the digestive system) and causing the generation of many diseases.' The *Ge Zhi Yu Lun* 格致余论 (c. 1347) by the same author further explained that this disorder was related to 'excessive desires and consumption of food, leading to retained phlegm and stagnation of blood, that can entangle and become deeper day after day and month after month, stagnating and binding to produce *ju* 聚, which can be like a walnut kernel (*he tao zhi rang* 核桃之穰). Long-term, *ji ju* 积聚 have a shape and are attached to the gastrointestinal tract in the thin parts, at the bends of the intestine. This *ji ju* 积聚 stays ('nests' *ke* 窠) a long time in this location, blocking the movement of the liquid and blood (*jin ye xue* 津液血), which 'steam and cook' (*xun zheng fan zhuo* 熏蒸燔灼), causing this disease.' A similar passage is found in *Yi Xue Gang Mu* 医学纲目 (c. 1556).

In the case of *zang du* 脏毒, the *Yan Shi Ji Sheng Fang* 严氏济生方 (c. 1253) section *Chang feng zang du lun zhi* 肠风脏毒论治 says that *chang feng* 肠风 and *zang du* 脏毒 are due to 'excessive eating, exhaustion from bedroom activity, exposure to drafts while sitting or sleeping, eating too much cold raw food or too much hot roasted food, excessive alcohol consumption, and/or deficiency of the *ying qi* and *wei qi* (*ying wei qi xu* 营卫气虚).'

In the *Yi Xue Ru Men* 医学入门 (c. 1575) section on blood (*xue lei* 血类), it says that 'it is important to distinguish whether blood in the stool (*bian xue* 便血) is due to internal or external causes. *Chang feng* 肠风 is external, the disease has a quick onset, the blood has a fresh appearance and most of the bleeding is before defaecation, it is from the *qi* division (*qi fen* 气分) of the large intestine. When the cause is internal, the disease is called *zang du* 脏毒, there has been accumulation for a long time, so the colour is dark, and most of the bleeding is after defaecation. It is from the Blood division (*xue fen* 血分) of the small intestine.'

The previously-mentioned passage from the *Ben Cao Gang Mu* 本草纲目 (c. 1578) said: '*zang du* 脏毒 was due to accumulation of heat, food and toxins, combined with dampness and heat.'

In the *Zheng Zhi Zhun Sheng — Za Bing* 证治准绳-杂病 (c. 1602) section on gastrointestinal bleeding (*xia xue* 下血), the author Wang Ken-tang 王肯堂 quoted the *Ying Ning Sheng Zhi Yan* 撄宁生厄言 by *Hua Bo-ren* 滑伯仁 saying: '*chang feng* 肠风 is due to long-term accumulation of heat in the foot *yang ming* (足阳明) generating wind; *zang du* 脏毒 is due to heat accumulated in the foot *tai yin* (足太阴), which over the long-term generates dampness which leads to bleeding.' The same quotation is included in the *Chi Shui Xuan Zhu* 赤水玄珠 (c. 1573) section on gastrointestinal bleeding.

Summary of Aetiology and Syndromes

In the earliest citation, the *Ling Shu* 灵枢 says that *ji ju* 积聚 is due to an external pathogen which enters the body when the body is weak and cannot resist it. It stays inside causing blockage. In both the *Zhu Bing Yuan Hou Lun* 诸病源候论 and *Bei Ji Qian Jin Yao Fang* 备急千金要方 it is implied that the nature of this pathogen is cold. The *Ren Zhai Zhi Zhi Fang Lun* 仁斋直指方论 expands this concept, saying that damage to the *luo* 络 vessels leads to bleeding and the cold coalesces this into a mass in the intestine.

Another explanation found in *San Yin Ji Yi Bing Zheng Fang Lun* 三因极一病证方论 is that accumulation of dampness deriving from excessive food and drink is the source of the stagnation which blocks the vessels leading to masses. *Zhu Dan-xi* 朱丹溪 provided more detail, saying that an unrestrained lifestyle and excessive indulgence in food and drink are what cause the stagnation of phlegm and stasis of Blood, which become severe and over a long period generate a mass that lodges in the intestine. The author also explained that the mass itself generated heat which transformed it into a hard mass like a walnut kernel which is difficult to treat.

In *Yan Shi Ji Sheng Fang* 严氏济生方, *zang du* 脏毒 could be due to a range of lifestyle factors such as excessive eating, as well as being due to external wind and cold, and weakness of the body. However, in later books it is identified as a disorder due to internal factors that develops over a long period. Notably, the *Ben Cao Gang Mu* 本草纲目 identifies accumulation of heat, food and toxins, combined with dampness and heat as the main causative factors leading to the bleeding, and later books tend to follow this explanation.

Chinese Herbal Medicine

In total, 409 citations mentioned an orally administered CHM treatment (Table 3.2). Most citations were located by the search term *zang du* 脏毒 (*n* = 366, 89.5%) followed by *ji ju* 积聚 (*n* = 40, 9.8%). None of the citations identified by *zang du* 脏毒 mentioned *ji ju* 积聚, so these were mutually exclusive categories. Twelve citations were for

Table 3.2 Dynastic Distribution of Citations of a Chinese Herbal Medicine Treatment

Dynasty	No. of Citations (%)
Before Tang dynasty (before 618)	1 (0.2)
Tang and 5 dynasties (618–960)	2 (0.5)
Song, Jin and Yuan dynasties (961–1368)	50 (12.2)
Ming dynasty (1369–1644)	230 (56.2)
Qing dynasty (1645–1911)	121 (29.6)
Min Guo/Republic of China (1912–1949)	5 (1.2)
Total	409 (100)

the terms associated with *zheng jia* 症/癥瘕 and *zheng* 症/癥 plus *chang* 肠 (one included both search terms) with nine of these also included for *ji ju* 积聚, so these were overlapping categories.

Frequency of Treatment Citations by Dynasty

The majority of citations (56.2%) were from books written in the Ming dynasty (c. 1369–1644), with close to a third (29.6%) from the Qing dynasty (c. 1645–1911). A small proportion (12.2%) were from the Song, Jin and Yuan dynasties (961–1368), and only three were from earlier periods.

The citations were located from 121 different books written between AD 363 (*Zhou Hou Bei Ji Fang* 肘后备急方) and 1938 (*Ben Cao Jian Yao Fang* 本草简要方). The books providing the most citations were *Pu Ji Fang* 普济方 (*n* = 63), *Ben Cao Gang Mu* 本草纲目 (*n* = 14), *Ji Yang Gang Mu* 济阳纲目 (*n* = 13), *Yi Xue Gang Mu* 医学纲目 (*n* = 11), *Qi Xiao Liang Fang* 奇效良方 (*n* = 11), and *Chi Shui Xuan Zhu* 赤水玄珠 (*n* = 11).

The 40 citations for *ji ju* 积聚 were from books written between c. 363 and c. 1884, while the 12 citations for *zheng jia* 症瘕/癥瘕 or *zheng* 症/癥 plus *chang* 肠 were each from different books written between c. 1196 and c. 1911. The 366 citations for *zang du* 脏毒 were from books written between c. 1061 and c. 1938. Therefore, the citations of *ji ju* 积聚 covered a longer period of time, compared to citations of *zheng jia* 症/癥瘕 and *zang du* 脏毒, which were from the Song Dynasty onwards.

Treatment with Chinese Herbal Medicine

Of the 409 citations, 143 (35%) did not have a formula name. Of these 36 (8.8%) were citations of single herbs for one of the conditions. In 15 citations (3.7%), multiple formula names were included, so the analysis of formulas was based on 266 citations of named formulas. The analysis of formula ingredients was based on 373 citations, with the 36 citations of single herbs being presented separately.

A number of formulas had the same name but somewhat different ingredients. For example, there were six versions of *Wen bai wan*

温白丸, three versions of *Huai hua san* 槐花散 and three versions of *Zang lian wan* 脏连丸. Some formulas that were the same had variant names. Therefore, the frequencies of formulas were based on those with the same or similar names and same ingredients. Overall, the most frequently mentioned formulas were *Huai hua san* 槐花散 no. 1 (n = 17), *Jie yin dan* 结阴丹 (n = 16), *Suan lian wan* 蒜连丸 (n = 9) and *Wen bai wan* 温白丸 no. 3 (n = 8).

To further explore the similarities and differences between the main terms, the 373 formula citations were analysed according to the mention of clinical symptoms that were relevant to CRC. Overall, the most frequent symptom was bleeding, which was mentioned in 88.5% of citations, followed by blockage of the gastrointestinal system (11.3%), distension of the abdomen (3.8%), pain (3.8%) and difficulty in consuming food and drink (3.8%). Weight loss/emaciation was mentioned in only four (1.1%) citations, only three mentioned constipation and none mentioned change in bowel habit.

In the 330 citations of formulas for *zang du* 脏毒, all mentioned bleeding which was associated with the intestine, while none mentioned a mass or blockage. Three also mentioned pain (0.9%), two mentioned distension, one mentioned emaciation and another one mentioned difficulty in consuming food and drink.

The 40 citations for *ji ju* 积聚 showed a different profile with none mentioning bleeding, 38 (95.0%) referring to a mass in the abdomen and three also mentioning the intestine. Blockage was mentioned in 39 citations (97.5%), distension in 12 (30.0%), and difficulty in consuming food and drink also in 12 citations, while 10 mentioned pain (25.0%). Constipation and emaciation were each mentioned in three citations.

The 12 citations for *zheng jia* 症/癥瘕 showed a similar profile to *ji ju* 积聚 with no mention of bleeding, 10 (83.3%) locating the mass in the abdomen, all mentioning blockage with four (33.3%) also mentioning distension. There were two mentions each for pain and emaciation, and one for difficulty in consuming food and drink.

Due to the small number of citations for *zheng jia* 症/癥瘕 and the similar profile to *ji ju* 积聚, these citations were analysed together, while *zang du* 脏毒 was analysed separately.

Most Frequent Formulas in Citations for *Ji Ju* and/or *Zheng Jia*

Due to the overlap between these terms and the relatively few citations, they were analysed together. In total, there were 43 citations for these terms with the majority for *ji ju* 积聚 (*n* = 40), nine for *ji ju* 积聚 plus *zheng jia* 症/癥瘕 and three just for *zheng jia* 症/癥瘕.

The majority of citations were from the Ming dynasty (*n* = 28, 65.1%), followed by the Qing dynasty (*n* = 7, 16.3%), with five (11.6%) from the Song, Jin and Yuan dynasties and three from the Tang dynasty or earlier (7.0%). The book providing the largest number of citations was *Pu Ji Fang* 普济方 (c. 1406) with 12 citations, followed by three citations from *Chi Shui Xuan Zhu* 赤水玄珠 (c. 1573). The earliest citation was one for *ji ju* 积聚 from *Zhou Hou Bei Ji Fang* 肘后备急方 (c. 363) with the most recent citation being one for *zheng jia* 癥瘕 from *Wu Ju Tong Yi An* 吴鞠通医案 (c. 1911). Each of the citations for *zheng jia* 症/癥瘕 was from a different book, with the earliest being from *Ye Shi Lu Yan Fang* 叶氏录验方 (c. 1186) which was for *ji ju zheng kuai* 积聚癥块.

Three formulas had no name. The most common formula name was *Wen bai wan* 温白丸 which appeared in 12 citations with eight of these being for *Wen bai wan* 温白丸 No. 3. The formula *Shen ming du ming yuan* 神明度命圆 appeared three times under slightly different names but with the same ingredients (Table 3.3). The formula *Wan ying zi wan wan* 万应紫菀丸 appeared twice but the ingredients were the same as in the citation of *Wan bing zi wan wan* 万病紫菀丸, so these were combined. *Jin ye dan* 金液丹 and *Jin lu wan* 金露丸 appeared in two citations each. There were also two citations of *Wu tou wan* 乌头丸 but the ingredients were different. None of the citations included combinations of multiple formulas and none were for single herbs for the disorder.

The three formulas *Wen bai wan* 温白丸 No. 3, *Wan ying zi wan wan* 万应紫菀丸 and *Jin lu wan* 金露丸 in Table 3.3 have overlapping ingredients and are illustrative of the formulas used for *ji ju* 积聚. They contained toxic ingredients which required processing prior to use such as *wu tou* 乌头, *wu zhu yu* 吴茱萸, *bai dou* 巴豆 and *gan sui* 甘遂, and many of the other ingredients were heat-processed or

Table 3.3   Most Frequent Formulas in Citations for *Ji Ju* and/or *Zheng Jia*

Formula Name	Herb Ingredients (Source Book)	No. of Citations
Wen bai wan 温白丸 No. 3	*Zi wan* 紫菀, *wu zhu yu* 吴茱萸, *chang pu* 菖蒲, *chai hu* 柴胡, *hou pu* 厚朴, *jie geng* 桔梗, *zao jia* 皂荚, *fu ling* 茯苓, *gui xin* 桂心, *gan jiang* 干姜, *huang lian* 黄连, *shu jiao* 蜀椒, *ba dou* 巴豆, *ren shen* 人参 and *wu tou* 乌头 (*Pu Ji Fang* 普济方 c. 1406)	8
Shen ming du ming yuan 神明度命圆[1]	*Da huang* 大黄 and *shao yao* 芍药 (*Bei Ji Qian Jin Yao Fang* 备急千金要方 c. 652, *Si Ku Quan Shu* 四库全书 edition)	3
Wan ying zi wan wan 万应紫菀丸 (*Wan bing zi wan wan* 万病紫菀丸)	*Zi wan* 紫菀, *chai hu* 柴胡, *chang pu* 菖蒲, *wu zhu yu* 吴茱萸, *hou pu* 厚朴, *jie geng* 桔梗, *fu ling* 茯苓, *zao jiao* 皂角, *huang lian* 黄连, *gui zhi* 桂枝, *gan jiang* 干姜, *chuan wu* 川乌, *qiang huo* 羌活, *du huo* 独活, *fang feng* 防风, *ba dou* 巴豆, *ren shen* 人参 and *shu jiao* 蜀椒 (*Qi Xiao Liang Fang* 奇效良方 c. 1470)	3
Jin lu wan 金露丸	*Cao wu tou* 草乌头, *huang lian* 黄连, *gui xin* 桂心, *gan jiang* 干姜, *jie geng* 桔梗, *fu ling* 茯苓, *chai hu* 柴胡, *shu jiao* 蜀椒, *wu zhu yu* 吴茱萸, *hou pu* 厚朴, *ren shen* 人参, *chang pu* 菖蒲, *zi wan* 紫菀, *bie jia* 鳖甲, *xiong qiong* 芎䓖, *zhi ke* 枳壳, *bei mu* 贝母, *gan sui* 甘遂, *gan di huang* 干地黄, *gan cao* 甘草, *fang feng* 防风 and *ba dou* 巴豆 (*Ye Shi Lu Yan Fang* 叶氏录验方 c. 1186)	2
Jin ye dan 金液丹	*Liu huang* 硫黄 and *chi shi zhi* 赤石脂 (*Shi Yi De Xiao Fang* 世医得效方 c. 1345)	2

[1]Also called *Shen ming du ming wan* 神明度命丸 and *Shen ming du ming dan* 神明度命丹.

Each of these formulas had detailed and complex processing requirements.

The use of some herbs/ingredients may be restricted in some countries. Readers are advised to comply with relevant regulations.

had other preparation requirements. In contrast, *Shen ming du ming yuan* 神明度命圆 was a simple two-ingredient formula with simple processing. *Jin ye dan* 金液丹 was an exception since it was a mineral preparation made by heat-processing sulphur (*shi liu huang* 石硫黄) with *chi shi zhi* 赤石脂 (red halloysite), salts, and other mineral ingredients for seven days and nights. It was used for a range of disorders including *ji ju* 积聚. See Sivin (1968)[39] and Needham (1976)[40] for discussions of these types of mineral preparations.

Most Frequent Herbs in Citations for *Ji Ju* and/or *Zheng Jia*

In the 43 citations of CHM treatments for *ji ju* 积聚 and/or *zheng jia* 症/癥瘕, there were 504 ingredients which included 118 different items of *materia medica* (Table 3.4). Of these, the most frequently used were *wu zhu yu* 吴茱萸 (processed; *n* = 21), *ba dou* 巴豆 (processed; *n* = 21), *ren shen* 人参 (*n* = 20), *huang lian* 黄连 (*n* = 20), *chuan jiao* 川椒 (*n* = 20), *jie geng* 桔梗 (*n* = 19), *gan jiang* 干姜 (*n* = 19), *wu tou* 乌头 (processed; *n* = 19), *fu ling* 茯苓 (*n* = 19), *hou po* 厚朴 (*n* = 19) and *rou gui* 肉桂 (*n* = 18).

When the 12 *zheng jia* 症/癥瘕 citations were considered separately (204 ingredients), the high-frequency herbs were very similar, with eight formulas containing *wu zhu yu* 吴茱萸, *ren shen* 人参 and/or *huang lian* 黄连, followed by seven with *chuan jiao* 川椒, *jie geng* 桔梗, *hou po* 厚朴 and/or *fu ling* 茯苓. Relatively less frequent were *wu tou* 乌头 (processed; *n* = 6) and *ba dou* 巴豆 (processed; *n* = 5).

Most Frequent Formulas in Citations for *Zang Du*

Of the 409 citations, 366 were for *zang du* 脏毒. None of these were also for *ji ju* 积聚 or *zheng jia* 症/癥瘕, but 176 were also used for *chang feng* 肠风. The citations were from 113 books written between 1061 and 1938 with the majority from the Ming dynasty (*n* = 202, 55.2%) and Qing dynasty (*n* = 114, 31.1%); 45 (12.3%) were from Song, Jin and Yuan dynasties (960–1368); and five (1.4%) were from the Min Guo period. The books that provided the most citations were *Pu Ji Fang* 普济方 (*n* = 51), *Ben Cao Gang Mu* 本草纲目

Table 3.4 Most Frequent Herbs in Citations for *Ji Ju* and/or *Zheng Jia*

Herb Name	Scientific Name	No. of Citations
Wu zhu yu 吴茱萸	*Euodia rutaecarpa* (Juss.) Benth.	21
Ba dou 巴豆	*Croton tiglium* L.	21
Ren shen 人参	*Panax ginseng* C. A. Mey.	20
Huang lian 黄连	*Coptis chinensis* Franch.	20
Chuan jiao 川椒	*Zanthoxylum* spp.	20
Jie geng 桔梗	*Platycodon grandiflorum* (Jacq.) A. DC.	19
Gan jiang 干姜[1]	*Zingiber officinale* Rosc.	19
Wu tou 乌头	*Aconitum* spp.	19
Fu ling 茯苓	*Poria cocos* (Schw.) Wolf	19
Hou po 厚朴	*Magnolia officinalis* Rehd. et Wils.	19
Rou gui 肉桂[2]	*Cinnamomum cassia* Presl	18
Chai hu 柴胡	*Bupleurum chinense* DC.	17
Zi wan 紫菀	*Aster tataricus* L. f.	17
Zao jia 皂荚	*Gleditsia sinensis* Lam.	17
Chang pu 菖蒲[3]	*Acorus* spp.	15
Da huang 大黄	*Rheum palmatum* L.	9
Mu xiang 木香	*Aucklandia lappa* Decne.	8
Chuan xiong 川芎	*Ligusticum chuanxiong* Hort.	7
Gan cao 甘草	*Glycyrrhiza uralensis* Fisch.	6
E zhu 莪术	*Curcuma* spp.	6
Xing ren 杏仁	*Prunus armeniaca* L.	6

[1]Plus *sheng jiang* 生姜 (*n* = 1).

[2]Plus *gui zhi* 桂枝 (*n* = 4).

[3]Plus *shi chang pu* 石菖蒲 (*n* = 3).

The use of some herbs may be restricted in some countries. Readers are advised to comply with relevant regulations.

(*n* = 13), *Ji Yang Gang Mu* 济阳纲目 (*n* = 12), *Yi Xue Gang Mu* 医学纲目 (*n* = 10) and *Qi Xiao Liang Fang* 奇效良方 (*n* = 10).

In 36 citations there was mention of a single herb for *zang du* 脏毒 and 330 citations were of a formula. In 104 citations there was no formula name and in 15 citations there were two or more formulas used in combination. Therefore, the analysis of formulas excludes the single-herb citations and includes all the unnamed formulas and each of the named formulas.

There were 259 mentions of a formula name (Table 3.5). The most frequently mentioned formulas were *Huai hua san* 槐花散 No. 1 (*n* = 17), *Jie yin dan* 结阴丹 (*n* =16), *Suan lian wan* 蒜连丸 (*n* = 9), *Wu jing wan* 乌荆丸 (*n* = 8) which was also called *Gu wu jing*

Table 3.5 Most Frequent Formulas for *Zang Du*

Formula Name	Herb Ingredients (Source Book)	No. of Citations
Huai hua san 槐花散 No. 1	*Huai hua* 槐花, *bai ye ce* 柏叶侧, *jing jie sui* 荆芥穗 and *zhi ke* 枳壳. (*Pu Ji Ben Shi Fang* 普济本事方 c. 1132)	17
Jie yin dan 结阴丹	Zhi ke 枳壳, wei ling xian 威灵仙, huang qi 黄芪, chen pi 陈皮, chun gen bai pi 椿根白皮, he shou wu 何首乌, and jing jie sui 荆芥穗. (*Ren Zhai Zhi Zhi Fang Lun* 仁斋直指方论(附补遗) c. 1264)	16
Suan lian wan 蒜连丸	*Ying zhua huang lian* 鹰爪黄连 and *du tou suan* 独头蒜. (*Pu Ji Ben Shi Fang* 普济本事方 c. 1132)	9
Wu jing wan 乌荆丸 (*Gu wu jing wan* 古乌荆丸 = 1)	*Chuan wu* 川乌 and *jing jie sui* 荆芥穗. (*Tai Ping Hui Min He Ji Ju Fang* 太平惠民和剂局方 c. 1107)	8
Shao yao tang 芍药汤 (*He jian shao yao tang* 河间芍药汤 = 1)	*Shao yao* 芍药, *dang gui* 当归, *huang lian* 黄连, *huang qin* 黄芩, *da huang* 大黄, *gui* 桂, *gan cao* 甘草, *bing lang* 槟榔 and *mu xiang* 木香. (*Su Wen Bing Ji Qi Yi Bao Ming Ji* 素问病机气宜保命集 c. 1186)	8
Xiang mei wan 香梅丸	*Wu mei* 乌梅, *xiang bai zhi* 香白芷 and *bai yao jian* 百药煎.[1] (*Yan Shi Ji Sheng Fang* 严氏济生方 c. 1253)	7
Wu huai wan 五槐丸	*Wu bei zi* 五倍子, *huai hua* 槐花 and *bai yao jian* 百药煎. (*Pu Ji Fang* 普济方 c. 1406)[2]	7

(Continued)

Table 3.5   (*Contiuned*)

Formula Name	Herb Ingredients (Source Book)	No. of Citations
Huai hua san 槐花散 No. 2	*Huai hua* 槐花, *sheng di huang* 生地黄, *qing pi* 青皮, *bai zhu* 白术, *jing jie sui* 荆芥穗, *chuan xiong* 川芎, *dang gui shen* 当归身 and *sheng ma* 升麻. (*Li Zhai Wai Ke Fa Hui* 立斋外科发挥 c. 1528)	6
Zang lian wan 脏连丸 No. 1	*Huang lian* 黄连, *huai hua mi* 槐花米, *zhi ke* 枳壳, *fang feng* 防风, *fen cao* 粉草, *huai jiao* 槐角, *xiang fu zi* 香附子, *zhu ya zao jiao* 猪牙皂角 and *mu xiang* 木香. (*Gu Jin Yi Tong Da Quan* 古今医统大全 c. 1556)	6
Ren shen chu pi san 人参樗皮散	*Ren shen* 人参 and *chu gen bai pi* 樗根白皮. (*Yi Fang Kao* 医方考 c. 1584)	5

[1]*Bai yao jian* 百药煎: *wu bie zi* 五倍子同茶叶 Mass Galla Chinensis et Camelliae Fermentata; *Fen cao* 粉草: *gan cao* 甘草; *Chu gen bai pi* 樗根白皮: *chun bai pi* 椿白皮; *Zhu ya zao jiao* 猪牙皂角: *zao jia* 皂荚, *zao jiao* 皂角.

[2]In *Pu ji fang* 普济方 the treatment is a combination of *Er qi dan* 二气丹, *Wu huai wan* 五槐丸, *huang lian* 黄连 and *sheng jiang* 生姜.

Each of these formulas had detailed and complex processing requirements.

The use of some herbs/ingredients may be restricted in some countries. Readers are advised to comply with relevant regulations.

wan 古乌荆丸 ('old *wu jing wan*'), and *Shao yao tang* 芍药汤 (*n* = 8) which was also called *He jian shao yao tang* 河间芍药汤 after the author of the book *Su Wen Bing Ji Qi Yi Bao Ming Ji* 素问病机气宜保命集 (by Liu Wan-Su 刘完素 aka He-jian 河间). The formula name *Zang lian wan* 脏连丸 appeared 13 times with six of these having the same ingredients. Six citations employed variations of *Si wu tang* 四物汤, including *Qin lian si wu tang* 芩连四物汤 and *Jie du si wu tang* 解毒四物汤.

Most Frequent Herbs in Citations for *Zang Du*

In the 366 citations of herbal treatments for *zang du* 脏毒, there were 1,593 herbal ingredients. Of these, 36 were for the 15 different single herbs not classified as formulas. The most frequent of these were *shi gan* 柿干 (*n* = 14), *chuan lian zi* 川棟子 (*n* = 4) and *mo han lian* 墨旱莲 (*n* = 3). When these were excluded, 1,557 herbal ingredients remained (Table 3.6). The ingredient most frequently included in a herbal formula was *huang lian* 黄连 (*n* = 110), followed by *huai hua* 槐花 (*n* = 98) and *zhi shi* 枳实/*zhi ke* 枳壳 (*n* = 72). In most cases the *huai hua* 槐花 was processed by dry frying (*chao* 炒) and the *zhi shi* 枳实/*zhi ke* 枳壳 was bran-fried till yellow (*fu chao huang se* 麸炒

Table 3.6   Most Frequent Herbs in Citations for *Zang du*

Herb Name	Scientific Name	No. of Citations
Huang lian 黄连	*Coptis chinensis* Franch.	110
Huai hua 槐花	*Sophora japonica* L.	98
Zhi shi 枳实/*zhi ke* 枳壳	*Citrus aurantium* L.	72
Jing jie 荆芥	*Schizonepeta tenuifolia* Briq.	60
Dang gui 当归	*Angelica sinensis* (Oliv.) Diels	58
Gan cao 甘草	*Glycyrrhiza uralensis* Fisch.	54
Zhu da chang 猪大肠	Pig intestine	40
Ce bai ye 侧柏叶	*Platycladus orientalis* (L.) Franco	38
Huang qi 黄芪	*Astragalus membranaceus* (Fisch.) Bge.	34
Huang qin 黄芩	*Scutellaria baicalensis* Georgi	34
Bai shao 白芍/*shao yao* 芍药	*Paeonia lactiflora* Pall.	32
Chun bai pi 椿白皮	*Ailanthus altissima* (Mill.) Swingle	30
Mu xiang 木香	*Aucklandia lappa* Decne.	29
Huang bo 黄柏	*Phellodendron amurense* Rupr.	29
Chuan xiong 川芎	*Ligusticum chuanxiong* Hort.	28
Wu mei 乌梅	*Prunus mume* (Sieb.) Sieb. et Zucc.	24
Da huang 大黄	*Rheum palmatum* L.	24
Di yu 地榆	*Sanguisorba officinalis* L.	22
Da suan 大蒜	*Allium sativum* L.	22
Ren shen 人参	*Panax ginseng* C. A. Mey.	20
Chen pi 陈皮	*Citrus reticulata* Blanco	20

The use of some herbs may be restricted in some countries. Readers are advised to comply with relevant regulations.

黄色). A number of formulas specified the type of *huang lian* 黄连 to be *ying zhao huang lian* 鹰爪黄连 which refers to roots in the shape of an eagle's claw which are characterised by being firm (i.e. not hollow in the interior) and a deep yellow colour.[41]

Discussion of Chinese Herbal Medicine for Colorectal Cancer

Although the terms *ji ju* 积聚 and *zheng jia* 症/癥瘕 appeared frequently in the classical literature, many were in the context of conditions unlikely to have been CRC, or did not provide sufficient information for a judgment to be made. Therefore, the included citations represent a sample of the formulas that are likely to have been used to treat abdominal masses associated with the intestines. Bleeding was seldom mentioned in relation to *ji ju* 积聚 and *zheng jia* 症/癥瘕. One explanation is that any tumours were located higher in the intestinal tract. It is also likely that the formulas that were used for these conditions were also for a wide variety of masses that were not CRC. Also, many citations were brief, so the authors did not list all of the symptoms of each condition, which made identification difficult. It is notable that while *ji ju* 积聚 was often accompanied by distension, constipation was seldom mentioned; however, purgative herbs such as *ba dou* 巴豆 and *da huang* 大黄 were frequent ingredients. This suggests that this symptom may have been present but not remarked upon.

Some citations mentioned a few symptoms, as in the case of *Shen ming du ming yuan* 神明度命圆 mentioned above, which were suggestive of an intestinal mass but were not sufficiently specific to identify CRC. In other citations, the formula could be used for multiple symptoms relevant to CRC, but it was unclear whether these symptoms appeared in combination, or whether the formula was intended for various symptoms and types of masses. This was the case for *Wen bai wan* 温白丸 and *Wan bing zi wan wan* 万病紫菀丸. Consequently, it is difficult to identify a citation in which the presentation was highly likely to have been CRC.

When the formula ingredients are considered, warming herbs such as *wu zhu yu* 吴茱萸, *gan jiang* 干姜, *wu tou* 乌头 and *rou gui*

肉桂 were frequently included, suggesting that cold was considered to be a major component of the aetiology.

In the case of *zang du* 脏毒, the condition was due to intestinal bleeding that may have been due to a neoplasm. Since the blood was not fresh, it was unlikely due to internal haemorrhoids which may have been a cause for *chang feng* 肠风.

In one citation from *Pu Ji Fang* 普济方 (c. 1406), *zang du* 脏毒 was associated with 'bleeding that does not stop and chronic weight loss' and in another there was 'blood in the stool, pain and vomiting'. However, in most citations there were too few symptoms to identify a subset likely to have been CRC. One hypothesis was that by excluding citations for *zang du* 脏毒 and/or *chang feng* 肠风 we could derive a more specific *zang du* 脏毒 group, but the list of most frequent herbal ingredients remained much the same. The presence of herbs for clearing heat and toxicity, such as *huang lian* 黄连, *huang qin* 黄芩 and *huang bai* 黄柏 is consistent with this condition being due to heat and dampness, while *huai hua* 槐花, *di yu* 地榆 and *ce bai ye* 侧柏叶 are typical herbs for stopping bleeding.

When the frequent herbs for *ji ju* 积聚 and *zheng jia* 症/癥瘕 were compared to those for *zang du* 脏毒, there was little overlap, although *huang lian* 黄连, *da huang* 大黄, *ren shen* 人参, *gan cao* 甘草 and *mu xiang* 木香 were frequent on both lists.

Acupuncture and Related Therapies

The searches identified 54 citations of treatments using acupuncture and/or moxibustion for at least one of the search terms. In 35 citations, the term was included in the list of clinical applications of the specific acupuncture point, while 19 citations were of acupuncture treatments for the particular disorder. Where possible, separate data are provided for these two types of citations. In 29 citations the use of moxibustion was mentioned and 18 mentioned needling, while the others did not mention how the point(s) should be stimulated.

The most common search term was *ji ju* 积聚 (*n* = 41), which appeared in 75.9% of the citations. *Zang du* 脏毒 (*n* = 13) appeared in 24.1% of citations and there was no overlap between these groups. The term *zheng jia* 症/癥瘕 only appeared in three citations and two of these also included *ji ju* 积聚. Therefore, citations for *ji ju* 积聚 and *zheng jia* 症/癥瘕 were combined in the analyses. Overall, bleeding was a feature of all citations for *zang du* 脏毒 but appeared in none of the citations for *ji ju* 积聚. *Zang du* 脏毒 was always associated with the intestine while *ji ju* 积聚 was always associated with the abdomen, with about 20% of citations also mentioning the intestine.

Frequency of Treatment Citations by Dynasty

The majority of the citations (55.6%) were derived from books written during the Ming dynasty (1369–1644), with nine (16.7%) from the Song, Jin and Yuan dynasties (961–1271), five (9.3%) from the Qing dynasty (1645–1911) and eight from the Tang dynasty or earlier (before 959) (Table 3.7).

The citations were derived from 25 different books with the earliest being *Zhen Jiu Jia Yi Jing* 针灸甲乙经 (c. 282) and the most recent being *Jin Zhen Mi Chuan* 金针秘传 (c. 1937). The most productive book was the acupuncture section of *Pu Ji Fang* 普济方 (c. 1406) with 10 (18.5%) citations, followed by *Zhen Jiu Zi Sheng Jing* 针灸资生经 (c. 1220) with five citations (9.3%), and *Zhen Fang Liu Ji* 针方六集 (c. 1618) and *Zhen Jiu Da Cheng* 针灸大成 (c. 1601) with four citations each.

Table 3.7 Dynastic Distribution of Citations of Acupuncture Therapies

Dynasty	No. of Treatment Citations(%)
Before Tang dynasty (before 618)	3 (5.6)
Tang and 5 dynasties (618–960)	5 (9.3)
Song, Jin and Yuan dynasties (961–1271)	9 (16.7)
Ming dynasty (1369–1644)	30 (55.6)
Qing dynasty (1645–1911)	5 (9.3)
Min Guo/Republic of China (1912–1949)	2 (3.7)
Total	54

Treatment with Acupuncture and Related Therapies

Overall, the 54 citations provided 72 mentions of 22 different acupuncture points and two citations provided non-point locations for moxibustion. The most frequently mentioned point was KI17 *Shangqu* 商曲 (*n* = 19), followed by SP12 *Chongmen* 冲门 (*n* = 8) and BL57 *Chengshan* 承山 (*n* = 7), with five mentions each for BL22 *Sanjiaoshu* 三焦俞 and GV1 *Changqiang* 长强, and four mentions of BL18 *Ganshu* 肝俞 (Table 3.8).

In the citations that focused on the applications of specific points, KI17 *Shangqu* 商曲 was again the most frequent (*n* = 15), followed by SP12 *Chongmen* 冲门 (*n* = 7), BL22 *Sanjiaoshu* 三焦俞 (*n* = 4) and BL57 *Chengshan* 承山 (*n* = 3). In the citations that mentioned acupuncture treatments for a particular condition, the points KI17 *Shangqu* 商曲, BL57 *Chengshan* 承山 and GV1 *Changqiang* 长强 were all mentioned four times, while BL17 *Geshu* 膈俞, BL18 *Ganshu* 肝俞 and BL20 *Pishu* 脾俞 were each mentioned three times. Therefore, the frequent points in these two subgroups were similar.

In the subgroup of 29 citations that mentioned moxibustion (*n* = 27 points), the most frequently mentioned point was KI17 *Shangqu* 商曲 (*n* = 10), with four mentions each for SP12 *Chongmen* 冲门 and BL22 *Sanjiaoshu* 三焦俞. In these citations, 17 (58.6%) also mentioned needling. Overall, the points used for moxibustion showed a

Table 3.8   Most Frequent Acupuncture Points for *Ji Ju*, *Zheng Jia* or *Zang Du*

Acupuncture Point	No. of Citations
KI17 *Shangqu* 商曲	19
SP12 *Chongmen* 冲门	8
BL57 *Chengshan* 承山	7
BL22 *Sanjiaoshu* 三焦俞	5
GV1 *Changqiang* 长强	5
BL18 *Ganshu* 肝俞	4
BL17 *Geshu* 膈俞	3
BL20 *Pishu* 脾俞	3

similar frequency profile to the above subgroup of citations for the applications of specific points. The main reason for this is, when the uses of a point are listed in a book, so are the methods of stimulation with needles and/or moxibustion.

In the following analyses, results are presented for the treatments for *ji ju* 积聚 and/or *zheng jia* 症/癥瘕 combined, and separately for treatments for *zang du* 脏毒.

Acupuncture Points in Citations for *Ji Ju* and/or *Zheng Jia*

The 42 citations of treatments for *ji ju* 积聚 and/or *zheng jia* 症/癥瘕 were derived from 19 different books written from c. 282 to c. 1937. The largest number of citations (*n* = 10) were from the acupuncture section of *Pu Ji Fang* 普济方 (c. 1406), followed by five citations from *Zhen Jiu Zi Sheng Jing* 针灸资生经 (c. 1220) and three each from *Bei Ji Qian Jin Yao Fang* 备急千金要方 (c. 652) and *Zhen Jiu Jia Yi Jing* 针灸甲乙经 (c. 282).

Almost all citations mentioned a form of blockage (*n* = 41, 97.6%) and pain was the most common associated symptom (*n* = 26, 61.9%), followed by digestive disturbance (*n* = 10, 23.8%) and distension (*n* = 8, 19.0%). Emaciation was mentioned in two citations and there was no mention of bleeding, constipation or change in bowel habit.

There were 46 mentions of 15 different points, with the most frequent being KI17 *Shangqu* 商曲 (*n* = 19), SP12 *Chongmen* 冲门 (*n* = 8) and BL22 *Sanjiaoshu* 三焦俞 (*n* = 5) (Table 3.9). Most citations related to uses of the specific points (*n* = 30) but 12 provided treatments for *ji ju* 积聚 and/or *zheng jia* 症/癥瘕. Of these, the earliest were from *Zhen Jiu Jia Yi Jing* 针灸甲乙经 (c. 282), which specified that for relieving pain associated with an abdominal mass (*fu zhong ji ju* 腹中积聚) a major point was KI17 *Shangqu* 商曲; and for lower abdominal mass (*shao fu ji ju* 少腹积聚) a major point was PC8 *Laogong* 劳宫. In the section on diseases of the intestines and abdominal distension it said that SP12 *Chongmen* 冲门 was a major point for abdominal mass with pain (*fu zhong ji ju teng tong* 腹中积聚疼痛).

Table 3.9 Most Frequent Acupuncture Points for *Ji Ju* and/or *Zheng Jia*

Acupuncture Point	No. of Citations
KI17 *Shangqu* 商曲	19
SP12 *Chongmen* 冲门	8
BL22 *Sanjiaoshu* 三焦俞	5
PC8 *Laogong* 劳宫	2
BL18 *Ganshu* 肝俞	2

Pu Ji Fang 普济方 (c. 1406) recommended BL20 *Pishu* 脾俞 for 'abdominal mass, pain in the intestines, and cannot eat.' It also recommended GV5 *Xuanshu* 悬枢 and moxibustion on BL22 *Sanjiaoshu* 三焦俞 for abdominal mass, and KI17 *Shangqu* 商曲 and moxibustion on *Weiwan* 胃脘 (aka CV13 *Shangwan* 上脘) for abdominal distension and mass. For upper abdomen mass, distension and pain (*xin fu ji ju pi teng tong* 心腹积聚痞疼痛) the *Qian Jin Yi Fang* 千金翼方 (c. 682) recommended moxibustion on BL18 *Ganshu* 肝俞.

Acupuncture Points in Citations for *Zang Du*

Of the 13 citations for *zang du* 脏毒 the earliest were two from *Bian Que Shen Ying Zhen Jiu Yu Long Jing* 扁鹊神应针灸玉龙经 (c. 1329) which was written during the Yuan dynasty, and the most recent was one from the Qing dynasty book *Jiu Fa Mi Chuan* 灸法秘传 (c. 1883). Of the nine different books that included citations, the most productive was *Zhen Fang Liu Ji* 针方六集 (c. 1618) with three citations. All 13 citations mentioned bleeding and three also mentioned pain (23.1%) but none mentioned change in bowel habit, distension, constipation, blockage, digestive disturbance or emaciation.

In total there were 27 mentions of 11 different points for acupuncture and/or moxibustion (Table 3.10). The most frequently mentioned points were BL57 *Chengshan* 承山 (*n* = 7) and GV1 *Changqiang* 长强 (*n* = 5). Another four points were mentioned twice each.

Seven citations were of treatments for *zang du* 脏毒. The following are illustrative examples. *Zhen Jiu Da Quan* 针灸大全 (c. 1439)

Table 3.10 Most Frequent Acupuncture Points for *Zang Du*

Acupuncture Point	No. of Citations
BL57 *Chengshan* 承山	7
GV1 *Changqiang* 长强	5
BL17 *Geshu* 膈俞	2
BL18 *Ganshu* 肝俞	2
BL20 *Pishu* 脾俞	2
BL52 *Zhishi* 志室	2

gave the combination of KI6 *Zhaohai* 照海, GV20 *Baihui* 百会 and TE6 *Zhigou* 支沟 for *zang du* 脏毒, swelling and pain (*zhong tong* 肿痛), and haemafecia that does not stop (*ben xue bu zhi* 便血不止). For the same combination of symptoms, the *Zhen Jiu Da Cheng* 针灸大成 (c. 1601) listed BL57 *Chengshan* 承山, BL18 *Ganshu* 肝俞 and BL17 *Geshu* 膈俞 as major points; for *zang du* 脏毒 with gastrointestinal bleeding (*xia xue* 下血) it listed BL57 *Chengshan* 承山, BL20 *Pishu* 脾俞 and BL52 *Zhishi* 志室 (aka Jinggong 精宫).

Of the later acupuncture books, *Zhen Jiu Yi Xue* 针灸易学 (c. 1798) gave the treatment for *zang du* 脏毒 with gastrointestinal bleeding as BL57 *Chengshan* 承山, BL20 *Pishu* 脾俞, BL52 *Zhishi* 志室 (精宫) and GV1 *Changqiang* 长强. A similar treatment was listed in *Zhen Jiu Feng Yuan* 针灸逢源 (c. 1822) for *zang du* 脏毒 with swelling, pain and haemafecia (*zhong tong ben xue* 肿痛便血) as follows: BL57 *Chengshan* 承山, BL17 *Geshu* 膈俞, BL18 *Ganshu* 肝俞 and GV1 *Changqiang* 长强.

The *Jiu Fa Mi Chuan* 灸法秘传 (c.1883) prescribed moxibustion on BL23 *Shenshu* 肾俞 for *zang du* 脏毒 with turbid blood in the stool and diarrhoea, and moxibustion on BL35 *Huiyang* 会阳 for *chang feng* 肠风 with fresh blood and knotted dry stool. For *chang feng* and *zang du* 肠风脏毒, the *Wan Shi Jia Chao Ji Shi Liang Fang* 万氏家抄济世良方 (c. 1609) gave the following moxibustion treatment: 'Have the person stand up, find the position on the spine that is level with the umbilicus, on this vertebra moxa with seven cones; in elderly people add two extra locations, one cun lateral on each side and moxa with seven cones on each.' This method was also included in *Wai Ke Da Quan* 外科大成 (c. 1665).

Discussion of Acupuncture for Colorectal Cancer

The citations of the use of acupuncture points for the search terms tended to be lists of diseases and symptoms for which the point could be used, so it was not possible to determine if symptoms appeared together. In the citations that specified treatments for one of the terms, a number mentioned multiple symptoms which could indicate CRC; however, the citations were brief and the treatments could also relate to other conditions with the same combination of symptoms. Consequently, it was not possible to select a subset of citations that were more likely to have been CRC.

Overall, *ji ju* 积聚 was the most frequent term and it was also the earliest term, appearing in *Zhen Jiu Jia Yi Jing* 针灸甲乙经 (c. 282) and multiple subsequent books. The most informative citations were the 12 that provided specific treatments for *ji ju* 积聚 (see above). These showed that the abdominal masses were mainly associated with pain, abdominal distension and/or digestive disturbance.

Acupuncture treatments for *zang du* 脏毒 appeared in the Yuan dynasty (c. 1271–1368) and in eight subsequent books. The citations of treatments specifically for *zang du* 脏毒 (see above) all mentioned bleeding and some mentioned pain and occasionally diarrhoea. These citations were the most relevant to CRC since people with these symptoms could be suspected of having CRC, but these symptoms could also have been due to other disorders.

Other Chinese Medicine Therapies

The searches located five citations that appeared relevant, one of which included two methods. The oldest was from *Zhu Bing Yuan Hou Lun* 诸病源候论 (c. 610) and the most recent was from *Li Yue Pian Wen* 理瀹骈文 (c. 1870). Three were related to the term *ji ju* 积聚, one was for *ji ju* 积聚 and *zheng jia* 癥瘕 and one was for *zang du* 脏毒.

In the *Zhu Bing Yuan Hou Lun* 诸病源候论 (c. 610), Roll 19 section on *ji ju bing* 积聚病, a *dao yin* 导引 exercise method to be done on waking was described as follows: 'Lie face upwards; stretch the arms and legs; close the eyes and mouth and hold the breath; expand the lower abdomen to maximum reaching to both feet; on the next breath, quickly breathe in and pull the abdomen inwards, lift the legs up and make fists of your hands; then gradually settle your breathing [and relax].' The exercise was performed regularly and according to the seasons (three times in Spring, five times in Summer, seven times in Autumn, nine times in Winter). Its effect was to cleanse the five solid organs and nourish and moisten the six hollow organs. The method was said to be effective for many diseases but made particular mention of *ji ju* 积聚 in the abdomen, saying that the out-and-in movements of the abdomen could scatter and break (*san po* 散破) the *zheng jia* 癥瘕. The same method also appears in the *zheng jia hou* 癥瘕候 section of the same book.

The *Bao Sheng Xin Jian* 保生心鉴 (c. 1592) included an illustrated sequence of 24 *qigong* 气功 methods called *Tai qing er shi wu qi shui huo ju san tu xu* 太清二十四气水火聚散图序. These include sitting (*zuo gong* 坐功) and moving (*xing gong* 行功) methods, each of which related to one of the 24 periods of the traditional calendar. All were for dissipating various types of accumulations (*ju* 聚) and for alleviating a range of symptoms. Exercise number 18 involved a series of actions combined with breathing to be performed every day between 1 am and 5 am (*chou yin shi* 丑寅时) at the beginning of winter (*li dong* 立冬). It was used for treating a range of symptoms including blood and pus in the stool (*bian nong xue* 便脓血), lower abdomen distension and pain (*xiao fu zhang tong* 小腹胀痛), *zang du* 脏毒, chronic haemorrhoids (*jiu zhi* 久痔) and rectal prolapse (*tuo gang* 脱肛).

The *Lu Di Xian Jing* 陆地仙经 (c. 1726) included a series of methods aimed at achieving longevity. One was described as an 'out and in disperse *ji ju* 积聚 method' (*gu he xiao ji ju* 鼓呵消积聚). This was conducted in the morning and involved a series of movements as follows: 'Place the hands on the opposite shoulders; breathe in, expand the abdomen and hold the breath; calm your mind and focus on the navel; until you cannot hold the breath any longer; gradually breathe out; repeat this nine times then hold your shoulders tightly and twist to the left and right; repeat seven times on each side; this is called *jiao lu* (搅轳).' It was used to dissolve *ji ju* 消积聚 and was for a number of other symptoms including abdominal pain and diarrhoea.

In *Dan Xi Xin Fa* 丹溪心法 (c. 1481) and *Ge Zhi Yu Lun* 格致余论 (c. 1347), which are both attributed to Zhu Dan Xi 朱丹溪, there are extended discussions on 'emptying the granary method' (*dao cang fa* 倒仓法) which was a dietary method for purging the stomach and intestines (i.e. the granary) followed by nourishing, which was aimed at expelling accumulations and treating multiple diseases including *ji ju* 积聚. Complete translations of the sections can be found in *Yang* (1993)[42] and *Yang* and *Duan* (1994),[43] so this section only paraphrases relevant parts. Dan Xi 丹溪 mentioned that in the past medicines such as *Wan bing wan* 万病丸 and *Wen bai wan* 温白丸 were used for these kinds of conditions but the *dao cang fa* 倒仓法 method was more effective. The method involved preparing a large amount of clear broth from bull's meat which was drunk in multiple small doses until it induced vomiting and/or diarrhoea. After the purging was completed, and after one or two days of sleep, the person would become hungry. Firstly, plain congee was given, then three days later they could eat vegetable soup. After 15 days, the person was said to feel full of energy and chronic diseases could be overcome.

In another section of the same book, following the explanation of the aetiology of *ji ju* 积聚 that was presented above, which described a condition consistent with a neoplasm in the intestine, Dan Xi 丹溪 made the following comment regarding the treatment of this condition: 'Short of using the miraculous method of cutting the intestine and scraping the bone, how can this disease be treated? How can a few doses of pills and powders penetrate the walls of the mass?' Here Dan Xi 丹溪 was clearly referencing the famous cases of Hua Tuo 华陀 performing surgery but it is unclear whether he was suggesting that *dao cang fa* 倒仓法 could be effective in such severe cases or whether he meant the only option was surgery when other methods had failed. A similar passage is found in *Yi Xue Gang Mu* 医学纲目 (c.1556).

In the *Li Yue Pian Wen* 理瀹骈文 (c. 1870), as part of an extended discussion, the author mentioned the surgical removal of *ji ju* 积聚 located in the gastrointestinal area and referenced the report from the *Wei Annals* (*Wei Zhi* 魏志 c. 300 AD) which included the cases of Hua Tuo 华陀 performing abdominal surgery using an anesthetic medicine called *Ma fei san* 麻沸散.[44] In this passage the author appears to imply that when the usual methods were ineffective, surgery may be the only option.

Discussion of Other Chinese Medicine Therapies

The use of exercises that involved breathing and physical movement was listed as applicable for abdominal masses in three citations. Such exercises would now be described as forms of *qi gong* 气功 or *dao yin* 导引. Each was used for a variety of conditions and was not specific for CRC, but each mentioned symptoms of signs that suggest it could have been used by people with CRC.

In Dan Xi's 丹溪 discussion of the aetiology of *ji ju* 积聚 we see a detailed description of the stages in the development of an intestinal neoplasm. Moreover, his description of the mass as being 'like a walnut kernal' suggests he may have observed such lumps. Although numerous dissections were carried out during the Song dynasty,[1, 45] it is unclear whether this practice continued during his time or whether he was reporting a description by someone else. He also confirms that formulas such as *Wen bai wan* 温白丸 would have been used for such conditions, but they may not have been effective. With regard to surgery, there are a number of mentions of surgery in the CM literature[1,45] but, other than military surgery, the practice was not widespread, so it is unclear whether Dan Xi 丹溪 would have had firsthand experience.

Classical Literature in Perspective

In classical CM there were no specific terms for CRC, but a number of disease and symptom names may have been applied to CRC. In our selection of terms, based on expert advice and the definition of

CRC in modern medicine, we excluded low-specificity search terms and citations unlikely to have referred to CRC. Consequently, the remaining citations had potential relevance to CRC. This approach resulted in the exclusion of many terms and citations that might have referred to some cases of CRC in the past but for which there was too little information for any decision to be made. It should be noted that classical citations tend to be brief and may only include the disease name without further details. Also, it was not possible to rule out the likelihood that the included citations referred to other conditions such as gastrointestinal bleeding, intestinal obstruction, enteritis, liver cancer or parasites. In pre-modern times the concept of CRC was not well defined although it was understood that neoplasms could develop in the intestines. A clinical diagnosis of CRC was beyond the technology of the times, so it is likely that treatments for palpable masses, such as *ji ju* 积聚 and *zheng jia* 症/癥瘕, were used for masses of diverse aetiology including CRC, but these treatments were not specific to CRC. Similarly, for *zang du* 脏毒, the clinical presentation of gastrointestinal bleeding with blood that was not fresh, could have been due to many types of lesions besides CRC. These limitations need to be considered when interpreting these results.

When compared to the modern approach to CRC in CM, as outlined in Chapter 2, there are some similarities with the classical approaches but also many differences. Whereas the classical formulas and acupuncture treatments were primary interventions, in modern practice western medicine approaches to treatment are usually combined with CM treatments to take advantage of the strengths and counter the weaknesses of both types of therapies. Modern CM treatment is used to extend life in patients with a tumour burden, improve the patient's quality of life, prolong survival time, speed up recovery after surgery, prevent recurrence and/or metastasis, and reduce the adverse effects and improve the efficacy of chemotherapy and/or radiotherapy.[8] Consequently, the formulas listed in clinical guidelines apply to the modern applications of CHM in CRC management.

In both classical and modern CM, the aetiology of CRC involves internal and external factors. The internal factors are internal damage due to disorder of the seven emotions, deficiency of the healthy *qi* and *yin-yang* disharmony. The external factors include external contraction of the six excesses, dietary irregularities and irregular lifestyle. The key feature in pathogenesis is the loss of the transporting function of the large intestine which leads to accumulation of dampness and heat, toxins and stasis, and producing obstruction and blockage of passage through the intestine. Over a long time, the obstructions undergo a pathological transformation into cancer (see Chapter 2).

In terms of specific herbal formulas, none of the formulas commonly used in the classical literature for *ji ju* 积聚 and *zheng jia* 症/癥瘕 (aggregation-accumulations) are listed in modern clinical guidelines. However for *zang du* 脏毒, versions of the classical formulas *Huai jiao wan* 槐角丸 and *Huai hua san* 槐花散 are still used to restrain gastrointestinal bleeding; *Liu jun zi tang* 六君子汤 is still used for Spleen deficiency (*pi xu* 脾虚); and dual deficiency of *qi* and Blood (*qi xue liang xu* 气血两虚) is still treated with formulas such as *Bu zhong yi qi tang* 补中益气汤 and *Si wu tang* 四物汤, all of which appeared in the classical data set.

For acupuncture, KI17 *Shangqu* 商曲 ($n = 19$) was the point most frequently mentioned for *ji ju* 积聚, but it is not mentioned in modern textbooks and guidelines for CRC (Chapter 2). However, other nearby points on the abdomen are still commonly used, such as CV10 *Xiawan* 下脘, CV12 *Zhongwan* 中脘 and ST25 *Tianshu* 天枢. Similarly, on the back the main point was BL22 *Sanjiaoshu* 三焦俞 ($n = 5$) in the classical data but modern books mention the nearby point BL21 *Weishu* 胃俞. Common to both classical and modern literature are BL20 *Pishu* 脾俞 ($n = 1$), BL17 *Geshu* 膈俞 ($n = 1$) and CV10 *Xiawan* 下脘 ($n = 1$). For *zang du* 脏毒, the most frequent point in the classical literature was BL57 *Chengshan* 承山 ($n = 7$), which is still a common point for blood in the stool, but the point GV1 *Changqiang* 长强 ($n = 5$) is no longer in common use due to its inconvenient location near the anus. The points BL17 *Geshu* 膈俞 ($n = 2$), BL20 *Pishu* 脾俞 ($n = 2$) and BL23 *Shenshu* 肾俞 ($n = 1$) are all still used in CRC.

With regard to other therapies, the *qi gong* 气功, *dao yin* 导引 and *gu he xiao ji ju* 鼓呵消积聚 methods had similar therapeutic aims to modern CM therapies (Chapter 2) including: soothing and freeing the channels and connecting vessels, promoting the flow of *qi* and Blood, strengthening the constitution, regulating mood and emotions, and building physique and improving health. In contemporary China, various *qi gong* 气功 methods are frequently used by cancer patients and reviews of clinical studies indicate improvements in immune function, quality of life and survival.[46,47] The 'Emptying the granary method' (*dao cang fa* 倒仓法) was a form of fasting and dietary therapy that aimed to firstly purge the body of accumulations, then nourish the body with a simple diet. Although this particular method does not appear in modern CM books, special diets and foods are suggested for cancer patients, and there is experimental and clinical evidence to suggest that fasting and caloric restriction can improve outcomes in cancer.[48–51]

From the point of view of modern CM clinical practice, the historical literature contains medical substances and formulas that are no longer in use and many of the methods included in the classical books have been replaced by more modern approaches. Consequently, this chapter is of historical interest and should not be used to guide clinical practice.

References

1. Needham J, Lu G. (2000) *Science and Civilisation in China*, Vol. 6. Part VI: Medicine. Cambridge University Press, Cambridge, UK.
2. Hu R, ed. (2014) *Zhong Hua Yi Dian* 中华医典 [*Encyclopaedia of Traditional Chinese Medicine*, 5th ed.] Hunan Electronic and Audio-Visual Publishing House, Changsha.
3. May BH, Lu CJ, Xue CCL. (2012) Collections of traditional Chinese medical literature as resources for systematic searches. *J Altern Complement Med* **18(12):** 1101–1107.
4. May BH, Lu YB, Lu CJ, *et al.* (2013) Systematic assessment of the representativeness of published collections of the traditional literature on Chinese medicine. *J Altern Complement Med* **19(5):** 403–409.
5. 中华中医药学会. (2008) 肿瘤中医诊疗指南. 北京: 中国中医药出版社.
6. 郁仁存. (1983) 中医肿瘤学. 北京: 科学出版社.

7. 刘嘉湘. (1996) 实用中医肿瘤手册. 上海: 上海科技教育出版社.

8. 吴万垠, 刘伟胜. (2013) 肿瘤科专病中医临床诊治 (第3版). 北京: 人民卫生出版社.

9. 罗云坚. (2007) 中医临床治疗特色与优势指南. 北京: 人民卫生出版社.

10. 林洪生. (2014) 恶性肿瘤中医诊疗指南. 北京: 人民卫生出版社.

11. 何裕民. (2005) 现代中医肿瘤学 (普通高等教育"十五"国家级规划教材面向21世纪课程教材). 北京: 中国协和医科大学出版社.

12. 陈锐深. (2003) 现代中医肿瘤学. 北京: 人民卫生出版社.

13. 李家庚, 屈松柏. (2001) 实用中医肿瘤学. 北京: 科学技术文献出版社.

14. 汪悦. (2002) 中医内科学. 上海: 上海中医药大学出版社.

15. 张蓓, 周志伟. (2004) 实用中西医结合肿瘤学. 广州: 广东人民出版社.

16. 周岱翰, 林丽珠. (2012) 中医肿瘤食疗学. 贵阳: 贵州科技出版社.

17. 徐振晔. (2013) 常见肿瘤的中医预防和护养. 上海: 复旦大学出版社.

18. 李家庚, 屈松柏. (1994) 中医肿瘤防治大全. 北京: 科学技术文献出版社.

19. 陈熠. (1999) 世界传统医学肿瘤学. 北京: 科学出版社.

20. 顾奎兴. (1998) 中医肿瘤学. 南京: 东南大学出版社.

21. 陈仁寿. (2006) 中医肿瘤科处方手册. 北京: 科学技术文献出版社.

22. 余桂清. (1989) 历代中医肿瘤案论选粹. 北京: 北京出版社.

23. 高淑萍. (1997) 高氏中医肿瘤诊疗精编(汉英对照). 北京: 中国中医药出版社.

24. 周宜强. (2006) 实用中医肿瘤学. 北京: 中医古籍出版社.

25. 邵梦扬, 宋光瑞. (1994) 中医肿瘤治疗学. 天津: 天津科技翻译出版公司.

26. 王希胜, 张亚密. (2011) 肿瘤病中医特色诊疗全书. 北京: 化学工业出版社.

27. 陈志强, 蔡炳勤, 招伟贤. (2008) 中西医结合外科学（第二版）. 北京: 科学出版社.

28. 沈英森, 赵长鹰, 王奕鸣. (1999) 常见肿瘤的中医防治. 广州: 暨南大学出版社.

29. 谢建兴. (2012) 中西医结合外科学. 北京: 人民卫生出版社.

30. 陈志强, 蔡光先. (2012) 中西医结合内科学（全国高等中医药院校规划教材 第九版）. 北京: 中国中医药出版社.

31. 王三虎. (2001) 肿瘤. 西安: 陕西科学技术出版社.

32. 潘敏求. (1996) 中华肿瘤治疗大成. 石家庄: 河北科学技术出版社.

33. 蒋玉洁, 李一明. (2001) 中国肿瘤秘方全书. 北京: 科学技术文献出版社.

34. 王英, 刘家卿. (1999) 肿瘤科病最新中医治疗. 北京: 中医古籍出版社.

35. May BH, Zhang A, Lu YB, *et al.* (2014) The systematic assessment of traditional evidence from the premodern Chinese medical literature: A text-mining approach. *J Altern Complement Med* **20(12):** 937–942.

36. Unschuld PU. (2016) *Huang Di Nei Jing Ling Shu* [*The Ancient Classic on Needle Therapy, the Complete Chinese Text with Annotated English Translation.*] University of California Press, Berkeley.

37. Wiseman N, Wilms S. (2013) *Jin Guì Yào Lüè:* [*Translation and Commentaries: Essential Prescriptions of the Golden Cabinet.*] Paradigm Publications, Taos.

38. Unschuld PU, ed. (1986) *Medicine in China: Nan Ching, the Classic of Difficulties.* University of California Press, Berkeley.

39. Sivin N. (1968) *Chinese Alchemy: Preliminary Studies.* Harvard University Press, Cambridge, MA.

40. Needham J, Ho PY, Lu GD. (1976) *Science and Civilisation in China*, Vol. 5. Part III: Spagyrical Discovery and Invention: Historical Survey, from Cinnabar Elixirs to Synthetic Insulin. Cambridge University Press, Cambridge.

41. State Administration of Traditional Chinese Medicine Chinese Materia Medica Committee, ed. (1998) *Zhong Hua Ben Cao: Jing Xuan Ben* [*Chinese Materia Medica*, abridged version.] Shanghai Scientific and Technical Publishers, Shanghai.

42. Yang SZ. (1993) *The Heart and Essence of Dan-Xi's Methods of Treatment: A Translation of Zhu Dan-Xi's Dan Xi Zhi Fa Xin Yao.* Blue Poppy Press, Boulder.

43. Yang SZ, Duan WJ. (1994) *Extra Treatises Based on Investigation and Inquiry: A Translation of Zhu Dan-Xi's Ge Zhi Yu Lun.* Blue Poppy Press, Boulder.

44. May B, Tomoda T, Wang M. (2000) The life and medical practice of Hua Tuo. *Pacific J of Oriental Medicine* **14:** 40–54.

45. Wong KC, Wu LT. (1936) *History of Chinese Medicine.* National Quarantine Service, Shanghai.

46. Sze DM, Chan V, Wu MB, *et al.* (2017) Critical review in qigong and immunity cancer research. *Int J Complement Altern Med* **7(3):** 00227.

47. Oh B, Butow P, Mullan B, *et al.* (2012) A critical review of the effects of medical qigong on quality of life, immune function, and survival in cancer patients. *Integr Cancer Ther* **11(2):** 101–110.

48. O'Flanagan CH, Smith LA, McDonell SB, Hursting SD. (2017) When less may be more: Calorie restriction and response to cancer therapy. *BMC Med* **15(1):** 106.

49. Lettieri-Barbato D, Aquilano K. (2018) Pushing the limits of cancer therapy: The nutrient game. *Front Oncol* **8:** 148.

50. Brandhorst S, Harputlugil E, Mitchell JR, Longo VD. (2017) Protective effects of short-term dietary restriction in surgical stress and chemotherapy. *Ageing Res Rev* **39:** 68–77.

51. Brandhorst S, Longo VD. (2016) Fasting and caloric restriction in cancer prevention and treatment. *Recent Results Cancer Res* **207:** 241–266.

4

Methods for Evaluating Clinical Evidence

OVERVIEW

This section describes the methods used to identify and evaluate clinical studies of Chinese medicine interventions for colorectal cancer. Studies were identified through a comprehensive search strategy and were screened against pre-defined eligibility criteria. The methodological quality of included studies was assessed using the risk of bias method. Results for the specified outcomes were evaluated using statistical methods to provide estimates of the effects of each type of Chinese medicine therapy.

Introduction

The use of Chinese medicine (CM) for colorectal cancer (CRC) has been extensively researched in clinical studies. In the following chapters the efficacy, effectiveness and safety of CM interventions have been evaluated using meta-analytic methods, where possible, for the controlled clinical trials, while a descriptive approach has been used for non-controlled clinical studies. The evidence is presented for the following main types of CM interventions:

- Chinese herbal medicine (CHM, Chapter 5);
- Acupuncture and related therapies (Chapter 7);
- Other CM therapies (Chapter 8);
- Combination CM therapies, e.g. CHM plus acupuncture (Chapter 9).

Published data on the clinical trials were obtained from databases and other sources and assessed by an expert review group including researchers, clinical physicians, CM experts and methodologists. All the included studies are referenced at the end of each chapter.

Randomised controlled trials (RCTs), non-randomised controlled clinical trials (CCTs) and non-controlled studies were evaluated separately. Meta-analyses were conducted for the RCTs and CCTs using the methods described below. This approach was not suitable for the evidence from the non-controlled studies. Therefore, the characteristics of the studies, details of the interventions and any adverse events were described and summarised.

References to included studies are indicated by a letter followed by a number. Studies of CHM are indicated by an 'H' e.g. H1; studies of acupuncture and related therapies are indicated by an 'A' e.g. A1; studies of other CM therapies are indicated by an 'O' e.g. O1; and studies of combinations of CM therapies are indicated by a 'C' e.g. C1.

Search Strategy

Comprehensive searches were conducted of multiple English- and Chinese-language databases using the methods outlined in the Cochrane Handbook of Systematic Reviews.[1] English-language databases included PubMed, Excepta Medica Database (Embase), Cumulative Index of Nursing and Allied Health Literature (CINAHL), Cochrane Central Register of Controlled Trials (CENTRAL) including the Cochrane Library, and Allied and Complementary Medicine Database (AMED). Chinese-language databases included China Biomedical Literature (CBM), China National Knowledge Infrastructure (CNKI), Chongqing VIP (CQVIP) and Wanfang. Databases were searched from their respective inceptions to August 2016. No restrictions were applied. Search terms were mapped to controlled vocabulary (where applicable) in addition to being searched as keywords.

Search terms were grouped into blocks of terms for (1) the disease (CRC and synonyms); (2) the CM intervention; and (3) the type of study (clinical trial, RCT, etc). The three search blocks were combined using 'AND' (or database-specific variant). Consequently, the following nine searches were conducted in each of the nine databases:

1. CHM — reviews;
2. CHM — controlled trials (randomised and non-randomised);
3. CHM — non-controlled studies;
4. Acupuncture and related therapies — reviews;
5. Acupuncture and related therapies — controlled trials (randomised and non-randomised);
6. Acupuncture and related therapies — non-controlled studies;
7. Other CM therapies — reviews;
8. Other CM therapies — controlled trials (randomised and non-randomised);
9. Other CM therapies — non-controlled studies.

Studies of combination CM therapies were identified from within the above searches.

In addition to the electronic databases, reference lists of systematic reviews and included studies were searched for additional publications. Clinical trial registries were searched to identify clinical trials which were ongoing or completed, and where required, trial investigators were contacted to obtain data. The searched trial registries included Australian New Zealand Clinical Trial Registry (ANZCTR), Chinese Clinical Trial Registry (ChiCTR), EU Clinical Trials Register (EU-CTR) and ClinicalTrials.gov.

Inclusion Criteria

Study Type

Controlled prospective studies, with or without randomisation (including parallel groups and crossover studies) and uncontrolled studies (cohort, case series and case studies) that employed a CM therapy as a test intervention and reported an outcome of relevance to CRC, were included.

Participants

Adults aged 18 years and over who had been diagnosed with CRC based on pathology tests. There was no restriction on cancer stage or performance status.

Interventions

Studies that employed a CM therapy as a test intervention including the following (Table 4.1):

- CHM: Administration routes included oral and/or topical application or enema;
- Acupuncture: With or without skin penetration, including ear acupuncture/acupressure and warm needling;
- Moxibustion: Direct or indirectly applied, using various heat sources;
- Manual therapies: Including *tui na* 推拿, *an mo* 按摩 (massage);
- Exercises: Including *tai chi* (*tai ji* 太极) and *qi gong* 气功;
- Dietary intervention.

Co-interventions were allowed provided the same intervention was used in at least two arms of the study.

Table 4.1   Chinese Medicine Interventions Included in Clinical Evidence Evaluation

Category	Included Intervention
Chinese herbal medicines	Orally administered CHM; topical CHM including fomentation (*yun tang* 熨烫), cataplasm (*yao gao* 药膏), hand and foot baths, or other topical delivery; and CHM enema.
Acupuncture and related therapies	Acupuncture, electroacupuncture, warm needling, acupressure, ear acupuncture, ear acupressure, moxibustion.
Other CM therapies	Chinese massage (*tui na* 推拿, *an mo* 按摩), *tai chi* 太極, other exercise therapy, CM dietary therapy.
Combination CM	Two or more CM interventions from different categories administered together. For example, oral CHM plus acupuncture, and combinations of other CM therapies.

Abbreviations: CHM, Chinese herbal medicine; CM, Chinese medicine.

Comparators in Controlled Trials (RCT, CCT)

The control interventions in RCTs and CCTs could include:

- No treatment, supportive care, placebo;
- Conventional therapy (using pharmacotherapies, radiotherapy and/or surgery aimed at treating CRC);

Studies could combine a CM intervention with a conventional therapy for CRC as an integrative medicine (IM) approach. Note that the combination of CM with usual supportive care and/or supportive care relating to surgery or chemotherapy and/or the co-administration of conventional therapy for non-CRC conditions, were not considered to be IM approaches.

Settings

In-patients or out-patients treated in hospitals or clinics. Patients treated in their own homes.

Outcomes

Studies reported at least one of the following pre-specified outcome measures:

- Primary outcome assessments: Studies reported at least one of the pre-specified outcome measures (Table 4.2);
- Secondary outcome assessments: Incidence and type of adverse events (AEs) relating to CM during the treatment.

The outcome measure instruments listed below are not the only scales used for assessing people with CRC. Describing every scale and variation is beyond the scope of this chapter. The included scales are ones that feature in the subsequent chapters. In addition to clinical scales, outcomes in cancer research include imaging and serological measures such as tumour markers, but these aspects are not assessed in the following meta-analyses.

Table 4.2 Main Clinical Outcome Measures

Outcome Categories	Outcome Measures	Units; Direction for Improvement
Survival	Overall survival (OS), median survival time (MST)	Time; longer is better
	Progression-free survival (PFS), median progression-free survival (mPFS)	Time; longer is better
	Time to progression (TTP), median time to progression (mTTP)	Time; longer is better
	Survival rate	Numbers at different time points (1–10 yrs)
	Recurrence and/or metastasis rates	Numbers at different time points (1–5 yrs)
Response to therapy	Complete response (CR)	Number of participants
	Partial response (PR)	Number of participants
	Objective response rate (ORR)/ tumour response rate (RR)	Number of participants, CR + PR
	Stable disease (SD)	Number of participants
	Progressive disease (PD)	Number of participants
Quality of life / performance status	Functional Assessment of Cancer Therapy-Colorectal (FACT-C)[2]	36 items; higher total score is better
	European Organisation for Research and Treatment of Cancer Quality of Life Questionnaire (EORTC QLQ-C30, version 3)[3]	30 items, the global health status/QOL scale; higher is better
	Chinese QOL scale[4]	12 items, total score is 60 points; higher is better
	Karnofsky Performance Scale (KPS)[5]	100 points; higher is better
	Edmonton Symptom Assessment System (ESAS)[6]	10 items; lower is better

(Continued)

Table 4.2 (*Continued*)

Outcome Categories	Outcome Measures	Units; Direction for Improvement
Immune function	T-cells: CD3+, CD4+, CD8+, NK cells, CD4+/CD8+, CD8+CD28+	Various
	Immunoglobulins: IgG, IgA, IgM, IgE	Various
Recovery of gastro-intestinal function	Time to first bowel sounds, time to first flatus, time to first defaecation, time to first liquid intake, time to first solid food intake, etc.	Time; shorter is better
Postoperative adverse reactions/ complications	Diarrhoea, abdominal distension, nausea and vomiting, intestinal obstruction, urinary retention, etc.	Number of participants
Adverse reactions to chemotherapy[7,8]	Chemotherapy-induced nausea and vomiting (CINV)	Grade, number of participants
	Diarrhoea	Grade, number of participants
	Constipation	Grade, number of participants
	Gastrointestinal reactions	Grade, number of participants
	Myelosuppression (including: leukopenia, neutropenia, erythropenia, decreased haemoglobin, and thrombocytopenia)	Grade, number of participants
	Chemotherapy-induced peripheral neurotoxicity (CIPN)	Grade, number of participants
	Hand-foot syndrome	Grade, number of participants
	Fatigue	Grade, number of participants
	Hepatotoxicity and/or nephrotoxicity	Grade, number of participants
	Heart function	Grade, number of participants

(*Continued*)

Table 4.2 (*Continued*)

Outcome Categories	Outcome Measures	Units; Direction for Improvement
	Oral mucositis	Grade, number of participants
	Fever	Grade, number of participants
	Alopecia	Grade, number of participants
	Skin rash	Grade, number of participants
Adverse reactions to radiotherapy	Radiation proctitis	Grade, number of participants
	Other adverse reactions to radiotherapy	Grade, number of participants
Adverse events (AE) associated with CM	Adverse events (as reported in studies)	Number and type of AEs and serious adverse events (SAE) in each group

Abbreviations: AE, adverse events; CD: cluster of differentiation (but cell names just use the acronym CD); CM, Chinese medicine; NK, natural killer (cells); Note: superscript numbers refer to the reference list at the end of the chapter.

Exclusion Criteria

Study Type

Clinical studies that used the following designs:

- CM versus other CM therapy;
- CM plus another therapy versus CM;
- CM plus pharmacotherapy versus CM.

Co-interventions were allowed provided the same intervention was used in at least two arms of the study. Retrospective RCTs and CCTs were not included in the meta-analysis or the counts for clinical trials. Such studies may be referred to in the text where relevant.

Participants

- The participant group included people with other cancers such as gastric cancer;
- The diagnosis of CRC was not clear.

Interventions

- Synthetic compounds or isolated chemical compounds, homeopathic preparations, nutritional supplements and plant-based products that are not used in CM;
- Integrative medicine studies that used different therapies in the intervention group compared to the control group.

Comparators in Controlled Trials

- Control groups that employed an intervention that was not used in the conventional care of CRC (in China or other countries);
- Controls using a superseded chemotherapy regimen;
- Controls using another CM intervention or other herbal product.

Outcomes

- Outcome measures based on instruments of unclear origin or validity;
- Outcomes that had missing data and/or data errors that could not be resolved after contacting authors or retrieving related articles. In such cases, the outcome was excluded.

Risk of Bias

Risk of bias was assessed for RCTs using the Cochrane Collaboration's tool.[1] Risk of bias was assessed for the following domains: sequence generation, allocation concealment, blinding of participants and personnel, blinding of outcome assessors, incomplete outcome data and selective reporting. Each domain was assessed to determine whether the risk of bias was 'low', 'high', or 'unclear'. Risk of bias assessment was verified by two dependent researchers and disagreement resolved by discussion and consultation with a third person.

Risk of bias is categorised using the following six domains:

- Sequence generation: The method used to generate the allocation sequence is given in sufficient detail to allow an assessment of whether it should produce comparable groups. 'Low' risk of bias refers to use of a random-number table or computerised randomisation. 'High' risk of bias includes studies that describe a non-random method of sequence generation such as odd or even date of birth or date of admission;
- Allocation concealment: The method used to conceal the allocation sequence is given in enough detail to determine whether intervention allocations could have been foreseen before or during enrolment. 'Low' risk of bias includes central randomisation or sealed envelopes and 'high' risk of bias includes open random sequence or date of birth, etc.;
- Blinding of participants and personnel: Measures used to describe if the study participants and personnel are blind to the intervention received. In addition, information relating to whether the blinding was effective is also assessed. Studies that ensure blinding of participants and personnel are at 'low' risk of bias. If the study is not blind, or incompletely blind, it is at 'high' risk of bias;
- Blinding of outcome assessors: Measures used to describe if the outcome assessors are blind to knowledge of which intervention a participant received. In addition, information relating to whether the blinding was effective is also assessed. Studies that ensure blinding of outcome assessors are at 'low' risk of bias. If the study is not blind, or incompletely blind, it is at 'high' risk of bias;
- Incomplete outcome data: Completeness of outcome data for each main outcome, including drop-outs, exclusions from the analysis with numbers missing in each group and reasons for drop-out or exclusions. Studies with 'low' risk of bias would include all outcome data; or if there is missing data, it is unlikely to relate to the true outcome or is balanced between groups. Studies at 'high' risk of bias would have unexplained missing data;
- Selective reporting: The study protocol is available and includes the pre-specified outcomes. Studies with a published protocol and

which include all pre-specified outcomes in their report would be at 'low' risk of bias. Studies at 'high' risk of bias would not include all pre-specified outcomes or the outcome data may be reported incompletely.

Statistical Analyses

Frequency of CM syndromes, CHM formulas, herbs and acupuncture points reported in included studies were presented using descriptive statistics. Chinese medicine syndromes reported in two or more studies were presented. In Chapter 5, the 20 most frequently reported CHM formulas and herbs were presented. In Chapter 7, the top ten acupuncture points used in CM are presented when available. Where data were limited, reports of single CM syndromes, formulas or acupuncture points are provided as a guide for the reader.

Definitions of statistical tests and results are described in the glossary. Meta-analysis of outcome measure data was performed when a sufficient number of comparable studies were available. Meta-analyses were based on reported data at the end of the treatment periods. Comparisons were between the CM intervention groups and the control groups at end of treatment (EoT).

Dichotomous data are reported as a risk ratio (RR) with 95% confidence intervals (CI), and continuous data are reported as mean difference (MD) or standardised mean difference (SMD) with 95% confidence intervals (CI). For dichotomous data, when the RR is greater than 1 and the upper and lower values of the 95% CI are both greater than 1, this indicates we can be 95% certain that there is a difference between the groups and the true effect lies within these CIs. The same is true for values less than 1. In such cases we say there is a 'significant difference' between the groups. For continuous data, when the MD is greater than zero and both the upper and lower values of the 95% CI are greater than zero, we say there is a 'significant difference' between the groups. The same is true on the negative side of the scale.[1]

Available case analysis with a random effects model was used in all analyses. This provides a conservative estimate of difference between groups and is applicable to data in which heterogeneity is present. Formal tests for heterogeneity were conducted using the I^2 statistic. An I^2 score greater than 50% was considered to indicate substantial heterogeneity.[1]

Sensitivity analysis was undertaken to explore potential sources of heterogeneity, based on low risk of bias for the domain of sequence generation. Where possible and appropriate, planned subgroup analyses included type of control medication, duration of treatment and/or CHM formula.

Assessment Using GRADE

The Grading of Recommendations, Assessment, Development and Evaluation (GRADE) approach was used.[9,10] The GRADE approach summarises and rates the strength and quality of evidence in systematic reviews using a structured process for presenting evidence summaries in terms of the 'certainty' of the evidence. The results are presented in summary of findings (SoF) tables. These provide an overview of the evidence reported by the RCTs for the main interventions, comparisons and outcome measures for CRC.

A panel of experts was established to evaluate the evidence. The panel included the systematic review team, CM practitioners, integrative medicine experts, research methodologists, and conventional medicine physicians. The experts were asked to rate the clinical importance of key interventions from CHM, acupuncture therapies, and other CM therapies, as well as comparators and outcomes. Results were collated and based on the rating scores and subsequent discussion, a consensus on the content for the SoF tables was achieved.

The certainty of evidence for each outcome was rated according to five factors outlined in the GRADE approach. The certainty of evidence might be rated down based on:

- Limitations in study design (risk of bias);
- Inconsistency of results (unexplained heterogeneity);
- Indirectness of evidence (interventions, populations and outcomes important to the patients with the condition);

- Imprecision (uncertainty about the results);
- Publication bias (selective publication of studies).

These five factors are additive and a reduction in one or more factors will reduce the quality of the evidence for that outcome.

These five factors are additive and a reduction in more than one factor will reduce the quality of the evidence for that outcome. The GRADE approach also includes three domains that can be rated up, including large magnitude of an effect, dose-response gradient and effect of plausible residual confounding. However, these three domains relate to observational studies including cohort, case-control, before-after, time series studies, etc. GRADE summaries in this monograph only include RCTs therefore these three domains for rating up were not assessed.

The GRADE approach also includes methods for assessing observational studies. In this monograph GRADE summaries only include RCTs. Treatment recommendations could also be assessed using the GRADE approach, however due to the diverse nature of CM practice, treatment recommendations were not included with the SoFs. Therefore, the reader should interpret the evidence with reference to the local practice environment. It should also be noted that the GRADE approach requires judgments about the strength and quality of evidence and some subjective assessment. However, the experience of the panel members suggests the judgments are reliable and transparent representations of the certainty of evidence.

The GRADE levels of evidence are grouped into four categories:

1) High certainty: We are very confident that the true effect lies close to that of the estimate of the effect;
2) Moderate certainty: We are moderately confident in the effect estimate: The true effect is likely to be close to the estimate of the effect, but there is a possibility that it is substantially different;
3) Low certainty: Our confidence in the effect estimate is limited: The true effect may be substantially different from the estimate of the effect;

4) Very low certainty: We have very little confidence in the effect estimate: The true effect is likely to be substantially different from the estimate of effect.

References

1. Higgins JPT, Green S, eds. (2011) Cochrane Handbook for Systematic Reviews of Interventions Version 5.1.0. The Cochrane Collaboration.
2. Ward WL, Hahn EA, Mo F, *et al.* (1999) Reliability and validity of the functional assessment of cancer therapy-colorectal (FACT-C) quality of life instrument. *Qual Life Res* **8(3):** 181–195.
3. Aaronson NK, Ahmedzai S, Bergman B, *et al.* (1993) The European-Organization-for-Research-and-Treatment-of-Cancer QLQ-C30: A quality-of-life instrument for use in international clinical-trials in oncology. *J Natl Cancer Inst* **85(5):** 365–376.
4. 孙燕. (2001) 内科肿瘤学. 北京: 人民卫生出版社, pp. 996–997.
5. Yates JW, Chalmer B, Mckegney FP. (1980) Evaluation of patients with advanced cancer using the Karnofsky performance status. *Cancer* **45(8):** 2220–2224.
6. Bruera E, Kuehn N, Miller MJ, *et al.* (1991) The Edmonton Symptom Assessment System (ESAS): A simple method for the assessment of palliative care patients. *J Palliative Care* **7(2):** 6–9.
7. National Institutes of Health and National Cancer Institute. (2008) Common Terminology Criteria for Adverse Events (CTCAE), Version 4. National Institutes of Health, Bethesda, MD.
8. Miller AB, Hoogstraten B, Staquet M, Winkler A. (1981) Reporting results of cancer treatment. *Cancer* **47(1):** 207–214.
9. Schunemann H, Brozek J, Guyatt G, Oxman A, eds. (2013) GRADE handbook for grading quality of evidence and strength of recommendations (the GRADE working group). Available from: http://www.guidelinedevelopment.org/handbook/.
10. Schünemann HJ, Higgins JPT, Vist GE, *et al.* Chapter 14: Completing 'summary of findings' tables and grading the certainty of the evidence. In: Higgins JPT, Thomas J, Chandler J, Cumpston M, Li T, Page MJ, *et al.*, editors (2019). Cochrane handbook for systematic reviews of interventions version 6.0 (updated july 2019), Cochrane; 2019. Available from www.training.cochrane.org/handbook

5

Clinical Evidence for Chinese Herbal Medicine

OVERVIEW

The searches identified 133 randomised controlled trials, 11 non-randomised controlled studies and 18 non-controlled studies of Chinese herbal medicine administered orally, as an enema, applied topically or inhaled for the management of colorectal cancer. In the majority of studies an integrative approach to therapy was used. The analyses of the study results are presented in four main sections depending upon the conventional therapy: (1) postoperative recovery; (2) chemotherapy; (3) radiotherapy or chemo-radiotherapy; and (4) supportive and/or palliative care. Most studies were for improving recovery after surgery for colorectal cancer or for alleviating the adverse effects of chemotherapy. The meta-analyses are grouped based on the main comparisons and subgrouped based on the particular conventional therapy. Due to the volume of the data, a detailed summary is presented at the end of the chapter.

Introduction

Interventions employing Chinese herbal medicine (CHM) have been evaluated in a large number of clinical trials for multiple outcomes in colorectal cancer (CRC). Chinese herbal medicine interventions typically comprise formulations made up of multiple ingredients of plant, animal or mineral origin. Details on these substances can be found in major pharmacopoeia and compendia of Chinese *materia medica*.[1-3] Chinese herbal medicines may be administered as a variety of preparation types including oral administration such as aqueous decoctions, liquid extracts, pills, capsules and powders, or topical applications including enemas. Injection products are beyond the scope of this chapter. Studies that combined a CHM with another Chinese medicine (CM) intervention are included in Chapter 9.

Previous Systematic Reviews

A number of reviews of CHMs for people with CRC have been published. A meta-analysis found CHM combined with chemotherapy increased survival rates, improved quality of life and had positive effects on immunoregulation.[4] Other meta-analyses of randomised controlled trials (RCTs) found that CHM combined with chemotherapy improved 0.5–5-year survival rate for medium and advanced CRC;[5] 1–3-year survival time for stage III-IV CRC;[6] improved quality of life and reduced chemotherapy-related adverse events (AEs);[7] and improved quality of life and immune function, as well as reduced chemotherapy-related AEs after surgery.[8] In advanced CRC, a meta-analysis found that FOLFOX4 (a chemotherapy regimen) combined with CHMs improved objective response rate, one-year survival rate and Karnofsky Performance Status (KPS), and reduced chemotherapy-related AEs.[9] The combination of CHM with oxaliplatin-based chemotherapies showed improvement in objective response rate,[10] reduced chemotherapy-related nausea and vomiting,[11] and reduced chemotherapy-related myelosuppression and neutropenia.[12]

A number of meta-analyses have focused on the type of CHM formula. Meta-analyses found that fortifying the Spleen (*jian pi* 健脾) CHMs combined with chemotherapy may reduce the incidence of grade I/II chemotherapy-related AEs, such as leucopenia, nausea and vomiting,[13] and may improve immune function.[14] In advanced CRC, a meta-analysis found that fortifying the Spleen CHMs plus chemotherapy improved objective response rate and quality of life, but there was no significant improvement in one-year survival rate.[15] Another review reported that herbs which fortify the Spleen and dispel dampness and stasis, and resolve toxins combined with chemotherapy increased survival rate and objective response rate, improved quality of life and decreased chemotherapy-related AEs.[16]

In a few reviews, specific formulas were the focus. *Jian pi bu shen fu fang* 健脾补肾复方 combined with chemotherapy was reported to improve tumour response rate, KPS and one-year, three-year and five-year survival rates;[17] and *Si jun zi tang* 四君子汤 plus chemotherapy improved quality of life and reduced chemotherapy-related AEs.[18]

Identification of Clinical Studies

The searches identified 133 RCTs, 11 controlled clinical trials (CCTs) and 18 non-controlled studies that met the inclusion criteria (Fig. 5.1). These tested oral CHM, topical CHM, CHM enemas and inhaled CHM for various outcomes in the management of CRC. Further details of the studies are provided at the beginning of each of the four main sections of this chapter.

Outline of the Data Analyses

The main types of CHM therapies tested in the clinical studies were oral CHMs, topical CHMs and CHM enemas. These were used at various stages during the treatment of CRC and in conjunction with a variety of conventional interventions.

The data analyses are organised in four main sections:

1. Chinese herbal medicine used during postoperative recovery (26 RCTs; three CCTs; five non-controlled studies);
2. Chinese herbal medicine used in association with chemotherapies (99 RCTs; eight CCTs; three non-controlled studies);
3. Chinese herbal medicine used in association with radiotherapy or chemo-radiotherapy (five RCTs; 0 CCTs; 0 non-controlled studies);
4. Chinese herbal medicine used for supportive and/or palliative care (three RCTs; 0 CCTs; ten non-controlled studies).

Within each section, descriptions of the included studies, risk of bias (RoB) assessments for the RCTs and meta-analyses of outcome

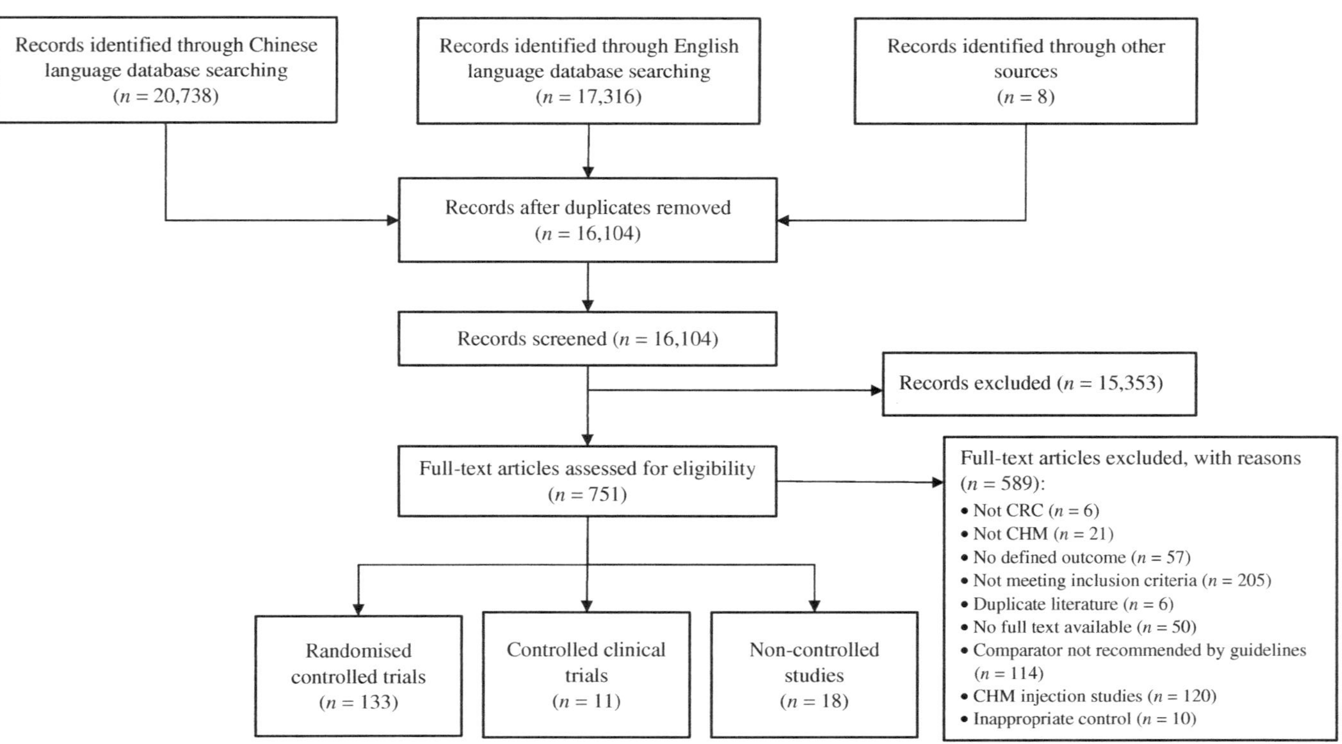

Fig. 5.1 Flowchart of Study Selection Process: Chinese herbal medicine.

data are presented separately for the type of CHM: oral CHMs, topical CHMs, CHM enemas and inhaled CHM (when available). Within each CHM type, any results of CCTs and non-controlled studies of the same type of CHM are presented following the RCTs. Meta-analyses of RCTs are organised according to the outcome measure and comparison. Any meta-analyses of CCTs are presented in a similar fashion after the RCTs. For non-controlled studies, results are descriptive summaries.

Section 1: Chinese Herbal Medicine During Postoperative Recovery

This section reports on studies that used a CHM treatment to assist in postoperative recovery. Twenty-six RCTs (H1–H26), three CCTs (H27–H29), and five non-controlled studies (H30–H34) reported outcomes. Oral CHM was tested in 19 RCTs, all three CCTs and all five non-controlled studies but one of these (H31) combined oral plus topical CHM. Topical CHM was used in six RCTs, no CCTs and in one non-controlled study that also used oral CHM (H31). One RCT (H26) used a CHM inhalation. No study used a CHM enema.

The main outcomes were recovery of gastrointestinal function, postoperative diarrhoea and other adverse reactions, KPS and immune function. Meta-analysis results are presented firstly for RCTs of oral CHM, next for RCTs of topical CHM and then for the single RCT of inhalation. Following this, results are reported for the CCTs, non-controlled studies and for safety of all studies in this section.

Randomised Controlled Trials of Oral Chinese Herbal Medicine for Postoperative Recovery

The 19 RCTs of oral CHM were all conducted in mainland China and enrolled 1,304 participants. The age of participants ranged from 18 to 83 years; however, age range was not reported in five studies

(H10–H12, H15, H18). Based on the reported means and standard deviations for ages, the majority of participants were aged between 46 and 78 years. Following drop-outs, 1,294 participants completed the studies.

Syndromes

Four studies used syndrome differentiation in the selection criteria. Each mentioned a different syndrome as follows:

- *Qi* deficiency failing to ensure containment – *qi xu shi she* 气虚失摄 (H7);
- Spleen deficiency and sunken *qi* – *pi xu xia xian* 脾虚下陷 (H9);
- Spleen deficiency with *qi* stagnation – *pi xu qi zhi* 脾虚气滞 (H3);
- Gastrointestinal *qi* stagnation – *wei chang qi zhi* 胃肠气滞 (H14).

There is considerable overlap between these syndromes, with the first three including *qi* deficiency and the last two including *qi* stagnation.

Formula and Herb Frequencies

The following three formulas, some with modifications, were each used in two studies:

- *Si mo tang* 四磨汤 (H2, H5);
- *Bu zhong yi qi wan/tang* 补中益气丸/汤 (H9, H19);
- Modified *Liu jun zi tang* 六君子汤 (H15, H17).

The herbs most frequently used in the 19 oral formulas were *bai zhu* 白术 (*n* = 13), *gan cao* 甘草 (*n* = 9), *huang qi* 黄芪 (*n* = 9), *chen pi* 陈皮 (*n* = 8) and *dang shen* 党参 (*n* = 8) (Table 5.1).

In accord with the syndromes mentioned above, four of the five most frequent herbs are typically used for *qi* deficiency (*bai zhu* 白术, *gan cao* 甘草, *huang qi* 黄芪 and *dang shen* 党参) while other herbs, such as *hou pu* 厚朴 and *mu xiang* 木香, can be used for *qi* stagnation.

Table 5.1 Frequently Used Herbs in Oral Formulas in Randomised Controlled Trials of Chinese Herbal Medicine for Postoperative Recovery

Herb Name	Scientific Name	Frequency of Use
Bai zhu 白术[1]	*Atractylodes macrocephala* Koidz.	13
Gan cao 甘草[2]	*Glycyrrhiza uralensis* Fisch.	9
Huang qi 黄芪	*Astragalus membranaceus* (Fisch.) Bge.	9
Chen pi 陈皮	*Citrus reticulata* Blanco	8
Dang shen 党参	*Codonopsis pilosula* (Franch.) Nannf.	8
Dang gui 当归	*Angelica sinensis* (Oliv.) Diels	6
Hou pu 厚朴	*Magnolia officinalis* Rehd. et Wils.	6
Mu xiang 木香	*Aucklandia lappa* Decne.	6
Da huang 大黄	*Rheum palmatum* L.; *R. tanguticum* Maxim. ex Balf.	5
Fu ling 茯苓	*Poria cocos* (Schw.) Wolf	5
Sha ren 砂仁	*Amomum villosum* Lour.	5
Zhi shi 枳实	*Citrus aurantium* L.	5
Bing lang 槟榔	*Areca catechu* L.	4
Lai fu zi 莱菔子	*Raphanus sativus* L.	4
Ren shen 人参[3]	*Panax ginseng* C. A. Mey.	4
Shan yao 山药	*Dioscorea opposita* Thunb.	4

[1]One RCT used *chao bai zhu* 炒白术.

[2]Three RCTs used *zhi gan cao* 炙甘草.

[3]One RCT used *sheng shai shen* 生晒参 and one used *hong shen* 红参.

The use of some herbs may be restricted in some countries. Readers are advised to comply with relevant regulations.

Risk of Bias

The risk of bias for sequence generation was judged 'low' in 11 RCTs since the method of randomisation was described (Table 5.2). The others were 'unclear' risk. Allocation concealment was not mentioned in any study, so all were judged 'unclear' risk. Five studies (H6, H10, H13, H14, H18) used inert fluids in the control group as a control for the CHM decoctions, but it was unclear whether these

Table 5.2   Risk of Bias of Randomised Controlled Trials of Oral Chinese Herbal Medicine for Postoperative Recovery

Risk of Bias Domain	Low Risk *n* (%)	Unclear Risk *n* (%)	High Risk *n* (%)
Sequence generation	11 (57.9)	8 (42.1)	0 (0)
Allocation concealment	0 (0)	19 (100)	0 (0)
Blinding of participants	0 (0)	0 (0)	19 (100)
Blinding of personnel	0 (0)	0 (0)	19 (100)
Blinding of outcome assessors	0 (0)	19 (100)	0 (0)
Incomplete outcome data	19 (100)	0 (0)	0 (0)
Selective outcome reporting	0 (0)	19 (100)	0 (0)

could be effective for blinding participants, so these were judged 'high' risk. The remaining studies were judged 'high' risk for blinding of participants and all studies were judged 'high' risk for blinding of personnel. Since most outcomes were based on routine assessments by hospital staff recorded in the patient's medical record, we judged 'unclear' risk for blinding of outcome assessors. Two studies reported there were drop-outs but reasons were given and the numbers were low so all studies were judged 'low' risk for incomplete outcome data. Although all studies reported the outcomes listed in the methods, no protocols could be located so all were judged 'unclear' risk for selective reporting.

Recovery of Gastrointestinal Function

Fifteen RCTs reported data for postoperative recovery of gastrointestinal function. In six RCTs the comparator was usual postoperative care alone. Five studies used the Fast Track Programme (FTP) of perioperative care in both groups and four used postoperative enteral nutrition (PEN) with, or without naso-gastric tube, in both groups. These groups were separated for the purpose of meta-analysis. Four RCTs (H2, H7, H9, H16) included rectal cancer patients only, two RCTs (H3, H17) included colon cancer only, three RCTs (H2, H12, H13) used laparoscopic surgery, and in one study (H3) all participants had gastrointestinal dysfunction at baseline. These differences were considered in the sensitivity analyses.

Three studies had three arms. In H12 the arms were CHM plus FTP, FTP alone and usual postoperative care. For this study, only the comparison CHM plus FTP versus FTP alone was included. In H15 the arms were CHM plus PEN, PEN alone and parenteral nutrition (i.e. injection), so only the comparison CHM plus PEN versus PEN alone was used. The number of participants were adjusted accordingly. One study (H5) included a warm needling arm which was included in Chapter 7.

Oral Chinese Herbal Medicine plus Usual Postoperative Care versus Usual Postoperative Care

Six RCTs reported on postoperative recovery of gastrointestinal function. Both groups received usual postoperative care but there was no CHM in the control group. In one study (H6), warm normal saline was used orally as a control for the CHM. All studies have been pooled together.

For time to first bowel sounds (Table 5.3), there was a significant reduction in the CHM groups in the pooled result, but the heterogeneity was considerable (mean difference [MD]: −6.09 [−11.20, −0.97] hours, I^2 = 87.6%). The single study of usual surgery for CRC showed no difference between groups (H5), whereas there was a significant reduction in the study of colon cancer that required that all participants were assessed as having gastrointestinal dysfunction (H3). There was a significant improvement in the study of rectal cancer that used a normal saline control (H6). Due to the differences between groups no sensitivity analysis was feasible.

For time to first flatus, data were available for six RCTs. The pooled result showed a significant reduction (MD: −24.42 [−34.36, −14.49] hours, I^2 = 95.7%) with considerable heterogeneity. In the sensitivity analyses, when the two studies of rectal cancer (H2, H6) were removed the result remained significant but heterogeneity was not reduced (MD: −29.99 [−50.81, −9.17] hours, I^2 = 97%). When the single study that used laparoscopic surgery (H2) was removed the result was similar (MD: −25.47 [−37.96, −12.97] hours, I^2 = 96%). When the single study of radical surgery (H4) was excluded from the pool, the mean recovery

Table 5.3 Oral Chinese Herbal Medicine for Recovery of Gastrointestinal Function

Outcome (Unit)	Cancer, Surgery (*N* Participants)[1]	Effect Size (MD [95% CI]), I^2	Included Studies
Time to first bowel sounds (hours)	Colon cancer[2] (64)	–6.10 [–8.43, –3.77]*	H3
	CRC, usual surgery (70)	–0.43 [–4.87, 4.01]	H5
	Rectal cancer (60)	–11.00 [–13.92, –8.08]*	H6
	Pooled result (194) 3 RCTs	–6.09 [–11.20, –0.97]*, 87.6%	All above
Time to first flatus (hours)	CRC, usual surgery (60)	–52.08 [–68.83, –35.34]*	H1
	Rectal cancer, laparoscopy (56)	–22.00 [–25.76, –18.24]*	H2
	Colon cancer[2] (64)	–18.10 [–23.81, –12.39]*	H3
	CRC, radical surgery (116)	–50.64 [–60.73, –40.55]*	H4
	CRC, usual surgery (70)	–3.09 [–7.10, 0.92]	H5
	Rectal cancer (60)	–14.40 [–23.42, –5.39]*	H6
	Pooled result (426) 6 RCTs	–24.42 [–34.36, –14.49]*, 95.7%	All above
Time to first defaecation (hours)	CRC, usual surgery (60)	–71.76 [–92.23, –51.29]*	H1
	Rectal cancer, laparoscopy (56)	–19.00 [–24.24, 13.76]	H2
	CRC, radical surgery (116)	–72.96 [–89.44, –56.48]*	H4
	CRC, usual surgery (70)	–2.25 [–7.90, 3.40]	H5
	Rectal cancer (60)	–14.88 [–18.56, –11.20]*	H6
	Pooled result (362) 5 RCTs	–32.41 [–47.44, –17.39]*, 95.9%	All above

[1]Comparator was usual care.

[2]All had gastrointestinal dysfunction.

*Statistically significant.

Abbreviations: CI, confidence interval; CRC, colorectal cancer; MD, mean difference; N, number; RCT, randomised controlled trial.

time was reduced but there was little reduction in heterogeneity (MD: –18.76 [–27.40, –10.12] hours, I^2 = 94.1%).

Five RCTs provided data for time to first defaecation. The pooled result was significant with considerable heterogeneity (MD: –32.41

hours). Removal of the study of radical CRC surgery (H4) reduced the mean time to defaecation (MD: –21.83 [–34.29, –9.37] hours, I^2 = 94.1%) but there was little effect on heterogeneity. After exclusion of the two studies of rectal cancer (H2, H6) the result was not significant (MD: –48.45 [–103.55, 6.65] hours, I^2= 97.9%) and the heterogeneity increased.

When the two studies of rectal cancer (H2, H6) were pooled separately, time to first flatus was significantly reduced in the CHM groups (MD: 17.52 [–26.15, –8.89] hours, I^2 = 92.2%), as was time to first defaecation (MD: –16.50 [–20.45, –12.56] hours, I^2 = 37%).

One study (H3) reported the incidence of complete recovery from gastrointestinal dysfunction and found no significant difference between groups (risk ratio [RR]: 2.50 [0.52, 11.96], *n* = 64).

Oral Chinese Herbal Medicine plus Fast Track Programme versus Fast Track Programme

In five RCTs FTP was used in both groups. All studies were of CRC; two studies (H12, H13) used laparoscopic surgery. Three studies (H10, H13, H14) used warm water as a control for the CHM.

Three RCTs reported data for time to first bowel sounds (Table 5.4). The pooled result showed no significant difference between groups (MD: –3.09 [–7.65, 1.48] hours, I^2 = 78.4%) with substantial heterogeneity. The differences between each of the studies precluded sensitivity analysis. It is notable that time to recovery in the control group in study H11 (usual surgery) was much longer than in the other two studies.

For time to first flatus, the pooled result of five RCTs showed a significant reduction in the CHM groups, with substantial heterogeneity (MD: –11.57 [–18.58, –4.74] hours, I^2 = 71.5%). When the two studies using laparoscopic surgery were removed, the result remained significant without heterogeneity (MD: –9.11 [–12.58, –5.64] hours, I^2 = 0%, *n* = 216).

For time to first defaecation the pooled result of three RCTs showed a significant reduction in the CHM groups

Table 5.4   Oral Chinese Herbal Medicine plus Fast Track Programme for Recovery of Gastrointestinal Function

Outcome (Unit)	Surgery (*N* Participants)[1]	Effect Size (MD [95% CI]), I^2	Included Studies
Time to first bowel sounds (hours)	Usual surgery (50)	−14.16 [−22.69, −5.63]*	H11
	Laparoscopy (75)	−1.10 [−3.38, 1.18]	H13
	Usual surgery (34)	−0.23 [−3.15, 2.69]	H14
	Pooled result (159) 3 RCTs	−3.09 [−7.65, 1.48], 78.4%	All above
Time to first flatus (hours)	Usual surgery (132)	−7.00 [−11.73, −2.27]*	H10
	Usual surgery (50)	−13.32 [−21.52, −5.13]*	H11
	Laparoscopy (61)	−2.50 [−13.44, 8.44]	H12
	Laparoscopy (75)	−38.40 [−55.89, −20.91]*	H13
	Usual surgery (34)	−10.47 [−17.03, −3.92]*	H14
	Pooled result (352) 5 RCTs	−11.57 [−18.58, −4.74]*, 71.5%	All above
Time to first defaecation (hours)	Usual surgery (50)	−12.16 [−19.52, −4.80]*	H11
	Laparoscopy (75)	−36.00 [−56.14, −15.87]*	H13
	Usual surgery (34)	−20.13 [−28.06, −12.20]*	H14
	Pooled result (159) 3 RCTs	−19.44 [−29.37, −9.50]*, 64.8%	All above
Time to food intake (hours)	Laparoscopy (61)	−1.60 [−4.68, 1.48]	H12

[1]Comparator was Fast Track Programme (FTP); all had colorectal cancer.

*Statistically significant.

Abbreviations: CI, confidence interval; MD, mean difference; N, number; RCT, randomised controlled trial.

(MD: −19.44 [−29.37, −9.50] hours, I^2 = 64.8%) with substantial heterogeneity. However, there were no clear grounds for sensitivity analysis.

For time to food intake, one RCT that used laparoscopy reported no difference between groups (MD: −1.60 [−4.68, 1.48]).

Oral Chinese Herbal Medicine plus Postoperative Enteral Nutrition versus Postoperative Enteral Nutrition

In four RCTs both groups received PEN. The control group only received PEN in three RCTs and one study (H18) also used normal saline as a control for the CHM. In one study (H17) all participants had colon cancer and in another study (H16) all had rectal cancer. All studies employed usual surgery. No study reported data for time to first bowel sounds.

For time to first flatus there was a significant reduction in the CHM groups (MD: -10.13 [-14.77, -5.49] hours, $I^2 = 92\%$) in the pooled result, but the heterogeneity was considerable (Table 5.5). When the study of rectal cancer was removed the result remained almost the same (MD: -9.18 [-14.95, -3.41] hours, $I^2 = 91\%$, $n = 258$).

For time to first defaecation, the reduction in the CHM groups was significant in the pooled result (MD: -9.42 [-13.19, -5.65]

Table 5.5 **Oral Chinese Herbal Medicine plus Postoperative Enteral Nutrition for Recovery of Gastrointestinal Function**

Outcome (Unit)	Cancer, (*N* Participants)[1]	Effect Size (MD [95% CI]), I^2	Included Studies
Time to first flatus (hours)	CRC (60)	-3.47 [-6.27, -0.67]*	H15
	Rectal cancer (40)	-12.88 [-14.93, -10.83]*	H16
	Colon cancer (158)	-8.45 [-10.42, -6.48]*	H17
	CRC (40)	-16.80 [-21.78, -11.82]*	H18
	Pooled result (298) 4 RCTs	-10.13 [-14.77, -5.49]*, 92%	All above
Time to first defaecation (hours)	CRC (60)	-4.53 [-7.89, -1.17]*	H15
	Rectal cancer (40)	-11.60 [-15.50, -7.70]*	H16
	Colon cancer (158)	-8.88 [-11.84, -5.92]*	H17
	CRC (40)	-14.30 [-20.07, -8.54]*	H18
	Pooled result (298) 4 RCTs	-9.42 [-13.19, -5.65]*, 74.3%	All above

[1]Comparator was enteral nutrition (PEN); all studies employed usual surgery.

* Statistically significant.

Abbreviations: CI, confidence interval; CRC, colorectal cancer; MD, mean difference; N, number; RCT, randomised controlled trial.

hours, I^2 = 74.3%) with substantial heterogeneity. Removal of the study of rectal cancer produced a similar result (MD: –8.75 [–13.46, –4.05] hours, I^2 = 77.8%, n = 258).

Postoperative Diarrhoea

Four studies reported data on this outcome. Two RCTs (H7, H8) compared CHMs to usual care, one RCT (H19) combined *Bu zhong yi qi wan* 补中益气丸 (three times a day) with loperamide for seven days or until diarrhoea stopped, and one study (H9) combined *Bu zhong yi qi tang* 补中益气汤 (one packet a day as two doses) with loperamide and montmorillonite for 14 days. In two studies (H7, H9) the diagnosis was rectal cancer and the other two (H8, H19) were of CRC. The studies used different standards for reporting results, but all reported the incidence of complete recovery.

For the two studies of CHM plus usual care compared to usual care alone (H7, H8), there was no significant difference between groups for complete recovery (RR: 2.47 [0.96, 6.37], I^2= 47.4%, n = 109) with moderate heterogeneity. The pooled result for the two studies (H9, H19) of *Bu zhong yi qi wan/tang* 补中益气丸/汤 combined with anti-diarrhoea medicines was not significant (RR: 1.28 [0.79, 2.08], I^2 = 3.4%, n = 108) with little heterogeneity.

Postoperative Abdominal Distension

The incidence of postoperative abdominal distension was reported in two RCTs. One study (H2) used laparoscopic surgery for rectal cancer and compared *Si mo tang* 四磨汤 (from one day after surgery, twice a day until recovery of gastrointestinal function) to usual care. It found the incidence of abdominal distension in the CHM group (n = 3) compared to the control (n = 11) was significantly lower (RR: 0.25 [0.08, 0.81], n = 56).

The other study (H12) used laparoscopic surgery for CRC and compared *Si jun zi tang jia wei* 四君子汤加味 plus FTP with FTP alone (n = 61). The CHM was administered once a day for three days before surgery, then again after surgery once the person could tolerate liquid intake for three to five days. There were no cases of abdominal distension in the CHM group and three cases in the control group. There was no significant difference between groups (RR: 0.13 [0.01, 2.41], *n* = 61).

Postoperative Nausea and Vomiting

Three RCTs reported data for postoperative nausea and vomiting. One study (H1), that compared a formula made by the author, called *Yi qi jian pi fang* 益气健脾方 (commenced one day after surgery, once a day for one month) plus usual care, to usual postoperative care alone reported the incidence of grades I to IV nausea and vomiting. There were no significant differences between groups for grades I+II combined (RR: 0.69 [0.39, 1.23], *n* = 60) and grades III+IV combined (RR: 0.33 [0.07, 1.52], *n* = 60). Another study (H4) also tested a formula called *Yi qi jian pi fang* 益气健脾方, which had eight ingredients in common with the previous formula plus four different herbs, and compared this formula (once a day for 30 days) to usual care after radical surgery for CRC. There was no significant difference between groups in total incidence of nausea and vomiting (RR: 0.62 [0.33, 1.16], *n* = 116).

The third study (H12) compared *Si jun zi tang jia wei* 四君子汤加味 (see above) plus FTP, with FTP alone, after laparoscopic surgery for CRC. There was no significant difference between groups (RR: 0.49 [0.27, 0.89], *n* = 61). The pooled result for the three studies showed a significant reduction in all grades (RR: 0.55 [0.38, 0.79], I^2 = 0%, *n* = 237).

Postoperative Intestinal Obstruction

Incidence of postoperative intestinal obstruction was reported in two RCTs. For rectal cancer (*n* = 60), *Jia wei da cheng qi tang* 加味大承气汤 (administered via naso-gastric tube twice a day until defaecation) was compared with usual care plus warm normal saline (H6). The study reported no cases in the treatment group versus four cases in the control group. In the other study (*n* = 132), which used FTP in both groups, a formula made by the author called *Tai gen yin* 太根饮

(*bai luo bo* 白萝卜, water and table salt *shi yan* 食盐) was administered from six to 24 hours after surgery with a dose of 100 ml every six hours. This was compared to warm water using the same administration method (H10). There were no cases of inflammatory bowel obstruction in the treatment group and two in the control group. These data could not be pooled since the conditions were different and there were no cases in the treatment groups.

Karnofsky Performance Scale

Five articles mentioned results for the Karnofsky Performance Scale (KPS). One article reported KPS scores (H16) and four provided the rates of participants who showed improvements of 10 points or more. The study that reported KPS scores was of rectal cancer and tested a herbal wine called *Ji chuan yang sheng zhu yan bu lao yao jiu* 济川养生驻颜不老药酒 (from 24 hours after surgery, 10 ml three times per day) combined with PEN, compared to PEN alone. There was significant improvement in KPS scores in the CHM group (MD: 17.25 [10.94, 23.56], *n* = 40).

In the four studies that reported the incidence of a 10-point or more increase in KPS (Table 5.6), three studies were comparisons with usual postoperative care alone and one study combined loperamide with *Bu zhong yi qi wan* 补中益气丸 (H19, see postoperative

Table 5.6 Oral Chinese Herbal Medicine for Postoperative Recovery: Karnofsky Performance Status (Improvements of 10 Points or More)

Cancer, Surgery (*N* Participants)	Comparator	Effect Size (RR [95% CI]), I²	Included Studies
CRC, usual surgery (60)	Usual care	1.29 [0.99, 1.67]	H1
CRC, radical surgery (116)	Usual care	1.21 [1.01, 1.45]*	H4
Rectal cancer, usual surgery (49)	Usual care	1.54 [0.88, 2.68]	H7
CRC (60), all had diarrhoea and took loperamide	Usual care plus loperamide	1.62 [1.01, 2.59]*	H19
Pooled result (285) 4 RCTs		1.28 [0.11, 1.47]*, 0%	All above

*Statistically significant.

Abbreviations: CI, confidence interval; CRC, colorectal cancer; MD, mean difference; N, number; RCT, randomised controlled trial; RR, risk ratio.

diarrhoea above for details). The pooled result showed a significantly higher incidence of KPS improvement in the oral CHM groups (RR: 1.28 [0.11, 1.47], $I^2 = 0\%$).

Postoperative Immune Function

Five studies reported data for immunoglobulin G (IgG), immunoglobulin A (IgA) and immunoglobulin M (IgM). Due to differences between the interventions, comparators and the way the units were reported in these studies, meta-analysis was conducted using standardised mean difference (SMD) (Table 5.7). One study (H11), that compared an unnamed CHM plus FTP with FTP alone for CRC, reported significant increases in IgG, IgA and IgM in the CHM group.

Four studies compared CHMs plus PEN to PEN alone. In one study (H18) normal saline was used in the control group. The pooled results found no significant differences between groups for IgG (SMD: 0.92 [–0.11, 1.94], $I^2 = 93.3\%$, $n = 298$) and IgM (SMD: 0.25

Table 5.7 Oral Chinese Herbal Medicine for Postoperative Recovery: Immunoglobulins

Cancer (Study) N Participants[1]	IgG; Effect Size (SMD [95% CI]), I^2	IgA; Effect Size (SMD [95% CI]), I^2	IgM; Effect Size (SMD [95% CI]), I^2
Fast Track Programme			
CRC (H11) 50	0.66 [0.09, 1.23]*	0.75 [0.17, 1.32]*	1.13 [0.53, 1.73]*
Postoperative enteral nutrition			
CRC (H15) 60	0.49 [–0.02, 1.01]	0.06 [–0.45, 0.56]	–0.16 [–0.67, 0.35]
Rectal cancer (H16) 40	0.04 [–0.58, 0.66]	5.77 [4.33, 7.20]*	–0.29 [–0.91, 0.33]
Colon cancer (H17) 158	2.17 [1.77, 2.56]*	0.73 [0.40, 1.05]*	0.72 [0.40, 1.05]*
CRC (H18) 40	0.91 [0.26, 1.56]*	0.82 [0.17, 1.46]*	0.63 [–0.00, 1.27]
Pooled result (4 RCTs) 298	0.92 [–0.11, 1.94], 93.3%	1.59 [0.36, 2.81]*, 94.5%	0.25 [–0.29, 0.79], 78.3%

[1]Comparators were Fast Track Programme or enteral nutrition.

*Statistically significant.

Abbreviations: CI, confidence interval; CRC, colorectal cancer; Ig, immunoglobulin; N, number; SMD, standardised mean difference; RCT, randomised controlled trial.

Table 5.8   Oral Chinese Herbal Medicine for Postoperative Recovery: Immune Cells

Cancer, Comparator (Study) *N* Participants	Cell Type	Effect Size (MD [95% CI])
CRC, usual care (H5) 70	CD4+	−0.61 [−3.64, 2.42]
	CD3+	1.05 [−2.93, 5.03]
	NK	1.24 [−0.32, 2.80]
	CD4+/CD8+	−0.02 [−0.28, 0.24]
Colon cancer, enteral nutrition (H17) 178	CD4+/CD8+	0.28 [0.15, 0.41]*

*Statistically significant.

Abbreviations: CD, cluster of differentiation; CI, confidence interval; CRC, colorectal cancer; MD, mean difference; N, number; NK, natural killer.

[−0.29, 0.79], I^2 = 78.3%), while there was a significant increase in IgA in the CHM groups (SMD: 1.59 [0.36, 2.81], I^2 = 94.5%) but the heterogeneity was considerable in all pools. The differences between studies made sensitivity analyses unfeasible.

Two studies reported on the counts of T cell subsets (cluster of differentiation [CD]4+, CD3+, CD4+/CD8+) and/or natural killer T cells (NK cells). In the study (H5) of *Si mo tang* 四磨汤 (one day after surgery, 20 ml three times per day for 10 days) versus usual postoperative care for CRC, there were no differences between groups for any cell type (Table 5.8). In the other study (H17), which compared *Xiang sha liu jun zi tang* 香砂六君子汤 (once a day for seven days) plus PEN versus PEN alone, data were only reported for the ratio CD4+/CD8+, which showed a significant difference between groups. Due to the different comparators, pooling data was not appropriate.

GRADE for Oral Chinese Herbal Medicine for Postoperative Recovery

Grading of Recommendations Assessment, Development and Evaluation (GRADE) assessments were conducted for the pooled results of six RCTs that reported data for measures of gastrointestinal recovery following surgery for the comparison of oral CHM plus usual postoperative care, versus usual postoperative care alone (see Table 5.3).

For time to first bowel sounds, these were detected an average of 6.09 hours sooner in the groups that received CHM in addition to usual postoperative care compared to those who received usual postoperative care alone. This difference reached statistical significance, but it was based on three unblinded RCTS (H3, H5, H6) with 195 participants. This is considered a small number, and the meta-analysis result had considerable statistical heterogeneity. Therefore, the GRADE of the evidence was rated down by three grades to 'very low' (Table 5.9).

On average, people in the groups that received the CHM passed their first flatus following surgery 24.42 hours sooner than people in the group that only received usual postoperative care. This result was statistically significant based on six RCTs (H1–H6) and a larger sample size (426 participants), but the studies were not blinded and there was considerable statistical heterogeneity in the meta-analysis, so the certainty of the evidence as a measure of the effect was downgraded by two grades to 'low'.

The time until the first defaecation following surgery was an average of 32.41 hours sooner in the CHM group (H1, H2, H4–H6). This difference was statistically significant, but the certainty of the evidence was downgraded to 'very low' because the five included RCTs were not blinded, the sample size was considered small (362 participants) and the statistical heterogeneity was considerable.

It should be noted that the issue of statistical heterogeneity in the pooled results indicates that we cannot be certain of the magnitude of reduction in the CHM groups due to variability in the results; however, all studies found a reduction, or a tendency towards a reduction, in average recovery time in the groups that received CHM compared to the control groups (see Table 5.3).

Table 5.9   GRADE for Recovery of Gastrointestinal Function: Oral Chinese Herbal Medicine plus Usual Postoperative Care versus Usual Postoperative Care

Outcome	Absolute Effect		Relative Effect (95% CI) N. Studies (N. Participants)	Certainty of Evidence GRADE
	With CHM	Without CHM		
Time to first bowel sounds	**28.41** hours	**34.5** hours	**MD −6.09*** (−11.20 to −0.97 hours) 3 (194)	⊕◯◯◯ VERY LOW[1,2,3]
	Average difference: 6.09 hours sooner (95% CI: 0.97 to 11.2 hours sooner)			
Time to first flatus	**18.58** hours	**43** hours	**MD −24.42*** (−34.36 to −14.49 hours) 6 (426)	⊕⊕◯◯ LOW[1,2]
	Average difference: 24.42 hours sooner (95% CI: 14.49 to 34.36 hours sooner)			
Time to first defaecation	**16.59** hours	**49** hours	**MD −32.41*** (−47.44 to −17.39 hours) 5 (362)	⊕◯◯◯ VERY LOW[1,2,4]
	Average difference: 32.41 hours sooner (95% CI: 17.39 to 47.44 hours sooner)			

[1]No blinding.

[2]Statistical heterogeneity was considerable.

[3]Three RCTs with small sample sizes.

[4]Five RCTs with small sample sizes.

Study references: H1–H6. See Table 5.3.

*Statistically significant result, random effect model.

Abbreviations: CHM, Chinese herbal medicine; CI, confidence interval; GRADE, Grading of Recommendations Assessment, Development and Evaluation; MD, mean difference; N, number.

Randomised Controlled Trial Evidence for Individual Oral Formulas for Postoperative Recovery

Three traditional oral CHMs were each used in two RCTs with the same comparisons and outcomes. All were used during postoperative recovery. In these studies, all participants received the same postoperative care, including postoperative PEN, usual postoperative care, or postoperative care including anti-diarrhoeic medications. These formulae provided data suitable for meta-analysis for recovery of gastrointestinal function, postoperative diarrhoea and/or levels of immunoglobulins.

Recovery of Gastrointestinal Function and Levels of Immunoglobulins

Two RCTs (H2, H5) compared *Si mo tang* 四磨汤 with usual postoperative care (details not provided) versus the same usual care. Both reported outcomes for time to first flatus and time to first defaecation (Table 5.10). In the study of rectal cancer treated with laparoscopic surgery (H2), there was a significant reduction in time to first flatus in the *Si mo tang* 四磨汤 group but there was no significant difference in the study of CRC with usual surgery (H5). The pooled result showed no significant difference between groups; however, the heterogeneity was considerable (MD: −12.56 [−31.09, 5.97], I^2 = 97.8%). For time to first defaecation there were no significant differences between groups in either study or in the pooled result (MD: −10.66 [−27.07, 5.76], I^2 = 94.5%).

Table 5.10 ***Si Mo Tang* for Recovery of Gastrointestinal Function**

Outcome	Cancer, Surgery (*N* Participants)[1]	Effect Size (MD [95% CI]), I^2	Included Studies
Time to first flatus (hours)	Rectal cancer, laparoscopy (56)	−22.00 [−25.76, −18.24]*	H2
	CRC, usual surgery (70)	−3.09 [−7.10, 0.92]	H5
	Pooled result (126) – 2 RCTs	−12.56 [−31.09, 5.97], 97.8%	All above
Time to first defaecation (hours)	Rectal cancer, laparoscopy (56)	−19.00 [−24.24, 13.76]	H2
	CRC, usual surgery (70)	−2.25 [−7.90, 3.40]	H5
	Pooled result (126) – 2 RCTs	−10.66 [−27.07, 5.76], 94.5%	All above

[1]Comparator was usual care.

*Statistically significant;.

Abbreviations: CI, confidence interval; CRC, colorectal cancer; MD, mean difference; RCT, randomised controlled trial.

Table 5.11   Modified *Liu Jun Zi Tang* for Recovery of Gastrointestinal Function and Immunoglobulins

Outcome	Cancer, (*N* Participants)[1]	Effect Size (MD [95% CI]), I^2	Included Studies
Time to first flatus (hours)	CRC, (60)	−3.47 [−6.27, −0.67]*	H15
	Colon cancer, (158)	−8.45 [−10.42, −6.48]*	H17
	Pooled result (218) – 2 RCTs	−6.06 [−10.94, −1.19]*, 87.7%	H15, H17
Time to first defaecation (hours)	CRC, (60)	−4.53 [−7.89, −1.17]*	H15
	Colon cancer, (158)	−8.88 [−11.84, −5.92]*	H17
	Pooled result (218) – 2 RCTs	−6.78 [−11.04, −2.52]*, 72.4%	H15, H17
IgG (g/L)	CRC, (60)	0.49 [−0.02, 1.01]	H15
	Colon cancer, (158)	2.17 [1.77, 2.56]*	H17
	Pooled result (218) – 2 RCTs	SMD 1.34 [−0.30, 2.98], 96.1%	H15, H17
IgA (g/L)	CRC, (60)	0.06 [−0.45, 0.56]	H15
	Colon cancer, (158)	0.73 [0.40, 1.05]*	H17
	Pooled result (218) – 2 RCTs	SMD 0.42 [−0.23, 1.08], 79.2%	H15, H17
IgM (g/L)	CRC, (60)	−0.16 [−0.67, 0.35]	H15
	Colon cancer, (158)	0.72 [0.40, 1.05]*	H17
	Pooled result (218) – 2 RCTs	SMD 0.30 [−0.56, 1.17], 88%	H15, H17

[1]Comparator was postoperative enteral nutrition (PEN); all studies used usual surgery.

*Statistically significant.

Abbreviations: CI, confidence interval; CRC, colorectal cancer; Ig, immunoglobulin; MD, mean difference; N, number; RCT, randomised controlled trial; SMD, standardised mean difference.

Two studies used modified *Liu jun zi tang* 六君子汤 plus PEN. One (H15) used *Chai shao liu jun zi tang* 柴芍六君子汤 in CRC and the other (H17) used *Xiang sha liu jun zi tang* 香砂六君子汤 in colon cancer (Table 5.11). In both studies usual surgery was employed. There was a significantly reduced time to first flatus in both studies and in the pooled result, with considerable heterogeneity (MD: −6.06 [−10.94, −1.19], I^2 = 87.7%). For time to first defaecation there were significant reductions in the modified *Liu jun zi tang* 六君子汤 groups in both studies and in the pooled result with substantial heterogeneity (MD: −6.78 [−11.04, −2.52],

I^2 = 72.4%). In addition, the results for IgG, IgA and IgM showed increases in one study (H15) but not in the other (H17). There were no significant differences between groups in the pooled results with considerable heterogeneity.

Postoperative Diarrhoea

One RCT combined *Bu zhong yi qi wan* 补中益气丸 (three times a day) with loperamide for diarrhoea following CRC surgery versus loperamide alone (H19). There was no significant difference between groups in the incidence of complete recovery (RR: 1.83 [0.78. 4.32], *n* = 60). The other RCT (H9) was of rectal cancer which combined *Bu zhong yi qi tang* 补中益气汤 (one packet a day as two doses) with loperamide plus montmorillonite for 14 days versus loperamide plus montmorillonite. The incidence of complete recovery was not significantly different between groups (RR: 1.09 [0.62, 1.92], *n* = 48). The pooled result for the two RCTs was not significant (RRL 1.28 [0.79, 2.08], I^2 = 3.4%, *n* = 108) with little heterogeneity (Table 5.12).

Table 5.12   *Bu Zhong Yi Qi Wan/Tang* for Postoperative Diarrhoea

Intervention	Cancer, (*N* Participants)[1]	Effect Size (RR [95% CI]), I^2	Included Studies
Bu zhong yi qi wan 补中益气丸 plus LOP versus LOP	CRC (60)	1.83 [0.78. 4.32]	H19
Bu zhong yi qi tang 补中益气汤 plus LOP and MON versus LOP and MON	Rectal cancer (48)	1.09 [0.62, 1.92]	H9
Pooled result	2 RCTs (108)	1.28 [0.79, 2.08]; 3.4%,	H9, H19

[1]All usual surgery, and all had diarrhoea.

*Statistically significant.

Abbreviations: CI, confidence interval; CRC, colorectal cancer; RR, risk ratio; LOP, loperamide; MON, montmorillonite; N, number; RCT, randomised controlled trial.

GRADE for Individual Oral Chinese Herbal Medicine Formulas

Measures of gastrointestinal recovery following surgery for CRC were selected for the GRADE assessments of the effects of individual formulas. Data were available for two orally administered formulas. For the formula *Si mo tang* 四磨汤 combined with usual care and compared to the same usual care, only one study (H5) reported on time to first bowel sounds and found no significant difference between groups. Data from two studies (H2, H5) and 126 participants found an average reduction of 12.56 hours in the combination therapy group for time to first flatus and an average reduction of 10.66 hours in time to first defaecation. However, the 95% confidence intervals were wide, so these differences between groups were not statistically significant. The certainty of the evidence was downgraded due to lack of blinding in both studies and small sample sizes for all comparisons. In addition, there was considerable statistical heterogeneity in the pooled results, so these two outcomes were further downgraded. Consequently, the GRADE assessments were 'low' for time to first bowel sounds and 'very low' for time to first flatus and defaecation (Table 5.13).

For modified *Liu jun zi tang* 六君子汤 combined with PEN (a form of postoperative care) compared to PEN alone, data were available for two RCTs (H15, H17) that assessed 218 participants (Table 5.14). The pooled effect showed an average reduction of 6.06 hours in the time to passing of first flatus in the combination therapy group, compared to the group that received PEN without the CHM. For time to first defaecation, there was an average reduction of 6.78 hours in the combination therapy group. These differences were statistically significant but the RCTs were not blinded; there was statistical heterogeneity in the pooled results; and the results were based on only two studies with relatively small sample sizes (310 participants in total), so the certainty of the evidence was downgraded to 'very low'.

Table 5.13 GRADE for Recovery of Gastrointestinal Function: *Si Mo Tang* plus Usual Care versus Usual Care

Outcome	Absolute Effect		Relative Effect (95% CI) N Studies (N Participants)	Certainty of Evidence GRADE
	With CHM	Without CHM		
Time to first bowel sounds	**46.7** hours	**47.1** hours	**MD −0.43** (−4.87 to 4.01 hours) 1 (70)	⊕⊕◯◯ LOW[1,2]
	Average difference: 0.43 hours sooner (95% CI: 4.87 hours sooner to 4.01 hours later)			
Time to first flatus	**30.44** hours	**43** hours	**MD −12.56** (−31.09 to 5.97 hours) 2 (126)	⊕◯◯◯ VERY LOW[1,3,4]
	Average difference: 12.56 hours sooner (95% CI: 31.09 hours sooner to 5.97 hours later)			
Time to first defaecation	**0.8** hours	**11.46** hours	**MD −10.66** (−27.07 to 5.76 hours) 2 (126)	⊕◯◯◯ VERY LOW[1,3,4]
	Average difference: 10.66 hours sooner (95% CI: 27.07 hours sooner to 5.76 hours later)			

*Statistically significant result, random effect model.

[1]No blinding.

[2]One RCT with small sample size.

[3]Statistical heterogeneity was considerable.

[4]Two RCTs with small sample sizes.

Study references: H2, H5. See Table 5.10.

Abbreviations: CHM, Chinese herbal medicine; CI, confidence interval; GRADE, Grading of Recommendations Assessment, Development and Evaluation; MD, mean difference; N, number.

Randomised Controlled Trials of Topical Chinese Herbal Medicine for Postoperative Recovery

Of the six RCTs of topical CHM, three (H20–H22) used a fomentation *yun tang* 熨烫, two (H24, H25) used a cataplasm *yao gao* 药膏

Table 5.14   GRADE for Recovery of Gastrointestinal Function: Modified *Liu Jun Zi Tang* plus Postoperative Enteral Nutrition Versus Postoperative Enteral Nutrition

Outcome	Absolute Effect		Relative Effect (95% CI) *N* Studies (*N* Participants)	Certainty of Evidence GRADE
	With CHM	Without CHM		
Time to first flatus	**49.94** hours	**56** hours	**MD −6.06*** (−10.94 to −1.19 hours) 2 (218)	⊕◯◯◯ VERY LOW[1,2,3]
	Average difference: 6.06 hours sooner (95% CI: 1.19 to 10.94 hours sooner)			
Time to first defaecation	**57.95** hours	**64.73** hours	**MD −6.78*** (−11.04 to −2.52 hours) 2 (218)	⊕◯◯◯ VERY LOW[1,3,4]
	Average difference: 6.78 hours sooner (95% CI: 2.52 to 11.04 hours sooner)			

*Statistically significant result, random effect model.

[1]No blinding.

[2]Statistical heterogeneity was considerable.

[3]Two RCTs with small sample sizes.

[4]Statistical heterogeneity was substantial.

Study references: H15, H17. See Table 5.11.

Abbreviations: CHM, Chinese herbal medicine; CI, confidence interval; GRADE, Grading of Recommendations Assessment, Development and Evaluation; MD, mean difference; N, number.

and one study (H23) used a specially developed ultrasound machine to facilitate absorption of the CHM by the skin. Results are reported separately for each of these three methods.

In one four-armed study (H20), one comparison was between the CHM fomentation and topical application of salt as a placebo, while the other comparison was with usual postoperative care alone. The fourth arm was CHM fomentation plus acupuncture, which is included in Chapter 9. Another study included four groups (H22): CHM fomentation plus usual perioperative care, CHM fomentation plus FTP, usual perioperative care, and FTP alone.

All six RCTs were conducted in mainland China. They enrolled 538 participants. The ages of participants ranged from 27 to 82 years, but the age range was not reported in one study (H22). Based on the reported means and standard deviations for ages, most participants were aged between 46 and 82 years. No study mentioned syndrome differentiation in the selection criteria.

The most frequently used topical herbs were *wu zhu yu* 吴茱萸 (*n* = 3), *da huang* 大黄 (*n* = 2), *mang xiao* 芒硝 (*n* = 2) and *zhi shi* 枳实 (*n* = 2).

Risk of Bias for Topical Chinese Herbal Medicine for Postoperative Recovery

Two studies were judged 'low' risk for sequence generation; two were judged 'high' risk, since they used order of surgery or patient arrival for allocation (Table 5.15). The others were 'unclear' risk. One (H20) was judged 'low' risk for allocation concealment since a centralised system was used and the others were 'unclear' risk. Blinding of participants was judged 'unclear' in one arm of the four-armed study (H20) since it was unclear whether salt would have been a convincing placebo. The other arm of this study and the remaining studies were judged 'high' risk for blinding of participants and personnel and 'unclear' risk for outcome assessors. One study (H20) was judged 'high' risk for incomplete outcome data since there were

Table 5.15   Risk of Bias of Randomised Controlled Trials of Topical Chinese Herbal Medicine for Postoperative Recovery

Risk of Bias Domain	Low Risk *n* (%)	Unclear Risk *n* (%)	High Risk *n* (%)
Sequence generation	2 (33.3)	2 (33.3)	2 (33.3)
Allocation concealment	1 (16.7)	5 (83.3)	0 (0)
Blinding of participants[1]	0 (0)	1 (14.3)	6 (85.7)
Blinding of personnel	0 (0)	0 (0)	6 (100)
Blinding of outcome assessors	0 (0)	6 (100)	0 (0)
Incomplete outcome data	5 (83.3)	0 (0)	1 (16.7)
Selective outcome reporting	0 (0)	6 (100)	0 (0)

Note: Based on seven groups.

eight drop-outs, but it was not clear which groups these were from and no reasons were given. No protocols could be located but all outcomes mentioned in the methods were reported so all studies were judged 'unclear' risk for selective reporting.

Recovery of Gastrointestinal Function

All six RCTs reported data for postoperative recovery of gastrointestinal function. One study (H20) included a comparison between a fomentation of *wu zhu yu* 吴茱萸 and a placebo, so this was assessed separately. The three studies of fomentations in which the comparator was usual care were assessed as a group. In one of these studies (H22) there was a comparison with FTP, which was assessed separately. The single studies of CHM cataplasm (H24) and CHM applied by ultrasound machine (H23) were assessed separately.

In the study that compared a fomentation of *wu zhu yu* 吴茱萸 with a salt placebo (H20), both were applied to the abdomen from one day after surgery for 30 minutes twice a day for six days. The CRC patients ($n = 40$) had received open, or laparoscopic, surgery plus usual care in both groups. There were no significant differences between groups for time to first bowel sounds (MD: 3.12 [–14.42, 20.66] hours, n = 40), first flatus (MD: 9.38 [–5.35, 24.11] hours, $n = 40$) or first defaecation (MD: –14.09 [–39.49, 11.31] hours, $n = 40$).

Three RCTs (H20–H22) compared a CHM fomentation plus usual postoperative or perioperative care versus usual postoperative or perioperative care alone. One study (H20) used *wu zhu yu* 吴茱萸, one study (H22) used *wu zhu yu* 吴茱萸 plus salt (*cu yan* 粗盐) and the other study (H21) used *zhi shi* 枳实 plus *bai zhu* 白术. All were applied to the abdomen. The pooled result for time to first bowel sounds found no difference between groups (MD: –1.43 [–8.28, 5.42] hours, $I^2 = 61.6\%$) with moderate heterogeneity, a significant reduction in the CHM groups for time to first flatus (MD: –6.33 [–20.49, –1.81] hours, $I^2 = 92.1\%$) with considerable heterogeneity, and no significant reduction in the CHM groups for time to first defaecation (MD: –4.74 [–21.10, 11.62] hours, $I^2 = 43.7\%$) with

Table 5.16   Chinese Herbal Medicine Fomentation for Recovery of Gastrointestinal Function

Outcome	Cancer, Surgery (*N* Participants)[1]	Effect Size (MD [95% CI]), I^2	Included Studies
Time to first bowel sounds (hours)	Colon cancer, usual surgery (60)	–3.83 [–4.72, –2.94]*	H21
	CRC, open or laparoscopic surgery (43)[2]	14.16 [–1.30, 29.62]	H20
	CRC, laparoscopy (78)	–4.48 [–12.66, 3.70]	H22
	Pooled result (181) – 3 RCTs	–1.43 [–8.28, 5.42], 61.6%	All above
Time to first flatus (hours)	Colon cancer, usual surgery (60)	–18.00 [–20.98, –15.02]*	H21
	CRC, open or laparoscopic surgery (43)[2]	11.47 [–0.42, 23.36]	H20
	CRC, laparoscopy (78)	–9.22 [–16.64, –1.81]*	H22
	Pooled result (181) – 3 RCTs	–6.33 [–20.49, –1.81]*, 92.1%	All above
Time to first defaecation (hours)	Colon cancer, usual surgery (60)	–9.64 [–16.92, –2.36] *	H21
	CRC, open or laparoscopic surgery (43)[2]	9.47 –17.66, 36.60]	H20
	Pooled result (103) – 2 RCTs	–4.74 [–21.10, 11.62], 43.7%	All above

[1]Comparator was usual care.

[2]Used salt placebo.

*Statistically significant.

Abbreviations: CI, confidence interval; CRC, colorectal cancer; MD, mean difference; N, number; RCT, randomised controlled trial.

moderate heterogeneity (Table 5.16). Sensitivity analyses were not feasible due to the multiple differences between studies.

Another study combined a fomentation of *wu zhu yu* 吴茱萸 plus salt (*cu yan* 粗盐) (H22) applied to the abdomen (for 30 minutes twice a day) with FTP, compared to FTP alone. There were no significant differences between groups for time to first bowel sounds (MD: -0.57 [-9.71, 8.57] hours, n=76) or time to first flatus (MD: 1.45 [-6.23, 9.13] hours, n=76).

In the two RCTs of CHM cataplasms, usual postoperative care was used in both groups. One study of colon cancer (H24) tested a cataplasm which combined the formulas *Si huang shui mi fang* 四黄

水蜜方 and *Mang xiao bing pian san* 芒硝冰片散 applied to ST36 *Zusanli* 足三里 and CV12 *Zhongwan* 中脘 (every night for 12 hours, repeated for five days). The other study (H25) used a mixture of *wu zhu yu* 吴茱萸 powder plus rice vinegar applied to CV8 *Shenque* 神阙 for rectal cancer (from 30 minutes after surgery for 24 hours, repeated until recovery of gastrointestinal functioning). The pooled result for time to first bowel sounds found a significant reduction in the CHM cataplasm groups (MD: −10.68 [−11.98, −9.38] hours, I^2 = 0%) with no heterogeneity and a significant reduction in time to first flatus in the CHM cataplasm groups (MD: −11.19 [−14.57, −7.81] hours, I^2 = 75.8%) with substantial heterogeneity (Table 5.17). For time to first defaecation, data were only available for one study (H25) which showed a significant reduction in time in the CHM group (MD: −14.88 [−18.56, −11.20] hours).

The single study of CHM applied by ultrasound machine (H23) used modified *Da cheng qi tang* 大承气汤 (from one day after surgery, for 30 minutes, twice a day) plus usual postoperative care for

Table 5.17 Chinese Herbal Medicine Cataplasm for Recovery of Gastrointestinal Function

Outcome	Cancer, (*N* Participants)[1]	Effect Size (MD [95% CI]), I^2	Included Studies
Time to first bowel sounds (hours)	Colon cancer, usual surgery (80)	−10.60 [−12.05, −9.15]*	H24
	Rectal cancer, usual surgery (60)	−11.00 [−13.92, −8.08]*	H25
	Pooled result (140) – 2 RCTs	−10.68 [−11.98, -9.38]*, 0%	All above
Time to first flatus (hours)	Colon cancer, usual surgery (80)	−9.70 [−11.19, −8.21]*	H24
	Rectal cancer, usual surgery (60)	−13.19 [−16.21, −10.17]*	H25
	Pooled result (140) – 2 RCTs	−11.19 [−14.57, −7.81]*, 75.8%	All above
Time to first defaecation (hours)	Rectal cancer, usual surgery (60)	−14.88 [−18.56, −11.20]*	H25

[1]Comparator was usual care; both studies used usual surgery.

*Statistically significant.

Abbreviations: CI, confidence interval; CRC, colorectal cancer; MD, mean difference; N, number; RCT, randomised controlled trial.

colon cancer versus the same postoperative care without the CHM. There was no difference between groups for time to first bowel sounds (MD: –0.20 [–1.36, 0.96] hours, n = 100) but there were significant reductions in time in the CHM group for time to first flatus (MD: –9.00 [–13.89, –4.11] hours, n = 100) and first defaecation (MD: –17.30 [–22.82, –11.78] hours, n = 100).

Postoperative Abdominal Distension

Only one study (H24) reported on postoperative abdominal distension. It found the incidence of this outcome was significantly lower in the CHM cataplasm group compared to the usual postoperative care group (RR: 0.27 [0.08, 0.91], *n* = 80).

Randomised Controlled Trial of Chinese Herbal Medicine Inhalation for Postoperative Recovery

One RCT (H26) (*n* = 47) tested an atomised inhalation of *Jia wei zhi zhu jian* 加味枳术煎 (*zhi shi* 枳实, *bai zhu* 白术, *hou po* 厚朴, *sha ren* 砂仁 and *da huang* 大黄) from six hours after surgery, three times a day for seven days, in people who had undergone surgery for cancer of the sigmoid colon and/or rectum. Both groups received usual postoperative care and the control group received no CHM. For gastrointestinal recovery, there were significant reductions in time to first bowel sounds (MD: –25.26 [–38.50, –12.02] hours, *n* = 47) and time to first flatus (MD: –25.00 [–42.21, –7.80] hours, *n* = 47).

Controlled Clinical Trials of Chinese Herbal Medicine for Postoperative Recovery

Three non-randomised CCTs of oral CHM that included 180 participants were identified. Two studies of CRC (H28, H29) were conducted in Japan and one CCT of stage IIIB/IV colon cancer (H27) was conducted in mainland China. The mean ages of participants ranged from 57 to 70 years. None of the studies mentioned syndrome differentiation.

Two studies (H28, H29) used *Da jian zhong tang* 大建中汤, although one of these (H28) combined it with *Gui zhi fu ling wan* 桂枝茯苓丸. The other study (H27) used *Si jun zi tang* 四君子汤. The most frequently used herbal ingredients in the three studies were *fu ling* 茯苓 (*n* = 2), *hua jiao* 花椒 (*n* = 2), *gan jiang* 干姜 (*n* = 2) and *ren shen* 人参 (*n* = 2).

Recovery of Gastrointestinal Function

Two CCTs reported data for postoperative recovery of gastrointestinal function in CRC. In both studies, usual postoperative care was provided in both groups. One study (H28) (*n* = 66) that used open surgery administered *Da jian zhong tang* 大建中汤 (*hua jiao* 花椒, *gan jiang* 干姜 and *ren shen* 人参) plus *Gui zhi fu ling wan* 桂枝茯苓丸 (*gui zhi* 桂枝, *fu ling* 茯苓, *dan pi* 丹皮, *tao ren* 桃仁 and *bai shao* 白芍) as granules from postoperative day one. There was a significant reduction in time to first flatus in the CHM group (MD: −31.30 [−44.82, −17.78] hours), and earlier tolerance of regular diet (MD: −3.80 [−4.64, −2.96] days) (Table 5.18).

The other study (H29) (*n* = 30) that used laparoscopic surgery administered *Da jian zhong tang* 大建中汤 granules from postoperative

Table 5.18 Oral Chinese Herbal Medicine versus Usual Care for Recovery of Gastrointestinal Function

Outcome	Cancer, Surgery (*N* Participants)[1]	Effect Size (MD [95% CI]), I^2	Included Studies
Time to first flatus (hours)	CRC, open surgery (66)	−31.30 [−44.82, −17.78]*	H28
	CRC, laparoscopic surgery (30)	−21.60 [−30.19, −13.01]*	H29
	Pooled result (96) – 2 CCTs	−24.99 [−34.05, −15.92]*, 29%	All above
Tolerance of regular diet (days)	CRC, open surgery (66)	−3.80 [−4.64, −2.96]*	H28

[1]Comparator was usual care.

*Statistically significant.

Abbreviations: CCT, non-randomised controlled clinical trial; CI, confidence interval; CRC, colorectal cancer; MD, mean difference; N, number; RCT, randomised controlled trial.

day one to day seven. Time to first flatus was shorter in the CHM group (MD: −21.60 [−30.19, −13.01] hours). The pooled result for time to first flatus showed a significant reduction in the CHM groups compared to the groups that received usual postoperative care alone (MD: −24.99 [−34.05, −15.92], I^2 = 29%) without important heterogeneity (Table 5.18).

Postoperative Nausea and Vomiting

One of the above CCTs (H28) reported the incidence of nausea and vomiting. For postoperative nausea, there were three cases in the CHM group versus five cases in the control group (RR: 0.72 [0.19, 2.77], *n* = 66) which was not a significant difference. For vomiting there were no cases in the CHM group and one case in the control group (too few for analysis).

Postoperative Immune Function

One CCT (H27) (*n* = 84) used *Si jun zi tang* 四君子汤 once a day via naso-gastric tube for one week plus PET, versus normal saline via naso-gastric tube (as a control for the CHM) plus PET. At eight days after surgery there were significant differences between groups in the T cell counts for CD3+, CD4+ and NK cells but not for CD8+ cells or the ratio CD4+/CD8+. The immunoglobulins IgG, IgA and IgM were all significantly higher in the CHM group (Table 5.19).

Non-controlled Clinical Studies of Chinese Herbal Medicine for Postoperative Recovery

Five non-controlled clinical studies that included 222 participants were identified. Four case series studies (H30–H33) were conducted in mainland China and one case study (H34) was from the United States of America. Three studies (H32–H34) reported the use of syndrome differentiation. The herbs used most frequently in the oral formulas were *bai zhu* 白术 (*n* = 2), *dang shen* 党参 (*n* = 2) *huang qi* 黄芪 (*n* = 2) and *mu xiang* 木香 (*n* = 2).

Table 5.19 Oral Chinese Herbal Medicine plus Postoperative Enteral Nutrition versus Saline plus Postoperative Enteral Nutrition: Immune Function

T cells (%)	Effect Size (MD[1] [95% CI]), I[2]
CD3+	−4.79 [−7.36, −2.22]*
CD4+	3.05 [1.49, 4.61]*
CD8+	−0.89 [−2.08, 0.30]
CD4+/CD8+	0.05 [−0.02, 0.12]
NK	1.11 [0.11, 2.11]*
Immunoglobulins (g/L)	
IgG	1.10 [0.69, 1.52]*
IgA	0.14 [0.003, 0.28]*
IgM	0.17 [0.08, 0.26]*

[1]Versus normal saline plus postoperative enteral nutrition.

*Statistically significant.

Abbreviations: CD, cluster of differentiation; CI, confidence interval; Ig, immunoglobulin; MD, mean difference; NK, natural killer.

Postoperative gastrointestinal function recovery was reported in two studies (H31, H33); KPS was reported in two studies (H30, H32); immune function was reported in one study (H32). Two studies (H30, H34) reported on survival.

One study (H31) reported the effect of a combination of oral *Jia wei da cheng qi tang* 加味大承气汤 once a day in two doses plus *chong bai* 葱白 mixed with vinegar (*shi cu* 食醋) applied to the abdomen as required in 56 people with early postoperative inflammatory ileus. The authors reported most patients recovered intestinal motility in 8–36 hours and defaecation in 20–52 hours. None required further surgery. In the other study (H33), all 73 patients had rectal cancer and postoperative diarrhoea, and all had the syndrome Sunken middle *qi* (*zhong qi xia xian* 中气下陷). They received *Bu zhong yi qi tang* 补中益气汤 once a day for three weeks. The authors reported there were improvements in diarrhoea and related symptoms.

For KPS, one study (H30) included 42 people with CRC who had received surgery for the CRC and subsequently had microwave ablation for liver metastases. They received *Yi qi jie du fang* 益气解毒方

(made by the authors) before, and after, the microwave ablation for at least one month. The authors reported an improvement in KPS scores after microwave ablation. In the other study (H32), 50 patients with CRC with symptoms of Spleen *qi* deficiency (*pi qi xu* 脾气虚) and dampness heat smouldering and binding (*shi re yun jie* 湿热蕴结) received *Chang yi jian* 肠益煎 (made by the authors) 35 ml twice a day for six months postsurgery. The authors reported that most of the symptoms improved and KPS improved by more than 10 points in 15 patients. The above study (H32) also reported on immune function. There were no significant differences in counts for CD4, CD3, CD8 and NK cells, or in the ratio CD4/CD8.

In the study of people who had microwave ablation for liver metastases (H30), the median survival time was 26 months, one-year survival rate was 84.4% and two-year survival rate was 57.9%.

In the case report from the United States (H34), a person with a family history of CRC had cancerous polyps and a section of colon removed followed by recurrence of pre-cancerous polyps. In order to avoid radical resection, CHM was administered and modified based on syndrome differentiation and symptoms, and the person received other supplements and dietary advice. The polyps were monitored by regular colonoscopy. After two years the polyps had not progressed. The author reported on changes in symptoms at various stages during treatment. There was some loose stool and abdominal bloating that may have been associated with the CHM which was resolved after formula modification. Contact with the author confirmed that the person was still stable and receiving treatment five years later.

Safety of Chinese Herbal Medicine for Postoperative Care

Six of the RCTs reported on AEs. Five of these mentioned there were no AEs from the CHMs. In one study (H14) two people who had severe abdominal distension dropped out since they had vomiting after taking the oral CHM. In the two CCTs conducted in Japan (H28, H29) there were no drop-outs, no increases in postoperative complications in the CHM groups and no differences in morbidity between groups, but there was no mention of minor AEs. The other CCT did not mention AEs (H27).

In the non-controlled studies, most did not report on AEs associated with CHM treatment; one (H32) reported there were no AEs and one (H34) reported minor AEs resolved by formula modification.

Section 2: Chinese Herbal Medicine in Conjunction with Chemotherapy

This section reports on studies that used a CHM treatment in conjunction with chemotherapy for CRC. Ninety-nine RCTs, eight CCTs, and three non-controlled studies either compared CHM with chemotherapy, combined CHM with chemotherapy or used a CHM for AEs associated with chemotherapy. Oral CHM was tested in 92 RCTs, one RCT used oral CHM or CHM enema, one RCT used CHM enema and five RCTs used topical CHM. All eight CCTs and all three non-controlled studies used oral CHM.

A number of chemotherapy regimens (see Chapter 1) were used in the studies. The following five regimens were similar in that they all used combinations of oxaliplatin, 5-fluorouracil (5-FU) plus leucovorin (LV): FOLFOX4, FOLFOX6, mFOLFOX6, FOLFOX and OLF. These were treated as a subgroup in meta-analysis where appropriate. The following two regimens both combine leucovorin and 5-fluorouracil: LF and Simplified bi-weekly infusional 5-FU/LV. The other regimens show distinct differences: FOLFIRI, XELOX, XELODA, XELIRI, tegafur gimeracil oteracil potassium (S-1) plus oxaliplatin, and hyperthermic intraperitoneal chemotherapy (HIPEC).

The main outcomes were objective response rate (ORR), survival, quality of life, KPS, immune function and chemotherapy-related AEs. Meta-analysis results of RCTs are presented firstly for oral CHM, oral CHM or CHM enema, CHM enema, and then for topical CHM. Following this, results are reported for the CCTs and non-controlled studies.

Randomised Controlled Trials of Oral Chinese Herbal Medicine in Conjunction with Chemotherapy

The 92 RCTs included two RCTs of oral CHM versus chemotherapy (H35, H36), three RCTs of oral CHM for postchemotherapy adverse reactions (H37–39) and 88 RCTs of oral CHM plus chemotherapy versus chemotherapy alone. One study (H35) included three groups so it is included in the comparisons CHM versus chemotherapy and CHM plus chemotherapy versus chemotherapy.

Syndromes

Of the studies of oral CHM, 35 RCTs used syndrome differentiation in the selection criteria and three studies (H36, H40, H41) used different CHMs according to the syndrome. In total 38 RCTs mentioned 56 syndromes. The syndrome names most frequently reported in the 38 RCTs were *pi qi xu* 脾气虚 (*n* = 5), *zheng qi kui xu, yu du ji zhi* 正气亏虚, 瘀毒积滞 (*n* = 2), *qi xue kui xu* 气血亏虚 (*n* = 2), *shi re yun jie* 湿热蕴结 (*n* = 2), *shen yang xu* 肾阳虚 (*n* = 2), *pi qi kui xu* 脾气亏虚 (*n* = 2), *pi shen liang xu* 脾肾两虚 (*n* = 2) , *pi xu shi yun* 脾虚湿蕴 (*n* = 2), *ai du* 癌毒 (*n* = 2), *qi zhi* 气滞 (*n* = 2), *xue xu* 血虚 (*n* = 2), *yin xu* 阴虚 (*n* = 2) and *yu xue* 瘀血 (*n* = 2).

Due to the syndrome names sharing similar features, these were separated to determine the most common components of the syndromes (Table 5.20). This analysis shows that Spleen deficiency (*pi xu* 脾虚)

Table 5.20 Frequency of Components of the Syndrome Names in Randomised Controlled Trials of Oral Chinese Herbal Medicines used in Conjunction with Chemotherapy

Syndrome Name	No. Studies
Spleen deficiency (*pi xu* 脾虚)	26
Stasis (*yu* 瘀)	16
Dampness (*shi* 湿)	14
Kidney deficiency (*shen xu* 肾虚)	8
Qi deficiency (*qi xu* 气虚)	6
Blood deficiency (*xue xu* 血虚)	5
Heat (*re* 热)	5
Qi stagnation (*qi zhi* 气滞)	3
Cancer toxin (*ai du* 癌毒)	2
Healthy *qi* deficiency (*zheng qi xu* 正气虚)	2
Phlegm (*tan* 痰)	2
Yin deficiency (*yin xu* 阴虚)	2

was the most common component followed by stasis (*yu* 瘀) and dampness (*shi* 湿). Kidney deficiency (*shen xu* 肾虚) was mentioned by eight RCTs. In the six RCTs that simply mentioned *qi* deficiency (*qi xu* 气虚), it is likely that this included Spleen deficiency and/or Kidney deficiency, indicating that forms of *qi* deficiency were typical of the participants in the RCTs included in this part.

Formula and Herb Frequencies

In the 92 RCTs there were 76 formula names. In some cases, formulas with the same name had different ingredients, so these were considered to be different formulas. The most frequently used formula was *Si jun zi tang* 四君子汤 which was tested in three RCTs (Table 5.21). In addition, three studies used modifications of *Liu jun zi tang* 六君子汤 including *Xiang sha liu jun wan* 香砂六君丸 (H42), *Gui qi liu jun tang* 归芪六君汤 (H45) and *Jia wei xiang sha liu jun zi tang* 加味香砂六君子汤 (H43). Another 12 formulas were tested in two studies each. Of these, four formulas were named by the authors or their hospital and one was a commercial product (*Fu fang ban mao jiao nang* 复方斑蝥胶囊). The other nine formulas were well-known formulas.

Many of the formula names included the words 'fortify the Spleen' *jian pi* 健脾 (16 formulas), 'replenish *qi*' *yi qi* 益气 (10 formulas), 'resist cancer' *kang ai* 抗癌 or 'repress tumour' *yi liu* 抑瘤 (15 formulas), 'resolve toxins' *jie du* 解毒 (7 formulas), and 'dissipate binds' *san jie* 散结 or 'disperse accumulations' *xiao ji* 消积 (7 formulas) to indicate their intended actions.

The herbs most frequently used in the oral formulas used in the 92 RCTs were *bai zhu* 白术 (*n* = 60), *huang qi* 黄芪 (*n* = 59), *fu ling* 茯苓 (*n* = 53), *yi yi ren* 薏苡仁 (*n* = 49) and *gan cao* 甘草 (*n* = 46) (Table 5.22).

Risk of Bias

A proper method of randomisation was reported in 37 studies; however 49 studies simply stated that the study was 'randomised' and six

Table 5.21 Frequently Used Formulas in Randomised Controlled Trials of Oral Chinese Herbal Medicines used in Conjunction with Chemotherapy

Formula Name	No. Studies	Main Ingredients (Studies)
Si jun zi tang[1] 四君子汤	3	*Ren shen* 人参, *fu ling* 茯苓, *gan cao* 甘草 and *bai zhu* 白术 (H36, H40, H44)
Modified *Liu jun zi tang*[1] 六君子汤	3	*Chen pi* 陈皮, *ban xia* 半夏, *fu ling* 茯苓, *gan cao* 甘草, *ren shen* 人参 and *bai zhu* 白术 (H42, H43, H45)
Ba zhen tang 八珍汤[1]	2	*Dang gui* 当归, *chuan xiong* 川芎, *bai shao* 白芍, *shu di* 熟地, *ren shen* 人参, *fu ling* 茯苓, *zhi gan cao* 炙甘草 and *bai zhu* 白术 (H46, H47)
Da chai hu tang[1] 大柴胡汤	2	*Chai hu* 柴胡, *huang qin* 黄芩, *shao yao* 芍药, *zhi gan cao* 炙甘草, *ban xia* 半夏, *da huang* 大黄, *zhi shi* 枳实 (H36, H40)
*Fu zheng xiao ji tang** 扶正消积汤	2	*Dang shen* 党参, *huang qi* 黄芪, *chao bai zhu* 炒白术, *fu ling* 茯苓, *yi yi ren* 薏苡仁, *shi jian chuan* 石见穿, *bai hua she she cao* 白花蛇舌草, *ban xia* 半夏, *ba qia* 菝葜 and *gan cao* 甘草 (H48, H49)
Fu fang ban mao jiao nang 复方斑蝥胶囊	2	*Ban mao* 斑蝥, *ren shen* 人参, *huang qi* 黄芪, *ci wu jia* 刺五加, *san leng* 三棱, *ban zhi lian* 半枝莲, *e zhu* 莪术, *shan zhu yu* 山茱萸, *nv zhen zi* 女贞子 and *gan cao* 甘草 (H50, H51)
Ling gui zhu gan tang[1] 苓桂术甘汤	2	*Fu ling* 茯苓, *gui zhi* 桂枝, *bai zhu* 白术 and *gan cao* 甘草 (H36, H40)
*Qi lian fu zheng jiao nang** 芪连扶正胶囊	2	*E zhu* 莪术, *lian qiao* 连翘, *ban xia* 半夏, *nan xing* 南星, *quan xie* 全蝎, *wu gong* 蜈蚣, *bi hu* 壁虎, *bai hua she she cao* 白花蛇舌草, *huang qi* 黄芪, *xian he cao* 仙鹤草 and *nv zhen zi* 女贞子 (H52, H53)
Si wu tang[1] 四物汤	2	*Bai shao* 白芍, *dang gui* 当归, *shu di* 熟地 and *chuan xiong* 川芎 (H36, H40)
Tao hong si wu tang[1] 桃红四物汤	2	*Dang gui* 当归, *shu di* 熟地, *chuan xiong* 川芎, *bai shao* 白芍, *tao ren* 桃仁 and *hong hua* 红花 (H36, H40)

(Continued)

Table 5.21   (*Continued*)

Formula Name	No. Studies	Main Ingredients (Studies)
*Wei tiao san hao fang** 微调3号方	2	*Dang shen* 党参, *zhu ling* 猪苓, *fu ling* 茯苓, *yi yi ren* 薏苡仁, *chao bai zhu* 炒白术, *fa ban xia* 法半夏, *chen pi* 陈皮 and *zhi pi pa ye* 炙枇杷叶 (H54, H55)
*Xiao liu tang** 消瘤汤	2	*Dang shen* 党参, *huang qi* 黄芪, *tian qi* 田七, *fu fang teng* 扶芳藤, *shan ci gu* 山慈菇, *zi he che* 紫河车, *ban zhi lian* 半枝莲, *yi yi ren* 薏苡仁 and *gan cao* 甘草 (H56, H57)
You gui wan[1] 右归丸	2	*Shu di* 熟地, *shan yao* 山药, *shan zhu yu* 山茱萸, *gou qi* 枸杞, *lv jiao jiao* 鹿角胶, *tu si zi* 菟丝子, *du zhong* 杜仲, *dang gui* 当归, *rou gui* 肉桂 and *zhi fu zi* 制附子 (H36, H40)
Zhi bai di huang tang[1] 知柏 地黄汤	2	*Shu di* 熟地, *shan zhu yu* 山茱萸, *shan yao* 山药, *mu dan pi* 牡丹皮, *fu ling* 茯苓, *ze xie* 泽泻, *zhi mu* 知母 and *huang bai* 黄柏 (H36, H40)

[1]Ingredients are referenced to the *Zhong Yi Fang Ji Da Ci Dian* 中医方剂大辞典.[19]

*Named by the authors or their hospital.

studies reported using patient visiting order or other inappropriate methods (Table 5.23). These studies were judged 'low', 'unclear' and 'high' risk respectively for sequence generation. Only three studies mentioned allocation concealment, and these used a proper method, so they were judged 'low' risk, and the remainder were judged 'unclear' risk. Only one study (H58) blinded participants using a placebo but blinding of personnel and outcome assessors was not mentioned. Therefore, it was judged 'unclear' risk for these domains. The remaining studies were judged 'high' risk for blinding of participants and personnel. Since most outcomes were based on laboratory reports or routine assessments by hospital staff recorded in the patient's medical record, we judged 'unclear' risk for blinding of outcome assessors. For incomplete outcome data, two studies had dropout rates of around 20% (H43, H59). When an intent to treat (ITT) approach was applied to the outcomes, the results did not change in terms of direction or significance, so these were judged

Table 5.22 Frequently Used Herbs in Randomised Controlled Trials of Oral Chinese Herbal Medicines used in Conjunction with Chemotherapy

Herb Name	Scientific Name	No. Studies
Bai zhu 白术[1]	*Atractylodes macrocephala* Koidz.	60
Huang qi 黄芪[2]	*Astragalus membranaceus* (Fisch.) Bge.	59
Fu ling 茯苓	*Poria cocos* (Schw.) Wolf	53
Yi yi ren 薏苡仁[3]	*Coix lacryma-jobi* L. var. *mayuen* (Roman.) Stapf	49
Gan cao 甘草[4]	*Glycyrrhiza uralensis* Fisch.	46
Dang shen 党参	*Codonopsis pilosula* (Franch.) Nannf.	36
She she cao 蛇舌草	*Hedyotis diffusa* Willd.	35
Ban zhi lian 半枝莲	*Scutellaria barbata* D. Don	29
Shao yao 芍药[5]	*Paeonia lactiflora* Pall.; *P. veitchii* Lynch	27
Ban xia 半夏[6]	*Pinellia ternata* (Thunb.) Breit.	23
E zhu 莪术	*Curcuma phaeocaulis* Val.	23
Chen pi 陈皮	*Citrus reticulata* Blanco	23
Shan yao 山药	*Dioscorea opposita* Thunb.	20
Dang gui 当归	*Angelica sinensis* (Oliv.) Diels	15
Ren shen 人参[7]	*Panax ginseng* C. A. Mey.	14
Xian he cao 仙鹤草	*Agrimonia pilosa* Ledeb.	13
Shu di 熟地	*Rehmannia glutinosa* Libosch.	12
Sha ren 砂仁	*Amomum villosum* Lour.	12
Tai zi shen 太子参	*Pseudostellaria heterophylla* (Miq.) Pax ex Pax et Hoffm.	11
Ji xue teng 鸡血藤	*Spatholobus suberectus* Dunn	11

[1]Fourteen RCTs used *chao bai zhu* 炒白术 and one used *jiao bai zhu* 焦白术.

[2]Eleven RCTs used *sheng huang qi* 生黄芪 and one used *zhi huang qi* 炙黄芪.

[3]Twelve RCTs used *sheng yi yi ren* 生薏苡仁 and one used *chao yi yi ren* 炒薏苡仁.

[4]Fourteen RCTs used *zhi gan cao* 炙甘草 and two used *sheng gan cao* 生甘草.

[5]Twenty-one RCTs used *bai shao* 白芍 and six RCTs used *chi shao* 赤芍.

[6]Seven RCTs used *fa ban xia* 法半夏, two used *jiang ban xia* 姜半夏, and one used *qing ban xia* 清半夏.

[7]Two RCTs used *sheng shai shen* 生晒参 and two used *hong shen* 红参.

The use of some herbs may be restricted in some countries. Readers are advised to comply with relevant regulations.

Table 5.23   Risk of Bias of Randomised Controlled Trials of Oral Chinese Herbal Medicine in Conjunction with Chemotherapy

Risk of Bias Domain	Low Risk *n* (%)	Unclear Risk *n* (%)	High Risk *n* (%)
Sequence generation	37 (40.2)	49 (53.3)	6 (6.5)
Allocation concealment	3 (3.3)	89 (96.7)	0 (0)
Blinding of participants	1 (1.1)	0 (0)	91 (98.9)
Blinding of personnel	0 (0)	1 (1.1)	91 (98.9)
Blinding of outcome assessors	0 (0)	92 (100)	0 (0)
Incomplete outcome data	89 (96.7)	3 (3.3)	0 (0)
Selective outcome reporting	0 (0)	91 (98.9)	1 (1.1)

'unclear' risk. In another study (H60), the group membership of the five drop-outs was not specified so it was judged 'unclear' risk. For selective outcome reporting, no protocols could be located which led to a judgement of 'unclear' risk, except in one study (H37) which specified it would report on safety and AEs in the method but omitted these results, so it was judged 'high' risk.

Oral Chinese Herbal Medicine Versus Chemotherapy

Two RCTs (H35, H36) provided comparisons between oral CHM without chemotherapy versus chemotherapy. In both studies XELODA was used in the control group as maintenance treatment. One study (H35) included three groups (45 participants per group), one of which was CHM plus XELODA. The results for this arm are reported in the following section. Both studies were conducted in mainland China. The total number of participants in this comparison was 215; all had stage IV CRC and their ages ranged from 40 to 75 years.

One study (H35) required all participants (*n* = 90) to have the syndrome of dual deficiency of *qi* and Blood (*qi xue liang xu* 气血两虚) and all people in the CHM group received a formula designed by the authors called *Zi bu tang* 滋补汤 (*dang shen* 党参, *bai zhu* 白术, *fu ling* 茯苓, *gan cao* 甘草, *shu di* 熟地, *bai shao* 白芍, *dang gui* 当归, *guan gui* 官桂, *chen pi* 陈皮, *mu xiang* 木香 and *da zao* 大枣),

one packet per day in two doses for two months. The control group received XELODA as two three-week cycles. There were no dropouts. Adverse events were not mentioned.

In the other study (H36) people with Stage IV CRC were allocated the CHMs according to eight syndromes as follows:

- Spleen deficiency (*pi xi xu* 脾气虚): *Si jun zi tang* 四君子汤;
- Kidney *yang* deficiency (*shen yang xu* 肾阳虚): *You gui wan* 右归丸;
- *Yin* deficiency (*yin xu* 阴虚): *Zhi bai di huang tang* 知柏地黄汤;
- Blood deficiency (*xue xu* 血虚): *Si wu tang* 四物汤;
- *Qi* stagnation (*qi zhi* 气滞): *Da chai hu tang* 大柴胡汤;
- Dampness obstruction (*shi zu* 湿阻): *Ling gui zhu gan tang* 苓桂术甘汤;
- Blood stasis (*yu xue* 瘀血): *Tao hong si wu tang* 桃红四物汤; and
- Cancer toxin (*ai du* 癌毒): *Long she yang quan tang* 龙蛇羊泉汤 (*long kui* 龙葵, *she mei* 蛇莓, *tu fu ling* 土茯苓 and *bai ying* 白英).

Each formula was taken once per day. The number of people with each syndrome was not reported. XELODA was administered as three-week cycles. There were 63 people in the CHM group, but three dropped out due to refusal to continue CHM. In the XELODA group there were 62 people and two dropped out due to AEs, so the final analysis was based on 120 participants. Treatment continued until tumour progression or intolerance appeared with the longest assessment being 18 months. In both studies, 80% or more consumption of the CHMs was a requirement for inclusion.

Both studies reported median progression-free survival (mPFS). In one study (H35), this was five months in the CHM group versus 4.5 months in the XELODA group (*n* = 90). In the other study (H36) mPFS was 5.4 months in the CHM group versus two months in the XELODA group (*n* = 120). This study also reported PFS which was 1.7 to 18 months in the CHM group and 1.5 to 12 months in the XELODA group.

For KPS (10 points or more improvement), in one study (H35) there was no significant difference between groups (RR: 1.69 [0.98, 2.93], *n* = 90) while in the other study (H36) there was a significant increase (RR: 1.85 [1.04, 3.27], *n* = 120). The pooled result showed a significant improvement in the CHM groups (RR: 1.76 [1.19, 2.62], $I^2 = 0\%$, $n = 210$).

One study (H36) reported results for immune function. There were significant differences between groups for NK cells (MD: 7.10 [4.22, 9.98], $n = 120$) and the ratio CD4/CD8 (MD: 0.59 [0.36, 0.82], $n = 120$).

In one study (H35) data were reported for incidence of hand-foot syndrome and reduced platelets, but it was unclear which criteria were used. The incidences were low in both groups and there were no statistical differences between groups for hand-foot syndrome (RR: 0.33 [0.04, 3.09], $n = 90$) or reduced platelets (RR: 0.50 [0.05, 5.32], $n = 90$).

Oral Chinese Herbal Medicine for Post-chemotherapy Adverse Reactions

In two studies (H37, H38) the CHM was for post-chemotherapy diarrhoea and one study (H39) was for chemotherapy-induced peripheral neurotoxicity (CIPN). All three studies reported on KPS.

Post-chemotherapy Diarrhoea

These two studies used different comparisons. One study (H38) compared an oral CHM with loperamide in people with diarrhoea due to mFOLFOX6 for CRC. All 126 participants had the syndrome of Spleen *qi* deficiency *pi qi kui xu* 脾气亏虚. Their ages ranged from 39 to 67 years. The CHM was made by the authors and called *Tong xie yi hao fang* 痛泄1号方 (*huang qi* 黄芪, *bai zhu* 白术, *cang zhu* 苍术, *fu ling* 茯苓, *ge gen* 葛根, *huang lian* 黄连, *mu xiang* 木香, *wu zhu yu* 吴茱萸, *gan cao* 甘草, *shen qu* 神曲, *shi liu pi* 石榴皮, *shan zhu yu* 山茱萸, *sha ren* 砂仁, *fa ban xia* 法半夏, *chao chai hu* 炒柴胡 and *huang qin* 黄芩). Participants received one packet per day in two doses. After seven days of treatment there was recovery in nine people in the CHM group versus three in the loperamide group, but the difference was not significant (RR: 2.73 [0.77, 9.61], $n = 126$).

In another RCT (H37), an oral CHM was combined with loperamide and compared to loperamide alone for diarrhoea due to FOLFIRI for CRC. All 36 participants were diagnosed with the syndrome Spleen deficiency with dampness encumbrance (*pi xu shi kun* 脾虚湿困). The mean age was 59.1 years in the CHM group and 56.8 in the control group. There were no drop-outs. All received *Fu zheng zhi xie tang* 扶正止泻汤 (*huang qi* 黄芪, *ren shen* 人参, *bai zhu* 白术, *fu ling* 茯苓, *yi yi ren* 薏苡仁, *ge gen* 葛根, *sheng ma* 升麻, *he zi* 诃子, *chi shi zhi* 赤石脂, *bai shao* 白芍, *fang feng* 防风 and *gan cao* 甘草), which was made by the author's teacher, one packet per day as three doses for seven days. Four participants recovered in the CHM plus loperamide group, compared to two in the loperamide alone group, but the difference was not significant (RR: 2.00 [0.42, 9.58], *n* = 36). For the number of diarrhoea events per day, there was significant improvement in the combination therapy group (MD: –1.05 [–1.96, –0.14], *n* = 36).

Chemotherapy-induced Peripheral Neurotoxicity

In one study (H39) all participants had CIPN due to oxaliplatin for CRC and all received monosialotetrahexosylganglioside sodium (GM-1) injection for the CIPN. The mean ages of the 64 participants was 61.1 years in the combination group and 60.8 years in the control group with no drop-outs. There was no syndrome differentiation. The unnamed CHM contained *dang shen* 党参, *huang qi* 黄芪, *chi shao* 赤芍, *bai shao* 白芍, *dang gui* 当归, *gui zhi* 桂枝, *chuan xiong* 川芎, *niu xi* 牛膝, *bai zhi* 白芷 and *gan cao* 甘草. It was administered once a day. Both treatments continued for 28 days. Based on modified World Health Organisation (WHO) criteria,[20] there was no significant difference in the incidence of grade III/IV CIPN (RR: 0.50 [0.05, 5.24], *n* = 64) or all grades of CIPN (RR: 0.83 [0.66, 1.04], *n* = 64).

Karnofsky Performance Scale

In the RCT of CHM versus loperamide (H38), more people improved 10 points or more on KPS in the CHM group (RR: 1.62 [1.12, 2.35], *n* = 126). In the RCT of CHM plus loperamide versus loperamide alone (H37), there was a significant improvement in scores in the combination therapy group (MD: 6.27 [4.96, 7.58], *n* = 36). In the study of CHM for CIPN (H39), the KPS scores were significantly higher in the combination therapy group at the end of treatment (MD: 9.08 [6.23, 11.93], *n* = 64).

None of the three RCTs mentioned AEs associated with the CHMs.

Oral Chinese Herbal Medicine plus Chemotherapy versus Chemotherapy

In 88 RCTs an oral CHM was combined with chemotherapy and compared to the same chemotherapy. In one study (H58) a placebo for the CHM was used in the control group. These studies enrolled 5,649 participants aged from 18 to 84 years, but the age range was not reported in 35 studies. Based on the reported means and standard deviations for ages, most participants were aged between 37 and 78 years. Eighty people dropped out, so 5,569 participants were assessed at end of treatment.

Results are reported for the main types of outcome measures including ORR, survival, progression, recurrence, metastasis rate, quality of life, KPS, immune function and chemotherapy-related AEs. The chemotherapies included FOLFOX4, FOLFOX6, mFOLFOX6, FOLFOX, OLF, LF, simplified bi-weekly infusional 5-FU/LV, FOLFIRI, XELOX, XELODA, XELIRI, tegafur gimeracil oteracil potassium (S-1) plus oxaliplatin and hyperthermic intraperitoneal chemotherapy (HIPEC). Results are subgrouped according to the chemotherapy. One study that presented results as ITT (H61) is reported separately.

Objective Response Rate

Objective response rate (ORR) is the sum of complete response (CR) and partial response (PR) of the tumour to treatment. Twenty five RCTs reported tumour size reduction as ORR based on the WHO criteria[21] and 23 RCTs used Response Evaluation Criteria in Solid Tumours (RECIST).[22] The results are presented separately.

For the studies that used the WHO criteria to assess ORR (CR+PR) most studies were of CRC (mainly stages III/V) with one study of rectal adenocarcinoma metastasis after radical surgery (H62) and one of advanced colon cancer (H63). There was no significant difference between groups for FOLFOX4, mFOLFOX6, FOLFOX or OLF separately; however, the pooled result for this group of similar regimens (14 RCTs) showed a significant benefit for combining CHM with chemotherapy (RR: 1.24 [1.06, 1.45], I^2 = 0%) without heterogeneity (Table 5.24). There was a significant increase in ORR for CHM combined with XELOX (RR: 1.43 [1.07, 1.91], I^2 = 0%) based on six RCTs but no differences for the other regimens. The pooled result for all chemotherapy regimens showed a significant benefit for CHMs combined with these chemotherapy regimens (RRL 1.30 [1.14, 1.47], I^2 = 0%) (Table 5.24).

For the studies that reported tumour ORR (CR+PR) using the RECIST criteria, most studies were of stage III/IV or stage IV CRC.

Table 5.24 Oral Chinese Herbal Medicine plus Chemotherapy versus Chemotherapy: Objective Response Rate (WHO criteria)

Chemotherapy Regimen[1]	*N* Studies (*N* Participants)	Effect Size (RR [95% CI]), I^2	Included Studies
FOLFOX4	9 (594)	1.17 [0.98, 1.41], 0%	H41, H54, H64–H70
mFOLFOX6	2 (143)	1.54 [0.94, 2.55], 36.2%	H62, H63
FOLFOX	1 (62)	1.11 [0.53, 2.35]	H71
OLF	2 (89)	1.41 [0.78, 2.55], 0%	H52, H53
Pool for similar Chemotherapy[2]	14 (888)	1.24 [1.06, 1.45] *, 0%	H41, H52–H54, H62–H71
FOLFIRI	2 (142)	1.43 [0.91, 2.23], 0%	H50, H72
XELOX	6 (389)	1.43 [1.07, 1.91]*, 0%	H45, H73–H77
XELODA	1 (95)	1.47 [0.57, 3.80]	H55
XFIIRI	2 (66)	1.35 [0.62, 2.91], 0%	H78, H79
Total pool	25 (1580)	1.30 [1.14, 1.47]*, 0%	All above

[1]Comparator was the same chemotherapy.

[2]These chemotherapy regimens all use oxaliplatin, 5-FU plus LV.

*Statistically significant.

Abbreviations: CI, confidence interval; N, number; RR, risk ratio; WHO, World Health Organisation.

There was one study of advanced or recurrent rectal cancer (H80), three RCTs of stage III/IV colon cancer (H49, H81, H82), one of advanced colon cancer (H48) and one of advanced or recurrent colon cancer (H83). There was a significant increase in tumour response rate for CHM combined with FOLFOX4 based on eight RCTs (RR: 1.21 [1.01, 1.45], I^2 = 0%) but there were no differences for FOLFOX6 or mFOLFOX6. For the pool of these similar regimens, there was significant benefit for the addition of CHM (RR: 1.25 [1.06, 1.46], I^2 = 0%). Of the other chemotherapy regimens, combining CHM with XELOX showed a significant benefit based on seven RCTs (RR: 1.47 [1.16, 1.86], I^2 = 0%). For the total pool of 23 RCTs of seven chemotherapy regimens, there was a significant increase in ORR in the CHM plus chemotherapy groups, compared to the chemotherapy alone groups (RR: 1.31 [1.16, 1.48], I^2 = 0%) without heterogeneity (Table 5.25).

Table 5.25 Oral Chinese Herbal Medicine plus Chemotherapy versus Chemotherapy: Objective Response Rate (RECIST criteria)

Chemotherapy Regimen[1]	N Studies (N Participants)	Effect Size (RR [95% CI], I^2)	Included Studies
FOLFOX4	8 (608)	1.21 [1.01, 1.45]*, 0%	H48, H49, H51, H80–H82, H84, H85
FOLFOX6	2 (136)	1.33 [0.88, 2.01], 0%	H44, H86
mFOLFOX6	1 (54)	1.46 [0.84, 2.53]	H87
Pool for similar chemo[2]	11 (798)	1.25 [1.06, 1.46]*, 0%	H44, H48, H49, H51, H80–H82, H84–C87
FOLFIRI	3 (154)	1.27 [0.85, 1.89], 0%	H43, H88, H89
XELOX	7 (417)	1.47 [1.16, 1.86] *, 0%	H59, H83, H90-H94
XELODA	1 (60)	1.25 [0.57, 2.73]	H95
XELIRI	1 (55)	1.38 [0.61, 3.09]	H96
Total pool	23 (1484)	1.31 [1.16, 1.48] *, 0%	All above

[1]Comparator was the same chemotherapy.

[2]These chemotherapy regimens all use oxaliplatin, 5-FU plus LV.

*Statistically significant.

Abbreviations: CI, confidence interval; N, number; RECIST, Response Evaluation Criteria in Solid Tumours; RR, risk ratio.

Survival Rate

Eight RCTs reported data on survival at various time-points ranging from 0.5 to five years (Table 5.26).

One study (H97) reported five-year survival in people with Dukes C CRC treated with LF (leucovorin, 5-fluorouracil) commencing four weeks after radical surgery (six 4-week cycles). The CHM treatment was in three stages: (1) from one to four weeks after surgery *Huang lian jie du kang ai tang* 莲花解毒抗癌汤 (*ban zhi lian* 半枝莲, *bai hua she she cao* 白花蛇舌草, *ban bian lian* 半边莲, *sheng huang qi* 生黄芪, *tai zi shen* 太子参, *ling zhi* 灵芝, *shan yao* 山药, *nv zhen zi* 女贞子, *gou qi* 枸杞, *san leng* 三棱, *e zhu* 莪术, *tian qi* 田七, *shi shang bai* 石上柏, *ba qia* 菝葜, and *zhi gan cao* 炙甘草) plus *Ba zhen tang* 八珍汤 were administered (both with modifications);

Table 5.26 Survival Rates at 0.5 to 5 Years for Chinese Herbal Medicine plus Chemotherapy versus Chemotherapy

Chemotherapy Regimen[1]	Included Studies: Cancer (*N* Participants T/C)	Survival Time	*N* Survivors T/C (%)
FOLFOX4	H98: Stage III colon cancer after radical laparoscopic surgery (25/25)	1 year	25/25 (100/100)
		2 years	22/16 (88/64)
		3 years	17/12 (68/48)
	H70: Stage III/IV advanced CRC (60/60)	0.5 year	52/45 (86.7/75)
		1 year	39/25 (65/41.7)
FOLFOX	H71: Advanced CRC (31/31)	1 year	24/21 (77.4/67.7)
		2 years	18/12 (58.1/38.7)
		3 years	15/5 (48.4/16.1)
FOLFIRI	H50: Stage III/IV CRC (47/40)	1 year	25/16 (53.2/40)
LF	H97: Dukes C CRC after radical surgery (46/44)	5 years	20/10 (43.5/22.7)
XELOX	H75: Advanced CRC (45/45)	1 year	37/24 (82.2/53.3)
	H45: Stage IV CRC (30/30)	1 year	25/17 (83.3/56.7)
XELODA	H55: Stage IV CRC with liver metastasis (48/48)	1 year	26/16 (54.2/34)

[1]Comparator was the same chemotherapy.

Abbreviations: CRC, colorectal cancer; T, treatment group; C, control group; N, number.

(2) From 4–24 weeks *Huang lian jie du kang ai tang* 莲花解毒抗癌汤 was combined with *Liu jun zi tang* 六君子汤 and *Zuo gui yin* 左归饮 (all with modifications); and (3) After half a year *Huang lian jie du kang ai tang* 莲花解毒抗癌汤 was used alone. The five-year survival rates were 43.5% in the CHM plus LF group versus 22.7% in the control group.

Two RCTs reported survival rates for one to three years. In one study (H98) people with stage III colon cancer received FOLFOX4 (six 2-week cycles) commencing within one month of radical laparoscopic surgery. The CHM, *Kang ai fang yi pian* 抗癌防移片, was made by the authors' hospital and contained 16 ingredients including *hong shen* 红参, *huang qi* 黄芪, *ban zhi lian* 半枝莲, *zao xiu* 蚤休, *jiang huang* 姜黄 and *e zhu* 莪术 (ten tablets, three times a day). It was administered with chemotherapy for three months. Survival rates were 100% versus 100% at one year, 88% versus 64% at two years, and 68% versus 48% at three years. In the other study (H71), people with advanced CRC were treated with FOLFOX (two 4-week cycles). The combination group also received *Jian pi kang ai fang* 健脾抗癌方 (*sheng huang qi* 生黄芪, *bai fu ling* 白茯苓, *jiao bai zhu* 焦白术, *sheng yi yi ren* 生薏苡仁, *tai zi shen* 太子参, *ba yue zha* 八月札, *teng li gen* 藤梨根, *xia ku cao* 夏枯草, *bai hua she she cao* 白花蛇舌草, *ba qia* 菝葜, *ye pu tao gen* 野葡萄根, *hong teng* 红藤 and *tian long* 天龙) which was made by the authors (one packet per day in two doses) for two months. The survival rates were 77.4% versus 67.7% at one year, 58.1% versus 38.7% at two years, and 48.4% versus 16.1% at three years.

In five RCTs (H45, H50, H55, H70, H75) the longest survival time-point reported was one year. All were of stage III and/or IV CRC, so one-year survival data were available for six RCTs of stage III and/or IV CRC. The survival rates in the CHM plus chemotherapy groups ranged from 53.2% to 83.3% and in the chemotherapy control groups one-year survival ranged from 34.0% to 67.7%.

Overall Survival and Median Survival Time

One RCT (H50) reported overall survival (OS) as a range and three RCTs reported median survival time (MST) (Table 5.27).

Table 5.27 Median Survival Time for Chinese Herbal Medicine plus Chemotherapy versus Chemotherapy

Chemotherapy Regimen[1]	Included Studies: Cancer (*N* Participants)	CHM plus Chemotherapy (Months)	Chemotherapy (Months)
FOLFIRI	H50: Stage III/IV CRC (87)	12.5	10.8
	H88: Stage IV CRC (66)	25.6	20.8
XELODA	H55: Stage IV CRC with liver metastasis (95)	13	8

[1]Comparator was the same chemotherapy.

Abbreviations: CHM, Chinese herbal medicine; CRC, colorectal cancer; N, number.

In one study (H50) people with stage III/IV CRC, who had recurrence after surgery or were not suitable for surgery, received FOLFIRI (four 2-week cycles). One group also received the commercial CHM product *Fu fang ban mao jiao nang* 复方斑蝥胶囊 (0.75 g, twice a day) administered for 60 days. The OS ranged from seven to 38 months in the CHM plus chemotherapy group (median 12.5 months) and from five to 31 months in the chemotherapy alone group (median 10.8 months).

In another RCT (H88) of 68 people with stage IV CRC who received FOLFIRI (four 2-week cycles), one group also received a CHM made by the authors called *Jian pi xiao ai fang* 健脾消癌方 (*ren shen* 人参, *bai zhu* 白术, *fu ling* 茯苓, *fa ban xia* 法半夏, *huang qi* 黄芪, *yin yang huo* 淫羊藿, *bai hua she she cao* 白花蛇舌草, *ban zhi lian* 半枝莲, *yu jin* 郁金, *chao zhi ke* 炒枳壳 and *gan cao* 甘草), one packet a day in two doses for eight weeks. Two people (1/1) were lost to follow-up. The MSTs were 25.6 months in the CHM plus chemotherapy group versus 20.8 months in the control group. In one RCT (H55), people with stage IV CRC and liver metastasis received XELODA (two 3-week cycles). One group also received a CHM manufactured by the authors' hospital called *Wei tiao san hao fang* 微调3号方 (*dang shen* 党参, *zhu ling* 猪苓, *fu ling* 茯苓, *yi yi ren* 薏苡仁, *chao bai zhu* 炒白术, *fa ban xia* 法半夏, *chen pi* 陈皮 and *zhi pi pa ye* 炙枇杷叶) 50 ml, twice a day for six weeks. The MST in the CHM plus chemotherapy group was 13 months compared to eight months in the group that received chemotherapy alone.

Median Progression-free Survival

Four RCTs reported on mPFS (Table 5.28). In one study (H87) of people with advanced CRC treated with mFOLFOX6 (four 2-week cycles) the CHM plus chemotherapy group also received *Jian pi yi qi jie du fang* 健脾益气解毒方 which was made by the authors and contained *huang qi* 黄芪, *bai zhu* 白术, *fu ling* 茯苓, *dang shen* 党参, *shan yao* 山药, *ban zhi lian* 半枝莲, *bai hua she she cao* 白花蛇舌草, *xian he cao* 仙鹤草, *e zhu* 莪术 and *shan ci gu* 山慈菇, one packet/day in two doses for at least eight weeks. In the combination therapy group, mPFS was 7.9 months compared to 6.7 months in the control group.

In two studies (H88, H91) all participants had stage IV CRC. The characteristics of one of these studies (H88) have been described above (see MST). In the other study (H91), all participants received XELOX (two 3-week cycles) and one group also received a CHM made by the authors: *Kang ai yi liu fang* 抗癌抑瘤方 (*tai zi shen* 太子参, *bai zhu* 白术, *fu ling* 茯苓, *hou pu* 厚朴, *bai tou weng* 白头翁, *bai jiang cao* 败酱草, *hong teng* 红藤, *teng li gen* 藤梨根, *ba yue zha* 八月札, *sheng yi yi ren* 生薏苡仁, *chao lai fu zi* 炒莱菔子, *er cha* 儿茶, *bai qu cai* 白屈菜, *bai hua she she cao* 白花蛇舌草, *huang jing* 黄精, *bie jia* 鳖甲, *gui ban* 龟板, *bai ying* 白英, *gan cao* 甘草 and *sha ren* 砂仁) one packet per day in two doses for two

Table 5.28   Median Progression-free Survival for Chinese Herbal Medicine plus Chemotherapy versus Chemotherapy

Chemotherapy Regimen[1]	Included Studies: Cancer (*N* Participants)	CHM plus Chemotherapy (Months)	Chemotherapy (Months)
mFOLFOX6	H87: Advanced CRC (54)	7.9	6.7
FOLFIRI	H88: Stage IV CRC (66)	11.6	8.8
XELOX	H91: Stage IV CRC (97)	11.2	8.9
XELODA	H35: Stage IV CRC maintenance treatment (90)	6.5	4.5

[1]Comparator was the same chemotherapy.

Abbreviations: CHM, Chinese herbal medicine; CRC, colorectal cancer; N, number.

weeks followed by a one-week break, then repeated once more. In these studies, the mPFS in the CHM plus chemotherapy groups were 11.6 and 11.2 months versus 8.8 and 8.9 months in the chemotherapy alone groups, respectively.

In one study (H35) XELODA was used as a maintenance treatment. This was a three-armed study and the characteristics have been described above (see oral CHM versus chemotherapy). In the CHM plus chemotherapy group the mPFS was 6.5 months versus 4.5 months in the group that received the chemotherapy alone.

Time to Progression

One study (H40) reported on time to progression (TTP) and median TTP (mTTP). In this study 150 participants with stage IV CRC were enrolled (75 people in each group) but eight dropped out during follow-up (five in CHM plus chemotherapy group; three in control group). All patients were treated with XELODA (three-week cycles) as a maintenance treatment. The CHM plus chemotherapy group also received 11 different CHMs (one packet per day in two doses) according to the following ten syndromes:

- Spleen deficiency (*pi qi xu* 脾气虚): *Si jun zi tang* 四君子汤;
- Kidney *yang* deficiency (*shen yang xu* 肾阳虚): *You gui wan* 右归丸;
- *Yin* deficiency (*yin xu* 阴虚): *Zhi bai di huang tang* 知柏地黄汤;
- Blood deficiency (*xue xu* 血虚): *Si wu tang* 四物汤;
- *Qi* stagnation (*qi zhi* 气滞): *Da chai hu tang* 大柴胡汤;
- Excess heat (*shi re* 实热): *Cheng qi tang lei* 乘气汤类;
- Dampness obstruction (*shi zu* 湿阻): *Ling gui zhu gan tang* 苓桂术甘汤;
- Dampness heat (*shi re* 湿热): *Bai tou weng tang* 白头翁汤;
- Blood stasis (*yu xue* 瘀血): *Tao hong si wu tang* 桃红四物汤 or *Ge xia zhu yu tang* 膈下逐瘀汤; and
- Cancer toxin (*ai du* 癌毒): *San gen tang* 三根汤.

The numbers of people with each syndrome were not reported. Treatment continued until tumour progression, with the longest treatment time being one year. Time to progression ranged from two to 12 months in the CHM plus chemotherapy group (median six months) and from two to 10 months in the chemotherapy alone group (median three months).

Recurrence and Metastasis Rates

Four RCTs reported on recurrence and/or metastasis rates when receiving adjuvant chemotherapy after radical surgery.

In one study (H99), 134 people with stage II/III CRC received FOLFOX4 (four 2-week cycles) with follow-up at one, two and three years. One group also received a formula made by the authors called *Jian pi xiao ai yin* 健脾消癌饮 (*dang shen* 党参, *huang qi* 黄芪, *bai zhu* 白术, *fu ling* 茯苓, *ling zhi* 灵芝, *yi yi ren* 薏苡仁, *dan shen* 丹参, *xian ling pi* 仙灵脾, *qi ye yi zhi hua* 七叶一枝花, *bai hua she she cao* 白花蛇舌草, *ban zhi lian* 半枝莲, *shi jian chuan* 石见穿, *fa xia* 法夏, *e zhu* 莪术, *gan cao* 甘草 and *mu xiang* 木香) one packet a day in two doses for eight weeks. At the one-year follow-up, no person had recurrence and/or metastasis in the combination therapy group versus four (5.7%) in the control group. The rates for the two-year follow-up were 6.1% versus 21.4% and the three-year follow-up rates were 17.1% versus 32.3%, respectively (Table 5.29).

In a study (H46) of 60 people with CRC (stage unspecified), all participants were diagnosed with the syndrome *qi* and Blood dual deficiency (*qi xue kui xu* 气血亏虚) and all received FOLFOX4 (twelve 2-week cycles) with a follow-up at six months after the end of treatment. One group also received *Ba zhen tang* 八珍汤 (*hong shen* 红参, *fu ling* 茯苓, *bai zhu* 白术, *gan cao* 甘草, *dang gui* 当归, *shou di* 熟地, *chuan xiong* 川芎 and *bai shao* 白芍) one packet a day in two doses for six months. At one year after the beginning of chemotherapy, the recurrence rates were 6.7% in the combination therapy group versus 13.3% in the control, and the metastasis rates were 3.3% and 13.3%, respectively.

The details of the other two studies (H97, H98) have been described above. In the study of people with stage III colon cancer (H98) who had undergone radical laparoscopic surgery and received FOLFOX4 adjuvant chemotherapy, the rates of recurrence and/or

Table 5.29 Recurrence and Metastasis Rate for Chinese Herbal Medicine plus Chemotherapy versus Chemotherapy

Chemotherapy Regimen[1]	Included Studies: Cancer (*N.* Participants T/C)	Time-point: Measure	CHM plus Chemo./ Chemo., *N* (%)
FOLFOX4 (adjuvant chemotherapy)	H99: Stage II/III CRC (67/67)	1 year: R/m	0/4 (0/5.7)
		2 years: R/m	3/9 (6.1/21.4)
		3 years: R/m	6/10 (17.1/32.3)
	H46: CRC (30/30)	1 year: Recurrence	2/4 (6.7/13.3)
		1 year: Metastasis	1/4 (3.3/13.3)
	H98: Stage III colon cancer after radical laparoscopic surgery (25/25)	3 years: R/m	5/12 (20/48)
LF (adjuvant chemotherapy)	H97: Dukes C CRC (46/44)	5 years: R/m	33/39 (71.7/88.6)

[1]Comparator was the same chemotherapy.

Abbreviations: C, control group; Chemo, chemotherapy; CHM, Chinese herbal medicine; CRC, colorectal cancer; LF, leucovorin and 5-fluorouracil; N, number; r/m, recurrence and/or metastasis; T, treatment group.

metastasis at three years were 20% in the combination therapy group versus 48% in the control group. In the study of people with Dukes C CRC who received LF adjuvant chemotherapy after radical surgery (H97), 71.7% of people had recurrence and/or metastasis at five years versus 88.6% in the control group that received LF alone.

Quality of Life

Sixteen RCTs reported on quality of life (QOL) but in six studies (H58, H73, H95, H100–H102) the results were not suitable for meta-analysis. Data from three different QOL scales were included in the meta-analysis.

The Functional Assessment of Cancer Therapy-Colorectal (FACT-C) is a 36 item self-report questionnaire that has versions in multiple languages including Chinese.[23] It includes five subscales, one of which is specific to CRC. To obtain total scores, some subscales are reverse-scored so that higher total scores indicate better QOL.[24]

The European Organisation for Research and Treatment of Cancer Quality of Life Questionnaire (EORTC QLQ-C30, version 3) is a 30-item questionnaire available in multiple languages that includes five functional scales, a scale for global health status/QOL and scales for multiple symptoms.[25] Scoring is normed at 100 with higher scores indicating better QOL for the first six scales with the reverse for the symptoms. In the following analysis, only the global health status/QOL scale was used.

In China, a 12-item QOL scale is frequently used.[26] The total score is 60 points with higher scores indicating better QOL. The meta-analysis results are presented separately for each questionnaire.

Two RCTs (H91, H103) reported on FACT-C. In one study (H103) of people with stage III/IV CRC all 41 participants were diagnosed with the syndrome Spleen and Kidney dual deficiency (*pi shen liang xu* 脾肾两虚) and all received mFOLFOX6 (two 2-week cycles) and one group also received an unnamed decoction (*sheng huang qi* 生黄芪, *dang shen* 党参, *chao bai zhu* 炒白术, *fu ling* 茯苓, *zhi gan cao* 炙甘草, *sha ren* 砂仁, *mu xiang* 木香, *chen pi* 陈皮, *ban xia* 半夏, *sang ji sheng* 桑寄生, *niu xi* 牛膝, *tu si zi* 菟丝子, *gou qi* 枸杞 and *nv zhen zi* 女贞子) that aimed to fortify the Spleen and replenish *qi* (*jian pi yi shen* 健脾益肾) at a dosage of one packet per day in two doses for four weeks. At the end of treatment there was a significant improvement in the combined treatment group (MD: 6.91 [3.39, 10.43], *n* = 41).

The other study (H91) has been described above (see mPFS). After six weeks of treatment, there was a significant improvement on FACT-C in the CHM plus chemotherapy group (MD: 12.90 [2.60, 23.20], *n* = 97). The pooled result for the two studies showed a significant improvement in QOL (MD: 7.87 [3.56, 12.17] I^2 = 14%, *n* = 138) without important heterogeneity.

Two studies assessed QOL using EORTC QLQ-C30 (version 3). In one study (H54), 45 people with stage IV CRC with liver metastases were all diagnosed with the syndrome Spleen deficiency with *qi* stagnation (*pi xu qi zhi* 脾虚气滞) and received FOLFOX4 (four

2-week cycles). One group also received a formula designed by the author's hospital called *Zhong yao wei tiao san hao fang* 中药微调三号方 (*dang shen* 党参, *chao bai zhu* 炒白术, *huai shan* 淮山, *chen pi* 陈皮, *jiang ban xia* 姜半夏, *fu ling* 茯苓, *fu shen* 茯神, *zhu ling* 猪苓, *yi yi ren* 薏苡仁, *gu ya* 谷芽, *mai ya* 麦芽, *pi pa ye* 枇杷叶 and *zhi gan cao* 炙甘草) one packet per day in two doses for eight weeks. On the global health status, there was a significant improvement at the end of treatment in the combined therapy group (MD: 12.40 [0.34, 24.46], *n* = 45).

In the other study (H94), 53 people with stage IV CRC who were diagnosed with the syndrome Spleen *qi* deficiency (*pi qi xu* 脾气虚) received modified XELOX (four 4-week cycles) with one group also receiving a three-stage CHM treatment (all one packet per day in two doses) as follows:

- Formula 1: *Dang shen* 党参, *zhu ling* 猪苓, *chao bai zhu* 炒白术, *huang qi* 黄芪, *mai dong* 麦冬, *nv zhen zi* 女贞子, *wu wei zi* 五味子, *sha ren* 砂仁, *yi yi ren* 薏苡仁, *zhi ji nei jin* 炙鸡内金 and *zhi gan cao* 炙甘草 taken during the first week of chemotherapy;

- Formula 2: *Xuan fu hua* 旋复花, *gan jiang* 干姜, *ding xiang* 丁香, *chao bai zhu* 炒白术, *fu ling* 茯苓, *jiang ban xia* 姜半夏, *chen pi* 陈皮, *shen qu* 神曲, *jiao gu ya* 焦谷芽, *jiao mai ya* 焦麦芽, *zhi gan cao* 炙甘草 and *da zao* 大枣 taken in weeks two and three;

- Formula 3: *Huang qi* 黄芪, *huang jing* 黄精, *dang gui* 当归, *ji xue teng* 鸡血藤, *shou di* 熟地, *rou gui* 肉桂, *chi shao* 赤芍, *bai shao* 白芍, *gou qi* 枸杞, *nv zhen zi* 女贞子, *chuan xiong* 川芎, *di long* 地龙, *san qi* 三七, *bu gu zhi* 补骨脂, *tu si zi* 菟丝子, *jiao gu ya* 焦谷芽 and *jiao mai ya* 焦麦芽 taken in the fourth week of chemotherapy.

At the end of the 16-week treatment, there was a significant improvement on EORTC QLQ-C30 in the combination therapy group (MD: 12.41 [1.26, 23.56], *n* = 53). The pooled result for the two studies showed a significant improvement in global health status (MD: 12.41 [4.22, 20.60], I² = 0%, *n* = 98).

Six RCTs reported results for QOL using the Chinese scale. These studies included one RCT of adjuvant chemotherapy for Dukes B/C

CRC after radical surgery (H104) and one RCT of adjuvant chemotherapy for colon cancer after radical surgery (H105) in people with the syndrome Spleen deficiency with dampness brewing (*pi xu shi yun* 脾虚湿蕴). In the other four RCTs all participants had stage IV CRC. In each of these studies the syndrome was reported (Table 5.30). The pooled result for all six studies, showed a significant improvement in the CHM plus chemotherapy groups (MD: 3.93 [1.27, 6.58], I^2 = 97%) but the heterogeneity was substantial. In the

Table 5.30 Quality of Life (Chinese Scale) for Chinese Herbal Medicine plus Chemotherapy versus Chemotherapy

Chemotherapy Regimen[1]	Cancer (*N* Participants), Syndrome	Effect Size (MD [95% CI,]) I^2	Included Studies
FOLFOX4	Dukes B/C CRC after radical surgery[2] (30), NA	1.20 [–3.70, 6.10]	H104
FOLFIRI	Stage IV CRC (36), *pi qi xu, yu du liu zhi* 脾气虚, 瘀毒留滞	4.78 [1.41, 8.15]*	H89
XELOX	Colon cancer after radical surgery[2] (60), *pi xu shi yun* 脾虚湿蕴	0.70 [0.34, 1.06]*	H105
	Stage IV CRC (40), *zheng qi kui xu, yu du ji zhi* 正气亏虚, 瘀毒积滞	4.20 [2.49, 5.91]*	H92
	Stage IV CRC (40), *zheng qi kui xu, yu du ji zhi* 正气亏虚, 瘀毒积滞	6.80 [4.99, 8.61]*	H93
Modified XELIRI	Stage IV CRC previously treated (36), *pi xu shi zhi yu du* 脾虚湿滞瘀毒	5.26 [4.57, 5.95]*	H78
Total pool	6 studies (242)	3.93 [1.27, 6.58]*, 97%	All above
Subgroup: Adjuvant chemotherapy.	2 studies: CRC, colon cancer (90)	0.70 [0.34, 1.06]*, 0%	H104, H105
Subgroup: Excluding adjuvant chemotherapy.	4 studies: stage IV CRC (152)	5.30 [4.38, 6.22]*, 30.8%	H78, H89, H92, H93

[1]Comparator was the same chemotherapy.

[2]Adjuvant chemotherapy.

*Statistically significant.

Abbreviations: CI, confidence interval; CRC, colorectal cancer; MD, mean difference; N, number.

subgroup of the two studies of adjuvant chemotherapy the result showed a small benefit for combined therapy (MD: 0.70 [0.34, 1.06], $I^2 = 0\%$). In the other four studies, which were all of participants with stage IV CRC, there was a significant improvement with moderate heterogeneity (MD: 5.30 [4.38, 6.22], $I^2 = 30.8\%$).

Karnofsky Performance Status

In total 71 RCTs reported data for KPS. Thirty-four RCTs reported KPS scores but data suitable for pooling in the meta-analyses were only available in 30 RCTs. One study, that reported data as ITT (H61), is reported separately. An additional 37 studies reported KPS as the incidence of improvements of ten points or more. These two forms of reporting are separated for meta-analysis.

For KPS scores, studies were grouped according to the type of chemotherapy. FOLFOX4 was the most commonly used chemotherapy (12 RCTs) followed by XELOX (11 RCTs) (Table 5.31). Most participants had advanced CRC or stage III/IV CRC. In one study (H106) all participants were treated with FOLFOX4 for rectal cancer and in four studies (H47, H81, H83, H105) all participants had colon cancer. In two studies all participants had stage IV CRC with liver metastases (H54, H55).

The pooled result for all FOLFOX4 studies showed improved KPS in the combined therapy groups (MD: 8.32 [7.14, 9.50], $I^2 = 0\%$) and there was a similar result in the subgroup of five studies in which FOLFOX4 was used as adjuvant chemotherapy after radical surgery (MD: 7.48 [5.61, 9.35], $I^2 = 0\%$). In the pooled result of 15 studies of similar chemotherapies (FOLFOX4, FOLFOX, FOLFOX6) there was a significant improvement in KPS scores (MD: 8.58 [7.54, 9.62], $I^2 = 0\%$) with no heterogeneity.

For the 11 studies that employed XELOX, the significant improvement in KPS (MD: 6.07 [3.60, 8.54], $I^2 = 82.6\%$) was associated with considerable heterogeneity, which was not resolved in the subgroups based on whether XELOX was administered after surgery or not. In the XELOX (after surgery) subgroup, one study (H105) was of colon cancer and used four cycles of XELOX, while the other study (H60)

Table 5.31 Oral Chinese Herbal Medicine plus Chemotherapy versus Chemotherapy: Karnofsky Performance Status (Score)

Chemotherapy Regimen[1]	N Studies (N Participants)	Effect Size (MD [95% CI]), I^2	Included Studies
FOLFOX4 (all)	12 (718)	8.32 [7.14, 9.50]*, 0%	H47, H54, H65, H66, H68, H69, H81, H84, H99, H104, H106, H107
FOLFOX4 (adjuvant, after radical surgery)	5 (290)	7.48 [5.61, 9.35]*, 0%	H47, H99, H104, H106, H107
FOLFOX6	2 (130)	10.22 [7.67, 12.77]*, 0%	H44, H108
FOLFOX	1 (62)	7.40 [3.20, 11.60]*	H71
Pool for similar chemotherapy[2]	15 (910)	8.58 [7.54, 9.62]*, 0%	H44, H47, H54, H65, H66, H68, H69, H71, H81, H84, H99, H104, H106–H108
XELOX (all)	11 (627)	6.07 [3.60, 8.54]*, 82.6%	H45, H59, H60, H76, H77, H83, H90, H92, H94, H105, H109
XELOX (after surgery)	2 (101)	1.67 [-0.41, 3.75], 92.8%	H60, H105
XELOX (no surgery)	9 (526)	6.32 [3.60, 9.03]*, 79.1%	H45, H59, H76, H77, H83, H90, H92, H94, H109
XELODA	1 (95)	4.28 [1.74, 6.82]*	H55
XELIRI	3 (106)	5.33 [4.06, 6.60]*, 0%	H78, H79, H102
Total pool	30 (1738)	7.05 [5.87, 8.23]*, 68.9%	All above
Sensitivity analysis	25 (1476)	7.43 [6.41, 8.45]*, 47.8%	Exclude H45, H83, H105; H81; H106

[1]Comparator was the same chemotherapy.

[2]These chemotherapy regimens all use oxaliplatin, 5-FU plus LV.

* Statistically significant.

Abbreviations: CI, confidence interval; MD, mean difference; N, number.

was of CRC and used two cycles of XELOX. These differences likely account for the heterogeneous result.

In the pool of nine studies of XELOX without surgery, the result also showed considerable heterogeneity (MD: 6.32 [3.60, 9.03], I^2 = 79.1%). In these studies, most participants were stage IV or advanced CRC with one study of advanced recurrent colon cancer (H83). Also, there were some inconsistencies in reporting of KPS in one study (H45). When these two studies (H45, H83) were removed in a sensitivity analysis the heterogeneity was reduced (MD: 6.75 [4.37, 9.13], I^2 = 58.7%, n = 507). In a sensitivity analysis of all XELOX studies following the removal of the above three studies (H45, H83, H105) the pooled result remained significant with reduced heterogeneity (MD: 7.06 [4.95, 9.16], I^2 = 56.8%, n = 447). In the three studies of XELIRI, all participants were stage IV CRC and the pooled result showed a benefit of adding the CHM (MD: 5.33 [4.06, 6.60], I^2 = 0%).

For all 30 RCTs, the pooled result showed a significant improvement in KPS score in the combination therapy groups (MD: 7.05 [5.87, 8.23], I^2 = 68.9%), but the heterogeneity was substantial. In a sensitivity analysis based on the removal of the three previously identified studies (H45, H83, H105) plus another study of colon cancer (H81) and the single study of rectal cancer (H106), the pooled result for the remaining studies of CRC showed a significant difference between groups with reduced heterogeneity (MD: 7.43 [6.41, 8.45], I^2 = 47.8%, n = 1,476).

One study used ITT analysis (H61). Eighty people with CRC, who had the syndrome of Spleen deficiency with dampness brewing (*pi xu shi yun* 脾虚湿蕴), were included. All received FOLFOX4 (one 2-week cycle) as adjuvant chemotherapy in people with stage II CRC, and adjuvant or palliative chemotherapy in people with stage III/IV CRC. Forty people also received the oral CHM *Wu jing gao* 芜菁膏 (*wu jing* 芜菁 and *feng mi* 蜂蜜) 60 g, three times per day for two weeks. There were two drop-outs in the CHM plus FOLFOX4 group and two drop-outs in the FOLFOX4 group. There was no significant difference in KPS scores between groups (MD: 1.94 [−3.44, 7.32], n − 76).

KPS was reported as incidence of improvement of ten points or more in 37 RCTs. Most studies (n = 15) were of FOLFOX4, followed by XELOX (n = 5) and FOLFIRI (n = 5) (Table 5.32). Four RCTs (H48, H49, H63, H82) were of colon cancer and the remainder were of CRC. In most studies participants had stage III/IV CRC. The pooled result for all 15 FOLFOX4 studies showed a significant improvement

Table 5.32 Oral Chinese Herbal Medicine plus Chemotherapy versus Chemotherapy: Karnofsky Performance Status (Improvements of 10 Points or More)

Chemotherapy Regimen[1]	N Studies (N Participants)	Effect Size (RR [95% CI]), I^2	Included Studies
FOLFOX4 (all)	15 (1,066)	1.67 [1.46, 1.91]*, 0%	H41, H46, H48, H49, H51, H64, H67, H70, H82, H85, H100, H110–H113
FOLFOX4 (adjuvant, after radical surgery)	2 (120)	1.66 [1.15, 2.39]*, 0%	H46, H110
FOLFOX6	2 (96)	2.00 [1.10, 3.65]*, 0%	H58, H86
mFOLFOX6	3 (170)	1.93 [1.35, 2.75]*, 0%	H63, H87, H103
OLF	2 (89)	3.09 [1.37, 6.95]*, 0%	H52, H53
Pool for similar chemotherapy[2]	22 (1,421)	1.73 [1.53, 1.95]*, 0%	H41, H46, H48, H49, H51–H53, H58, H63, H64, H67, H70, H82, H85–H87, H100, H103, H110–H113
FOLFIRI	5 (296)	1.76 [1.33, 2.35]*, 0%	H43, H50, H72, H88, H89
SI + Oxaliplatin	1 (66)	1.64 [1.04, 2.59]*	H101
XELOX (all)	5 (279)	2.09 [1.51, 2.91]*, 0%	H42, H74, H75, H93, H114
XELOX (after surgery)	1 (40)	2.00 [0.94, 4.27]*	H114
XELOX (no surgery)	4 (239)	2.12 [1.47, 3.05]*, 0%	H42, H74, H75, H93
XELODA	1 (90)	1.85 [1.08, 3.15]*	H35[4]
XELIRI	1 (55)	14.48 [0.87, 241.82][3,] *	H96
HIPEC	2 (164)	2.10 [1.42, 3.10]*, 0%	H56, H57
Total pool	37 (2,371)	1.79 [1.62, 1.97]*, 0%	All above

[1]Comparator was the same chemotherapy.

[2]These chemotherapy regimens all use oxaliplatin, 5-FU plus LV.

[3]The large figure is due to zero events in the control group.

[4]This is a three-armed study; see the oral CHM versus chemotherapy section for further results of this study.

*Statistically significant.

Abbreviations: CI, confidence interval; HIPEC: hyperthermic intraperitoneal chemotherapy; MD, mean difference; N, number.

in KPS in the combination CHM plus FOLFOX4 groups (RR: 1.67 [1.46, 1.91], I^2 = 0%). The result was similar in the subgroup of studies of FOLFOX4 as adjuvant chemotherapy following radical surgery. The pooled result for 22 studies that used similar chemotherapy regimens (FOLFOX4, FOLFOX6, mFOLFOX6, OLF) showed a significant benefit for the combination therapy groups (RR: 1.73 [1.53, 1.95], I^2 = 0%) without heterogeneity. In the five studies of FOLFIRI, there was a significant improvement in KPS in the CHM plus chemotherapy groups (RR: 1.76 [1.33, 2.35], I^2 – 0%). For XELOX, the pooled result for all five studies showed a benefit for the combination therapy groups (RR: 2.09 [1.51, 2.91], I^2 = 0%) and the result was similar for the subgroups of studies in which XELOX was used after surgery and without surgery. In the pooled result of two studies of hyperthermic intraperitoneal chemotherapy (HIPEC), addition of the CHMs improved KPS (RR: 2.10 [1.42, 3.10], I^2 = 0%). The total pool of 37 RCTs found a significant improvement in KPS in the CHM plus chemotherapy groups compared to chemotherapies alone (RR: 1.79 [1.62, 1.97], I^2 = 0%) without heterogeneity.

Immune Function

Thirty RCTs reported measures of immune function including T cells (a type of lymphocyte) and immunoglobulins, but data suitable for pooling in the meta-analysis were available for 28 studies. For the T cells, these were mainly reported as percentages of CD3+ (18 RCTs), CD4+ (22 RCTs), CD8+ (19 RCTs) and NK cells (17 RCTs), and the ratio CD4+/CD8+ (19 RCTs), which are reported separately. One study (H115) reported percentage of CD8 + CD28 + T cells. One study (H61), that reported data as ITT, is reported separately. Immunoglobulin levels were reported for IgG (two RCTs), IgA (two RCTs), IgM (two RCTs) and IgE (one RCT).

CD3+ Cells

For CD3+ cells (%) (Table 5.33), the results for the group of eight studies that used FOLFOX4 showed a significant increase in the percentage

Table 5.33 Oral Chinese Herbal Medicine plus Chemotherapy versus Chemotherapy: CD3+ cells (%)

Chemotherapy Regimen[1]	N Studies (N Participants)	Effect Size (MD [95% CI]), I^2	Included Studies
FOLFOX4 (all)	8 (503)	11.99 [6.58, 17.41]*, 96.6%	H47, H68, H82, H84, H98, H100, H104, H117
FOLFOX4 (adjuvant, after radical surgery)	3 (125)	12.76 [–2.30, 27.81] 97.4%	H47, H98, H104
FOLFOX6	1 (30)	7.76 [2.31, 13.21]*	H58
FOLFOX	1 (62)	10.64 [7.96, 13.32]*	H71
OLF	1 (40)	3.24 [0.54, 5.94]*	H53
Pool for similar chemotherapy[2]	11 (635)	10.67 [6.71, 14.63]*, 95.5%	H47, H53, H58, H68, H71, H82, H84, H98, H100, H104, H117
Simplified bi-weekly infusional 5-FU/LV	1 (83)	–12.50 [–13.93, –11.07]*	H116
XELOX (all no surgery)	5 (329)	10.81 [5.06, 16.56]*, 93.8%	H45, H75, H77, H94, H115
FOLFIRI	1 (55)	3.55 [1.16, 5.94]*	H72
Total pool	18 (1102)	9.01 [4.50, 13.52]*, 98.3%	All above

[1]Comparator was the same chemotherapy.

[2]These chemotherapy regimens all use oxaliplatin, 5-FU plus LV.

[3]The large figure is due to zero events in the control group;

[4]This is a three-armed study, see the oral CHM versus chemotherapy section for further results of this study.

*Statistically significant.

Abbreviations: CI, confidence interval; MD, mean difference; N, number.

of CD3+ cells in the combination therapy groups (MD: 11.99 [6.58, 17.41], I^2 = 96.6%), but the result showed considerable heterogeneity. The heterogeneity remained in the subgroup of studies of FOLFOX4 as adjuvant chemotherapy after radical surgery (three RCTs) but there was no difference between groups. One of these studies (H98) was distinctive since it employed laparoscopic surgery for stage III colon cancer (see survival rate for details) and showed a much larger difference between groups (MD: 28.60 [23.80, 33.41], *n* = 50). When this study was removed in the sensitivity analysis, the pooled result for FOLFOX4 as adjuvant chemotherapy after radical surgery (two RCTs) was significant without heterogeneity (MD: 4.42 [1.93. 6.91], I^2 = 0%, *n* = 75). Further sensitivity analyses were not conducted since clear criteria were not evident. Significant increases were evident in the single studies of FOLFOX6, FOLFOX and OLF. The pooled result for similar chemotherapies was similar to that for the total FOLFOX4 pool with considerable heterogeneity (MD: 10.67 [6.71, 14.63], I^2 = 95.5%).

In the single study (H116) of simplified bi-weekly infusional 5-FU/LV (six times within 12 weeks) as adjuvant chemotherapy for people with stage II/III rectal cancer (*n* = 83) after radical surgery, which used the authors' formula *Fu zheng gu yuan tang* 扶正固元汤 (*huang qi* 黄芪, *dang shen* 党参, *e zhu* 莪术, *ji xue teng* 鸡血藤, *bie jia* 鳖甲, *zi cao* 紫草, *ling zhi* 灵芝, *chuan xiong* 川芎, *zang hong hua* 藏红花, *shan yu rou* 山萸肉, *bai zhu* 白术, *fu ling* 茯苓 and *yi yi ren* 薏苡仁) one packet per day as two doses for 12 weeks, there was a significant reduction in CD3+ cell percentage (MD: –12.50 [–13.93, –11.07]).

For the five RCTs that employed XELOX without surgery, there was a significant increase in the combination therapy groups (MD: 10.81 [5.06, 16.56], I^2 = 93.8%) with considerable heterogeneity, but there was no clear basis for sensitivity analyses. The pooled result for all studies was similar to that for FOLFOX4 and the heterogeneity remained considerable.

CD4+ Cells

For percentage of CD4+ cells (Table 5.34), the pooled result for nine studies of FOLFOX4 found a significant but heterogeneous result (MD: 6.55 [3.62, 9.48], I^2 = 94.7%). In the subgroup of three studies of FOLFOX4 as adjuvant chemotherapy after radical surgery the result remained significant without heterogeneity (MD: 7.30 [5.20, 9.40], I^2 = 0%) and there was a similar result when the study of laparoscopic surgery (H98) was removed (MD: 6.62 [4.14, 9.10], I^2 = 0%, *n* = 75).

Table 5.34 Oral Chinese Herbal Medicine plus Chemotherapy versus Chemotherapy: CD4+ cells (%)

Chemotherapy Regimen[1]	N Studies (N Participants)	Effect Size (MD [95% CI]), I^2	Included Studies
FOLFOX4 (all)	9 (594)	6.55 [3.62, 9.48]*, 94.7%	H47, H49, H68, H82, H84, H98, H100, H104, H117
FOLFOX4 (adjuvant, after radical surgery)	3 (125)	7.30 [5.20, 9.40]*, 0%	H47, H98, H104
FOLFOX6	1 (30)	10.40 [5.08, 15.72]*	H58
mFOLFOX6	1 (60)	8.31 [5.69, 10.93]*	H119
FOLFOX	1 (62)	3.26 [1.42, 5.10]*	H71
OLF	1 (40)	3.04 [1.23, 4.85]*	H53
Pool for similar chemotherapy[2]	13 (786)	6.36 [4.06, 8.65]*, 93.8%	H47, H49, H53, H58, H68, H71, H82, H84, H98, H100, H104, H117
LF	1 (60)	0.93 [–2.35, 4.21]	H118
Simplified bi-weekly infusional 5-FU/LV	1 (83)	9.40 [8.22, 10.59]*	H116
XELOX (all no surgery)	6 (415)	6.26 [4.15, 8.38]*, 78.8%	H45, H75–H77, H94, H115
FOLFIRI	1 (55)	2.94 [1.09, 4.79]*	H72
Total pool	22 (1399)	6.08 [4.54, 7.63]*, 92.1%	All above

[1]Comparator was the same chemotherapy.

[2]These chemotherapy regimens all use oxaliplatin, 5-FU plus LV.

*Statistically significant.

Abbreviations: CI, confidence interval; LF, leucovorin and 5-fluorouracil; MD, mean difference; N, number.

In the single studies of FOLFOX6, mFOLFOX6, FOLFOX and OLF there were significant increases in percentages of CD4+ cells in the combination therapy groups. The pooled result for the subgroup of similar chemotherapies produced a similar result to the FOLFOX4 pool. In the six studies that used XELOX without surgery, there was a significant increase in the combined groups (MD: 6.26 [4.15, 8.38], I^2 = 78.8%) with considerable heterogeneity, but sensitivity analyses were not feasible. In the single study of LF (H118), there was no difference between groups but there were significant differences in the single studies of simplified bi-weekly infusional 5-FU/LV (H116) and FOLFIRI (H72). The pooled result for all 22 studies showed a significant increase in CD4+ percentage in the combined therapy groups (MD: 6.08 [4.54, 7.63], I^2 = 92.1%) with considerable heterogeneity.

CD8+ Cells

For CD8+ cells (%), the results were mixed with increases in some studies and reductions in others (Table 5.35). For the pool of nine studies of FOLFOX4, there was no significant difference between groups (MD: 0.46 [–4.52, 5.45], I^2 = 98.4%) with considerable heterogeneity. There was a similar result in the subgroup of three studies of FOLFOX4 as adjuvant chemotherapy after radical surgery (MD: 0.39 [–3.83, 4.62], I^2 = 84.1%) with considerable heterogeneity, which could not be resolved by sensitivity analysis. The pooled result for 12 studies that used similar chemotherapy also showed no difference between groups with considerable heterogeneity (MD: –0.31 [–4.46, 3.84], I^2 = 98.2%). For the five studies of XELOX without surgery, three studies showed significant reductions in the percentage of CD8+ cells in the combination therapy groups and the pooled result showed a significant reduction (MD: –2.48 [–4.05, –0.91], I^2 = 69.4%) with substantial heterogeneity. There was a significant reduction in the study of LF (H118), but there was a significant increase in the study of simplified bi-weekly infusional 5-FU/LV (H116). In the pooled result for all 19 RCTs, there was no difference between groups (MD: –1.28 [–4.30, 1.73], I^2 = 98.2%), but heterogeneity was considerable.

Ratio of CD4+/CD8+ Cells

For the ratio of CD4+/CD8+ (Table 5.36), the pooled result for all eight studies of FOLFOX4 found a significant increase (MD: 0.28 [0.12, 0.44], I^2 = 87.3%) in the combination therapy groups. In the subgroup

Table 5.35 Oral Chinese Herbal Medicine plus Chemotherapy versus Chemotherapy: CD8+ Cells (%)

Chemotherapy Regimen[1]	N Studies (N Participants)	Effect Size (MD [95% CI]), I^2	Included Studies
FOLFOX4 (all)	9 (594)	0.46 [–4.52, 5.45], 98.4%	H47, H49, H68, H82, H84, H98, H100, H104, H117
FOLFOX4 (adjuvant, after radical surgery)	3 (125)	0.39 [–3.83, 4.62], 84.1%	H47, H98, H104
mFOLFOX6	1 (60)	–0.97 [–5.66, 3.71]	H119
FOLFOX	1 (62)	–2.73 [–4.87, –0.59]*	H71
OLF	1 (40)	–1.23 [–3.18, 0.72]	H53
Pool for similar chemotherapy[2]	12 (756)	–0.31 [–4.46, 3.84], 98.2%	H47, H49, H53, H68, H71, H82, H84, H98, H100, H104, H117
LF	1 (60)	–10.28 [–11.91, –8.65]*	H118
Simplified bi-weekly infusional 5-FU/LV	1 (83)	1.90 [0.89, 2.91]*	H116
XELOX (all no surgery)	5 (353)	–2.48 [–4.05, –0.91]*, 9.4%	H45, H75–H77, H94
Total pool	19 (1252)	–1.28 [–4.30, 1.73] 98.2%	All above

[1]Comparator was the same chemotherapy.

[2]These chemotherapy regimens all use oxaliplatin, 5-FU plus LV.

*Statistically significant.

Abbreviations: CI, confidence interval; LF, leucovorin and 5-fluorouracil; MD, mean difference; N, number.

of three studies of FOLFOX4 as adjuvant chemotherapy after radical surgery, the result was similar with greatly reduced heterogeneity (MD: 0.35 [0.18, 0.52], I^2 = 8.8%) and the sensitivity analysis, which removed one study (H49) of colon cancer, found a similar result (MD: 0.41 [0.25, 0.57], I^2 = 0%, n = 75). The single studies of FOLFOX6 and OLF found significant increases. The pooled result for the subgroup of

Table 5.36 Oral Chinese Herbal Medicine plus Chemotherapy versus Chemotherapy: Ratio of CD4+/CD8+ Cells

Chemotherapy Regimen[1]	N Studies (N Participants)	Effect Size (MD [95% CI]), I^2	Included Studies
FOLFOX4 (all)	8 (483)	0.28 [0.12, 0.44]*, 87.3%	H47, H49, H64, H68, H98, H100, H104, H117
FOLFOX4 (adjuvant, after radical surgery)	3 (125)	0.35 [0.18, 0.52]*, 8.8%	H47, H98, H104
FOLFOX6	1 (30)	0.59 [0.13, 1.05]*	H58
OLF	1 (40)	0.15 [0.07, 0.23]*	H53
Pool for similar chemotherapy[2]	10 (553)	0.28 [0.15, 0.40]*, 84.6%	H47, H49, H53, H58, H64, H68, H98, H100, H104, H117
LF	1 (60)	0.36 [0.30, 0.42]*	H118
Simplified bi-weekly infusional 5-FU/LV	1 (83)	0.31 [0.19, 0.43]*	H116
XELOX (all no surgery)	4 (289)	0.35 [0.15, 0.55]*, 73.2%	H45, H75, H76, H94
FOLFIRI	1 (55)	0.14 [0.04, 0.24]*	H72
XELODA	1 (142)	0.51 [0.27, 0.75]*	H40
HIPEC	1 (104)	0.32 [0.23, 0.41]*	H57
Total pool	19 (1286)	0.30 [0.22, 0.38]*, 84.8%	All above

[1]Comparator was the same chemotherapy.

[2]These chemotherapy regimens all use oxaliplatin, 5-FU plus LV.

*Statistically significant.

Abbreviations: CI, confidence interval; HIPEC: hyperthermic intraperitoneal chemotherapy; LF, leucovorin and 5-fluorouracil; MD, mean difference; N, number.

ten studies that used similar chemotherapy was very similar to that for the pool of all FOLFOX4 (MD: 0.28 [0.15, 0.40], I^2 = 84.6%). The pooled result for four studies of XELOX without surgery showed a significant increase (MD: 0.35 [0.15, 0.55], I^2 = 73.2%), but the heterogeneity was substantial since one study (H45) showed no difference between groups. There were significant increases in all the single studies of FOLFIRI, LF, simplified bi-weekly infusional 5-FU/LV, XELODA and HIPEC. The pooled result for all 19 RCTs showed a significant increase in the ratio CD4+/CD8+ cells (MD: 0.30 [0.22, 0.38], I^2 = 84.8%) but the heterogeneity was considerable.

Natural Killer Cells

For NK cells (%) (Table 5.37), the pooled result for all seven studies of FOLFOX4 found a significant percentage increase (MD: 9.65 [7.66,

Table 5.37 Oral Chinese Herbal Medicine plus Chemotherapy versus Chemotherapy: Natural Killer Cells (%)

Chemotherapy Regimen[1]	N Studies (N Participants)	Effect Size (MD [95% CI]), I^2	Included Studies
FOLFOX4 (all)	7 (507)	9.65 [7.66, 11.63]*, 79.5%	H47, H65, H70, H82, H84, H98, H100
FOLFOX4 (adjuvant, after radical surgery)	2 (95)	14.34 [6.62, 22.06]*, 90.3%	H47, H98
FOLFOX6	1 (30)	1.71 [–2.71, 6.13]	H58
FOLFOX	1 (62)	2.16 [0.29, 4.04]*	H71
OLF	2 (89)	4.44 [–0.11, 8.99] 88.5%	H52, H53
Pool for similar chemotherapy[2]	11 (688)	7.37 [5.09, 9.64]*, 91%	H47, H52, H53, H58, H65, H70, H71, H82, H84, H98, H100
XELOX (all no surgery)	3 (240)	3.88 [2.50, 5.26]*, 0%	H75–H77
FOLFIRI	1 (55)	4.83 [2.68, 6.98]*	H72
XELODA	1 (142)	5.10 [2.50, 7.70]*	H40
HIPEC	1 (104)	9.40 [6.04, 12.76]*	H57
Total pool	17 (1,229)	6.56 [4.87, 8.26]*, 88.9%	All above

[1]Comparator was the same chemotherapy.

[2]These chemotherapy regimens all use oxaliplatin, 5-FU plus LV.

*Statistically significant.

Abbreviations: CI, confidence interval; HIPEC: hyperthermic intraperitoneal chemotherapy; MD, mean difference; N, number.

11.63], I^2 = 79.5%) with considerable heterogeneity. The heterogeneity was even higher in the subgroup of two studies of FOLFOX4 as adjuvant chemotherapy after radical surgery (H47, H98), although both studies showed significant increases. There was no difference between groups in the single study of FOLFOX6 (H58) and one of the studies of OLF (H53). The result for the 11 studies of similar chemotherapy showed a significant improvement (MD: 7.37 [5.09, 9.64], I^2 = 91%) with considerable heterogeneity. The pooled result for the three studies of XELOX without surgery showed a significant increase in the percentage of NK cells (MD: 3.88 [2.50, 5.26], I^2 = 0%) without heterogeneity, and the single studies of FOLFIRI, XELODA and HIPEC all showed significant increases. For all 17 RCTs, the total pooled result showed a significant increase in NK cells in the combined therapy groups, compared to controls (MD: 6.56 [4.87, 8.26], I^2 = 88.9%), but the heterogeneity was considerable.

The single study that used ITT analysis (H61) also reported data on T cells (a type of lymphocyte). There was a significant increase in CD4+ cells in the CHM plus FOLFOX4 group (MD: 8.02 [4.85, 11.19] %, n = 76), and no differences between groups for CD8+ cells (MD: 1.61 [–2.28, 5.50] %, n = 76), the ratio of CD4+/CD8+ cells (MD: 0.21 [–0.03, 0.45], n = 76) or for NK cells (MD: 1.35 [–3.17, 5.87] %, n = 76).

CD8+ CD28+ T Cells

In the single RCT of 62 people with advanced CRC that reported the percentage of CD8+ CD28+ T cells (H115) there was a significant increase in the combined therapy group (MD: 6.52 [5.11, 7.93] %, n = 62) which received XELOX (two 3-week cycles) without surgery plus a formula made by the authors called *Teng long bu zhong tang* 藤龙补中汤 (*teng li gen* 藤梨根, *long kui* 龙葵, *she mei* 蛇莓, *bai zhu* 白术, *fu ling* 茯苓, *yi yi ren* 薏苡仁, *ban zhi lian* 半枝莲 and *xie ji sheng* 槲寄生) one packet a day as two doses for six weeks.

Immunoglobulins

In the two studies (H47, H100) that reported on immunoglobulins, there were no differences between groups for IgA (MD: –0.11 [–0.32,

Table 5.38 Oral Chinese Herbal Medicine plus Chemotherapy versus Chemotherapy: Immunoglobulins

Immunoglobulins[1]	*N* Studies (*N* Participants)	Effect Size (MD [95% CI]), I^2	Included Studies
IgA (g/L)	2 (95)	–0.11 [–0.32, 0.10] 0%	H47, H100
IgG (g/L)	2 (95)	1.65 [–0.13, 3.43] 54%	H47, H100
IgM (g/L)	2 (95)	0.52 [0.27, 0.78]*, 0%	H47, H100
IgE (mg/L)	1 (45)	0.03 [–0.08, 0.14]	H47

[1]Comparator was the same chemotherapy.

*Statistically significant.

Abbreviations: CI, Confidence Interval, Ig, Immunoglobulin; MD, mean difference; N, number.

0.10], I^2 = 0%), IgG (MD: 1.65 [–0.13, 3.43], I^2 = 54%) or IgE (MD: 0.03 [–0.08, 0.14]), but there was a significant increase in IgM (MD: 0.52 [0.27, 0.78], I^2 = 0%) (Table 5.38).

Chemotherapy-related Adverse Events

In total, 77 RCTs reported on chemotherapy-related AEs; however, two studies (H59, H82) reported number of events rather than number of participants who experienced the event. In three RCTs (H51, H102, H113) there was insufficient detail for the data to be usable and there was a data error in one study (H52), so the data from these studies were not suitable for pooling. Eight RCTs (H35, H46, H50, H57, H62, H64, H97, H119) did not specify which criteria were used, so these were pooled separately for all grades only (since the criteria for grade III and grade IV may be different, whereas all grades were consistent across criteria). Therefore, 71 RCTs were included in the meta-analysis. One study (H61) that reported data as ITT is reported separately. The chemotherapy-related AEs are reported under the following categories:

- Nausea/vomiting (CINV): 52 RCTs;
- Diarrhoea: 44 RCTs;
- Constipation: 2 RCTs;

- Gastrointestinal reactions: 4 RCTs;
- Myelosuppression: 61 RCTs, but one RCT (H74) had a data error in the results table, and one study (H117) only reported one number for grades II and above, so these were excluded from the meta-analysis, which included 59 RCTs;
- Chemotherapy-induced peripheral neurotoxicity (CIPN): 41 RCTs;
- Hand-foot syndrome (HFS): 9 RCTs;
- Fatigue: 4 RCTs;
- Hepatotoxicity or/and nephrotoxicity: 32 RCTs;
- Abnormal heart function: 3 RCTs;
- Oral mucositis: 12 RCTs;
- Fever: 4 RCTs;
- Alopecia: 4 RCTs;
- Skin rash: 2 RCTs.

Nausea and/or Vomiting

Fifty-two RCTs reported data on chemotherapy-induced nausea and vomiting (CINV). Of these, 41 RCTs used the WHO criteria, five RCTs used the National Cancer Institute-Common Terminology Criteria for Adverse Events (NCI-CTCAE) and six RCTs did not specify the criteria. These six were analysed separately for all grades only.

For combined grade III plus IV, according to the WHO criteria, data were available for 35 RCTs. However, when there were zero events in both groups, meta-analysis was not feasible. Since 13 studies reported zero events in both groups, only 22 RCTs contributed to the pooled meta-analysis results. The total number of studies including those with zero events is noted in column one of Table 5.39 and column two shows the number of studies in the meta-analysis.

In studies that combined a CHM with FOLFOX4, there was a significant reduction in grade III and IV CINV in the combination therapy groups (RR: 0.33 [0.14, 0.79], I^2 = 0%). There was no difference between groups for FOLFOX6, mFOLFOX6, FOLFOX and OLF. For the subgroup of similar chemotherapies, there was a significant reduction in the CHM plus chemotherapy groups (RR: 0.43 [0.26, 0.71], I^2 = 0%). There was a significant reduction in the CHM plus

Table 5.39 Oral Chinese Herbal Medicine plus Chemotherapy versus Chemotherapy: Chemotherapy-induced Nausea and Vomiting (WHO Grade III+IV)

Chemotherapy Regimen:[1] *N* Studies (*N* Participants); *N* Studies with 0 Events in Both Groups	*N* Studies (*N* Participants) in Meta-analysis	Effect Size (RR [95% CI]), I^2	Included Studies (Studies with 0 Events in Both Groups)
FOLFOX4: 14 (854); 9	5 (258)	0.33 [0.14, 0.79]*, 0%	H47, H54, H66, H67, H85 (H41, H65, H70, H99, H100, H104, H107, H110, H112)
FOLFOX6: 2 (136); 0	2 (136)	0.67 [0.09, 5.12], 39.4%	H44, H86
mFOLFOX6: 2 (129); 0	2 (129)	0.43 [0.14, 1.36], 22.3%	H63, H87
FOLFOX: 1 (62); 0	1 (62)	0.50 [0.17, 1.49]	H71
OLF: 1 (40); 0	1 (40)	0.20 [0.01, 3.92]	H53
Pool for similar chemotherapy[2]: 20 (1221); 9	11 (625)	0.43 [0.26, 0.71]*, 0%	H44, H47, H53, H54, H63, H66, H67, H71, H85, H87 (H41, H65, H70, H99, H100, H104, H107, H110, H112)
XELOX: 8 (413); 2	6 (313)	0.31 [0.16, 0.62]*, 0%	H60, H74, H75, H92–H94 (H83, H114)
FOLFIRI: 3 (159); 0	3 (159)	0.60 [0.26, 1.42] 28.1%	H72, H88, H89
LF: 1 (60); 1	0 (0)	Both groups = 0 events	(H118)
S1+oxaliplatin: 1 (66); 0	1 (66)	0.33 [0.04, 3.04]	H101
XELIRI: 2 (66); 1	1 (36)	0.22 [0.01, 4.33]	H78 (H79)
Total pool: 35 (2045); 13	22 (1,199)	0.42 [0.30, 0.60]*, 0%	All above

[1]Comparator was the same chemotherapy.

[2]These chemotherapy regimens all use oxaliplatin, 5-FU plus LV.

*Statistically significant.

Abbreviations: CI, Confidence Interval; LF, leucovorin and 5-fluorouracil; N, number; RR, risk ratio; WHO, World Health Organisation.

XELOX groups (RR: 0.31 [0.16, 0.62], I^2 = 0%) but no difference between groups for the other chemotherapies. The total pool of 22 RCTs found a significant reduction in grade III and IV CINV in the CHM plus chemotherapy groups without heterogeneity (RR: 0.42 [0.30, 0.60], I^2 = 0%).

For all grades of CINV (WHO grades I to IV), there were significant reductions in the total FOLFOX4 group (RR: 0.64 [0.42, 0.97], I^2 = 91%) (Table 5.40). The considerable heterogeneity was due to one study (H66) that reported that all participants had at least grade I nausea and vomiting. When this study was removed from the pool, the result was similar but with greatly reduced heterogeneity (RR: 0.66 [0.55, 0.78], I^2 = 4.9%, n = 794). A similar result was found in the subgroup of studies of FOLFOX4 as adjuvant chemotherapy after radical surgery (RR: 0.51 [0.37, 0.71], I^2 = 0%). There were no differences between groups for the studies of FOLFOX6 and mFOLFOX6, but the heterogeneity was substantial. There were significant reductions in the single studies of FOLFOX and OLF. For the pool of 20 RCTs that used similar chemotherapies, there was a significant reduction in all grades of CINV (RR: 0.69 [0.55, 0.85], I^2 = 93%) but the heterogeneity was considerable. The main cause of heterogeneity was the two studies (H63, H66) in which all participants had grade I or higher CINV. When removed from the pooled results for this subgroup, the significant reduction remained with reduced heterogeneity (RR: 0.68 [0.59, 0.78], I^2 = 21%, n = 1,086).

In the eight studies that used XELOX, there was a significant reduction in CINV (RR: 0.64 [0.50, 0.83], I^2 = 61.7%), which was also found in the subgroups for XELOX after surgery and XELOX without surgery. There were no differences between groups for XELODA, FOLFIRI, S1 plus oxaliplatin, and XELIRI. The total pool showed a significant reduction in the combination therapy groups (RR: 0.64 [0.54, 0.76], I^2 = 92%) but heterogeneity was considerable. When the two studies that reported CINV for all participants were removed from the pool, the heterogeneity was reduced while the result still showed a reduction in all grades of CINV in the CHM plus chemotherapy groups (RR: 0.64 [0.57, 0.73], I^2 = 59.4%).

Table 5.40 Oral Chinese Herbal Medicine plus Chemotherapy versus Chemotherapy: Chemotherapy-induced Nausea and Vomiting (WHO All Grades)

Chemotherapy Regimen[1]	N Studies (N Participants)	Effect Size (RR [95% CI], I^2)	Included Studies
FOLFOX4 (all)	14 (854)	0.64 [0.42, 0.97]*, 91%	H41, H47, H54, H65, H66, H67, H70, H85, H99, H100, H104, H107, H110, H112
FOLFOX4 (adjuvant, after radical surgery)	5 (309)	0.51 [0.37, 0.71]*, 0%	H47, H99, H104, H107, H110
FOLFOX6	2 (136)	0.77 [0.44, 1.35], 72.5%	H44, H86
mFOLFOX6	2 (129)	0.83 [0.32, 2.15], 96%	H63, H87
FOLFOX	1 (62)	0.67 [0.45, 0.98]*	H71
OLF	1 (40)	0.53 [0.32, 0.89]*	H53
Pool for similar chemotherapy[2]	20 (1,221)	0.69 [0.55, 0.85]*, 93%	H41, H44, H47, H53, H54, H63, H65, H66, H67, H70, H71, H85–H87, H99, H100, H104, H107, H110, H112
XELOX (all)	8 (413)	0.64 [0.50, 0.83]*, 61.7%	H60, H74, H75, H83, H92–H94, H114
XELOX (after surgery)	2 (81)	0.51 [0.36, 0.72]*, 0%	H60, H114
XELOX (without surgery)	6 (332)	0.69 [0.51, 0.93]*, 63.3%	H74, H75, H83, H92–H94
XELODA	1 (60)	0.33 [0.04, 3.03]	H95
FOLFIRI	4 (209)	0.61 [0.32, 1.16], 92.1%	H43, H72, H88, H89
LF	1 (60)	0.50 [0.28, 0.88]*	H118
S1+oxaliplatin	1 (66)	0.60 [0.35, 1.02]	H101
XELIRI	3 (121)	0.63 [0.30, 1.34], 61.9%	H78, H79, H96
HIPEC	1 (60)	0.39 [0.19, 0.79]*	H56
Total pool	39 (2,210)	0.64 [0.54, 0.76]*, 92%	All above
Sensitivity	37 (2,075)	0.64 [0.57, 0.73]*, 59.4%	Excluding H63, H66

[1]Comparator was the same chemotherapy.

[2]These chemotherapy regimens all use oxaliplatin, 5-FU plus LV.

*Statistically significant.

Abbreviations: CI, confidence interval; HIPEC, hyperthermic intraperitoneal chemotherapy; LF, leucovorin and 5-fluorouracil; N, number; RR, risk ratio; WHO, World Health Organisation.

Two RCTs (H68, H111) reported separate data on vomiting. For WHO grade III plus IV vomiting, one study (H111) of people with stage II/III/IV CRC who received FOLFOX4 after surgery reported zero events in both groups, while there was a significant reduction in all grades in the combination therapy group (RR: 0.48 [0.33, 0.70], $n = 85$). In the other study (H68) of FOLFOX4 in people with advanced CRC without surgery, there was an increase in grade III plus IV vomiting in the combination therapy group (RR: 2.33 [1.01, 5.37], $n = 70$), but no difference between groups for all grades since all participants had grade I vomiting or higher. This study (H68) also reported separate data for nausea. WHO grade III plus IV nausea was significantly increased in the combination therapy group (RR 2.80 [1.13, 6.94], $n = 70$). For all grades, all participants experienced at least grade I nausea and there was no difference between groups.

Five RCTs reported CINV using the NCI-CTCAE criteria. The single study that used ITT analysis (H61) was not pooled with the others. For grade III plus IV events, each study used a different chemotherapy (FOLFOX6, mFOLFOX, XELOX). There were no differences between groups for the individual studies, but the pooled result showed a significant reduction in the combination therapy groups (RR: 0.24 [0.07, 0.78], I^2 = 0%). For all grades, there were significant reductions in two studies (H58, H103), but no differences in the others. The pooled result showed no difference between groups (RR: 0.56 [0.24, 1.29], I^2 = 88.9%) with considerable heterogeneity (Table 5.41).

In the single study that used ITT analysis (H61) all 80 participants received FOLFOX4 for stage II CRC as adjuvant chemotherapy, or stage III/IV as adjuvant or palliative chemotherapy for CRC. For NCI-CTCAE grade III plus IV there was no difference between groups (RR: 0.50 [0.05, 5.29], $n = 76$). There was a significant reduction in the combination therapy group for all grades of CINV (RR: 0.53 [0.28, 0.98], $n = 76$).

In the six RCTs (H46, H50, H57, H62, H64, H119) that did not specify whether WHO or NCI-CTCAE criteria were used, five studies (of FOLFOX4, mFOLFOX6, FOLFIRI or HIPEC) reported nausea and vomiting and one (H64) reported only vomiting. For all grades of CINV there was a significant reduction in the combination therapy

Table 5.41 Oral Chinese Herbal Medicine plus Chemotherapy versus Chemotherapy: Chemotherapy-induced Nausea and Vomiting (NCI-CTCAE)

Chemotherapy Regimen[1]	*N* Studies (*N* Participants)	Effect Size (RR [95% CI]), I^2	Included Studies
Grade III+IV			
FOLFOX6	1 (30)	0.14 [0.01, 2.55]	H58
mFOLFOX6	1 (41)	0.32 [0.01, 7.38]	H103
XELOX	1 (60)	0.25 [0.06, 1.08]	H42
Total pool	3 (131)	0.24 [0.07, 0.78]*, 0%	H42, H58, H103
All grades			
FOLFOX6	1 (30)	0.40 [0.16, 0.996]*	H58
mFOLFOX6	1 (41)	0.40 [0.17, 0.92]*	H103
XELOX	2 (122)	0.74 [0.33, 1.67], 85.9%	H42, H90
Total pool	4 (193)	0.56 [0.24, 1.29], 88.9%	H42, H58, H90, H103

[1]Comparator was the same chemotherapy.

*Statistically significant.

Abbreviations: CI, confidence interval; N, number; NCI-CTCAE, National Cancer Institute-Common Terminology Criteria for Adverse Events; RR, risk ratio.

groups (RR: 0.61 [0.48, 0.78], I^2 = 0%, *n* = 379). In the single study that reported data on vomiting, there were five cases in the FOLFOX4 alone group and zero cases in the combination therapy group (RR: 11.34 [0.65, 196.88], *n* = 63) which was not a significant difference.

Diarrhoea

In the 44 RCTs that reported data for chemotherapy-related diarrhea, 31 used the WHO criteria, seven used the NCI-CTCAE criteria, six did not specify the criteria used and one study (H120) also reported mean duration of diarrhoea.

In total, 27 studies reported data for WHO grade III plus IV events, but eight studies had zero events in both groups (seven of

Table 5.42 Oral Chinese Herbal Medicine plus Chemotherapy versus Chemotherapy: Chemotherapy-related Diarrhoea (WHO Grade III+IV)

Chemotherapy Regimen:[1] N Studies (N Participants); N Studies with 0 Events in Both Groups	N Studies (N Participants) in Meta-analysis	Effect Size (RR [95% CI]), I^2	Included Studies (Studies with 0 Events in Both Groups)
FOLFOX4: 12 (759); 7	5 (332)	0.49 [0.17, 1.41], 0%	H65, H70, H85, H107, H112 (H47, H54, H67, H99, H100, H104, H111)
FOLFOX6: 2 (136); 0	2 (136)	0.52 [0.09, 2.87], 0%	H44, H86
mFOLFOX6: 1 (54); 0	1 (54)	0.20 [0.01, 3.98]	H87
FOLFOX: 1 (62); 0	1 (62)	0.40 [0.08, 1.91]	H71
Pool for similar chemotherapy[2]: 16 (1011); 7	9 (584)	0.44 [0.21, 0.95]*, 0%	H44, H65, H70, H71, H85–H87, H107, H112 (H47, H54, H67, H99, H100, H104, H111)
XELOX: 5 (264); 0	5 (264)	0.28 [0.08, 0.99]*, 0%	H60, H75, H92–H94
FOLFIRI: 2 (104); 0	2 (104)	0.16 [0.03, 0.88]*, 0%	H88, H89
LF: 1 (60); 1	0 (0)	Both groups = 0 events	(H118)
S1+oxaliplatin: 1 (66); 0	1 (66)	1.00 [0.15, 6.68]	H101
XELIRI: 2 (66); 0	2 (66)	0.44 [0.08, 2.25], 0%	H78, H79
Total pool: 27 (1,571); 8	19 (1084)	0.39 [0.23, 0.68]*, 0%	All above

[1]Comparator was the same chemotherapy.

[2]These chemotherapy regimens all use oxaliplatin, 5-FU plus LV.

*Statistically significant.

Abbreviations: CI, confidence interval; LF, leucovorin and 5-fluorouracil; N, number; RR, risk ratio; WHO, World Health Organisation.

FOLFOX4, one of LF), so they could not be included in the meta-analysis pools (Table 5.42). For FOLFOX4 the pooled result for five RCTs found no significant difference between groups (RR: 0.49 [0.17, 1.41], I^2 = 0%) and there was a similar result for the two studies of FOLFOX6 (RR: 0.52 [0.09, 2.87], I^2 = 0%). However, in the subgroup of nine RCTs of similar chemotherapies there was a significant difference between groups in favour of the combined therapy groups (RR: 0.44 [0.21, 0.95], I^2 = 0%). In the five studies of XELOX there was a significant reduction in incidence of diarrhoea in the

CHM plus XELOX groups (RR: 0.28 [0.08, 0.99], I^2 = 0%), and also in the two studies of CHM plus FOLFIRI (RR: 0.16 [0.03, 0.88], I^2 = 0%). There was no difference between groups in the two studies of XELIRI (RR: 0.44 [0.08, 2.25], I^2 = 0%). The pooled results for 19 RCTs showed a significant reduction in diarrhoea in the CHM plus chemotherapy groups (RR: 0.39 [0.23, 0.68], I^2 = 0%) without heterogeneity.

For all WHO grades (Table 5.43), there was a significant reduction in incidence of chemotherapy-related diarrhoea in the pool of 12 RCTs of CHM plus FOLFOX4 (RR: 0.65 [0.51, 0.83], I^2 = 0%). The result was similar in the subgroup of four RCTs in which FOLFOX4 was an adjuvant chemotherapy after radical surgery (RR: 0.48 [0.32, 0.73], I^2 = 0%), but there was no difference between groups in the two studies of FOLFOX6 (RR: 0.91 [0.72, 1.16], I^2 = 0%). In the pooled result for 16 studies of similar chemotherapies there was a significant reduction in diarrhoea in the CHM plus chemotherapy groups (RR: 0.73 [0.62, 0.86], I^2 = 3.1%).

The five RCTs of XELOX showed a significant benefit for the CHM plus XELOX groups (RR: 0.52 [0.38, 0.70], I^2 = 0%) with a similar result for the subgroup of four RCTs of XELOX without surgery (RR: 0.46 [0.31, 0.70], I^2 = 0%). The pooled result for three studies of XELIRI showed a significant benefit for the CHM plus XELIRI groups (RR: 0.66 [0.46, 0.95], I^2 = 0%), but there was no difference in the three studies of FOLFIRI (RR: 0.51 [0.15, 1.70], I^2 = 93.3%) with considerable heterogeneity due to one study (H89) that had equally high incidences (16/18) in both groups. The total pooled result for 31 RCTs showed a significant reduction in chemotherapy-related diarrhoea in the combination therapy groups (RR: 0.64 [0.55, 0.74], I^2 = 36.7%) with moderate heterogeneity.

Six RCTs reported results for chemotherapy-related diarrhoea using the NCI-CTCAE criteria. Five of these studies reported data for grade III plus IV events, but there were zero events in both groups in one study (H103) (Table 5.44). For the pool of four studies, there was no significant difference between groups (RR: 0.33 [0.10, 1.10], I^2 = 0%). For all grades, there was no difference in the three studies of

Table 5.43 Oral Chinese Herbal Medicine plus Chemotherapy versus Chemotherapy: Chemotherapy-related Diarrhoea (WHO All Grades)

Chemotherapy Regimen[1]	N Studies (N Participants)	Effect Size (RR [95% CI]), I^2	Included Studies
FOLFOX4 (all)	12 (759)	0.65 [0.51, 0.83]*, 0%	H47, H54, H65, H67, H70, H85, H99, H100, H104, H107, H111, H112
FOLFOX4 (adjuvant, after radical surgery)	4 (249)	0.48 [0.32, 0.73]*, 0%	H47, H99, H104, H107
FOLFOX6	2 (136)	0.91 [0.72, 1.16], 0%	H44, H86
mFOLFOX6	1 (54)	0.63 [0.35, 1.12]	H87
FOLFOX	1 (62)	0.50 [0.25, 0.99]*	H71
Pool for similar chemotherapy[2]	16 (1,011)	0.73 [0.62, 0.86]*, 3.1%	H44, H47, H54, H65, H67, H70, H71, H85–H87, H99, H100, H104, H107, H111, H112
XELOX (all)	5 (264)	0.52 [0.38, 0.70]*, 0%	H60, H75, H92–H94
XELOX (after surgery)	1 (41)	0.58 [0.38, 0.90]*	H60
XELOX (without surgery)	4 (223)	0.46 [0.31, 0.70]*, 0%	H75, H92–H94
XELODA	1 (60)	0.20 [0.01, 4.00]	H95
FOLFIRI	3 (154)	0.51 [0.15, 1.70], 93.3%	H43, H88, H89
LF	1 (60)	0.62 [0.30, 1.27]	H118
S1+oxaliplatin	1 (66)	0.55 [0.23, 1.30]	H101
XELIRI	3 (121)	0.66 [0.46, 0.95]*, 0%	H78, H79, H96
HIPEC	1 (60)	0.93 [0.53, 1.63]	H56
Total pool	31 (1,796)	0.64 [0.55, 0.74]*, 36.7%	All above

[1]Comparator was the same chemotherapy.

[2]These chemotherapy regimens all use oxaliplatin, 5-FU plus LV.

*Statistically significant.

Abbreviations: CI, confidence interval; HIPEC: hyperthermic intraperitoneal chemotherapy; LF, leucovorin and 5-fluorouracil; N, number; RR, risk ratio; WHO, World Health Organisation.

Table 5.44 Oral Chinese Herbal Medicine plus Chemotherapy versus Chemotherapy: Chemotherapy-related Diarrhoea (NCI-CTCAE)

Chemotherapy Regimen[1]	N Studies (N Participants)	Effect Size (RR [95% CI]), I^2	Included Studies
Grade III+IV			
FOLFOX6	1 (30)	1.00 [0.07, 14.55]	H58
mFOLFOX6	1 (41)	Both groups = 0 events	H103
FOLFIRI	1 (44)	0.33 [0.04, 2.96]	H120
XELOX	2 (157)	0.20 [0.04, 1.14], 0%	H42, H91
Total pool	4 (231)	0.33 [0.10, 1.10], 0%	H42, H58, H91, H120
All grades			
FOLFOX6	1 (30)	0.50 [0.15, 1.64]	H58
mFOLFOX6	1 (41)	0.48 [0.10, 2.32]	H103
FOLFIRI	1 (44)	0.50 [0.25, 1.00]	H120
XELOX	3 (219)	0.69 [0.41, 1.16], 34.6%	H42, H90, H91
Total pool	6 (334)	0.61 [0.44, 0.85]*, 0%	H42, H58, H90, H91, H103, H120

[1]Comparator was the same chemotherapy.

*Statistically significant.

Abbreviations: CI, confidence interval; N, number; NCI-CTCAE, National Cancer Institute-Common Terminology Criteria for Adverse Events; RR, risk ratio.

CHM plus XELOX (RR: 0.69 [0.41, 1.16], I^2 = 34.6%), but there was a significant improvement in the total pool (RR: 0.61 [0.44, 0.85], I^2 = 0%) in favour of the combination therapy groups.

In the single study that used ITT analysis (H61) for NCI-CTCAE criteria there was no difference between groups for grade III plus IV (RR: 0.33 [0.01, 7.93], n = 76) and the result was similar for all grades (RR 0.44 [0.15, 1.32], n = 76).

In the six RCTs (H46, H50, H57, H62, H64, H119) that did not specify whether WHO or NCI-CTCAE criteria were used, five studies (of FOLFOX4, mFOLFOX6, FOLFIRI or HIPEC) reported diarrhoea, and one (H119) reported abdominal distention and diarrhoea. For the five RCTs that reported on all grades of diarrhoea there was no difference between groups (RR: 0.73 [0.45, 1.16], I^2 = 23.9%, n = 382). In the single study of mFOLFOX6 for CRC following radical surgery that reported data on abdominal distention and diarrhoea, there was significant reduction in the CHM plus mFOLFOX6 groups (RR: 0.33 [0.12, 0.92], n = 60).

Another study (H120) also reported the duration of diarrhoea following FOLFIRI for stage IV CRC. The result showed there was a significant decrease in the combined group (MD: −2.22 [−4.19, −0.25] days, n = 44) which received *Huang qin tang* 黄芩汤 (*huang qin* 黄芩, *bai shao* 白芍, *gan cao* 甘草 and *da zao* 大枣) as a liquid (20 ml, three times per day) taken from one day before chemotherapy until the chemotherapy finished.

Constipation

Two studies reported data on chemotherapy-related constipation. One used the WHO criteria (H47) and the other used the NCI-CTCAE criteria (H103). For grades III plus IV, both studies had zero events in both groups. For all grades, there was no significant difference between groups in the study of FOLFOX4 as adjuvant chemotherapy (H47) after radical surgery for stage IIA to IIIC colon cancer using the WHO criteria (RR: 0.48 [0.13, 1.74], n = 55). Similarly, in the study of mFOLFOX6 for stage III/IV CRC (see QOL for details) there was no difference between groups for all grades of constipation based on the NCI-CTCAE criteria (RR: 0.95 [0.22, 4.18], n = 41).

Gastrointestinal Reactions

Four studies reported data for chemotherapy-related gastrointestinal reactions. Two studies used the WHO criteria and two used NCI-CTCAE (Table 5.45).

In the two studies of FOLFOX4 (H69, H80) that reported the WHO criteria, there was no difference between groups for grade III plus IV (RR: 0.69 [0.32, 1.49], I^2 = 0%) or for all grades (RR: 0.91 [0.81, 1.02], I^2 = 0%). For the two studies that used the NCI-CTCAE criteria (H91, H116), there was a reduction in grade III plus IV events

Table 5.45 Oral Chinese Herbal Medicine plus Chemotherapy versus Chemotherapy: Chemotherapy-related Gastrointestinal Reactions

Chemotherapy Regimen[1]	N Studies (N Participants)	Effect Size (RR [95% CI]), I^2	Included Studies
WHO grade III+IV			
FOLFOX4	2 (117)	0.69 [0.32, 1.49], 0%	H69, H80
WHO all grades			
FOLFOX4	2 (117)	0.91 [0.81, 1.02], 0%	H69, H80
NCI-CTCAE grade III+IV			
XELOX, advanced/recurrent stage IV CRC	1 (97)	0.33 [0.04, 3.03]	H91
Simplified bi-weekly infusional 5-FU/LV, rectal cancer	1 (83)	0.16 [0.05, 0.49]	H116
Total (NCI-CTCAE grade III+IV)	2 (180)	0.18 [0.07, 0.50]*, 0%	H91, H116
NCI-CTCAE all grades			
XELOX advanced/recurrent stage IV CRC	1 (97)	0.77 [0.60, 0.97]*	H91
Simplified bi-weekly infusional 5-FU/LV, rectal cancer	1 (83)	0.16 [0.05, 0.49]*	H116
Total (NCI-CTCAE all grades)	2 (180)	0.46 [0.15, 1.46], 93.9%	H91, H116

[1]Comparator was the same chemotherapy.

*Statistically significant.

Abbreviations: CI, confidence interval; CRC, colorectal cancer; N, number; NCI-CTCAE, National Cancer Institute-Common Terminology Criteria for Adverse Events; RR, risk ratio; WHO, World Health Organisation.

in the study of simplified bi-weekly infusional 5-FU/LV (H116) for stage II/III rectal cancer after radical surgery (RR: 0.16 [0.05, 0.49]) but there was no difference in the study of XELOX without surgery (H91) in advanced or recurrent stage IV CRC (RR: 0.33 [0.04, 3.03]). The pooled result for the two studies showed a significant reduction in grade III plus IV gastrointestinal reactions in the combination therapy groups (RR: 0.18 [0.07, 0.50], I^2 = 0%). For all NCI-CTCAE grades, there were significant reductions for the studies of simplified bi-weekly infusional 5-FU/LV (H116) and XELOX without surgery (H91), but there was no significant difference between groups in the pooled result (RR: 0.46 [0.15, 1.46] I^2 = 93.9%) with considerable heterogeneity.

Myelosuppression

Sixty-one RCTs reported data on chemotherapy-related myelosuppression. One RCT (H74) had a data error in the results table and one study (H117) only reported one number for grades II and above, so these were excluded from the meta-analysis. Forty-eight RCTs used WHO criteria, six RCTs used NCI-CTCAE criteria and five RCTs did not specify the criteria used. Because the content of the WHO and NCI-CTCAE criteria are the same for myelosuppression, these were pooled together. The single study that used ITT analysis (H61) was not pooled with the others. The results were separated as follows: leukocytes (43 RCTs), neutrophils (ten RCTs), red blood cells (six RCTs), haemoglobin (32 RCTs), platelets (44 RCTs) and myelosuppression (type not specified) (eight RCTs).

Leukocytes

Thirty-nine RCTs reported data for chemotherapy-related reduction in leukocytes (leukopenia) using the WHO or NCI-CTCAE criteria, but one study (H54) had a data error in the results table and was excluded from this meta-analysis. For grade III+IV, six RCTs reported zero events in both groups so the meta-analysis results were based on 29 studies (Table 5.46). The nine studies of FOLFOX4 showed reduced incidence of grade III+IV leukopenia (RR: 0.40 [0.17, 0.94], I^2 = 50.8%) in the CHM plus FOLFOX4 groups with moderate heterogeneity. There was no difference between groups in the pool of two studies of FOLFOX6 (RR: 0.31 [0.05, 1.89], I^2 = 0%). The pooled result for 14 studies that used similar chemotherapies found a significant reduction in grade III+IV leukopenia in the CHM plus chemotherapy groups (RR: 0.43 [0.25, 0.75], I^2 = 28.9%). In the eight studies of XELOX, there was a significant reduction in the combination

Table 5.46 Oral Chinese Herbal Medicine plus Chemotherapy versus Chemotherapy: Chemotherapy-related Leukopenia (Grade III+IV)

Chemotherapy Regimen:[1] N Studies (N Participants); N Studies with 0 Events in Both Groups	N Studies (N Participants) in Meta-analysis	Effect Size (RR [95% CI]), I^2	Included Studies (Studies with 0 Events in Both Groups)
FOLFOX4: 13 (727); 4	9 (497)	0.40 [0.17, 0.94]*, 50.8%	H65–H69, H80, H85, H107, H112 (H47, H104, H110, H111)
FOLFOX6: 2 (96); 0	2 (96)	0.31 [0.05, 1.89], 0%	H58, H86
mFOLFOX6: 2 (95); 1	1 (54)	0.31 [0.12, 0.82]*	H87 (H103)
FOLFOX: 1 (62); 0	1 (62)	0.50 [0.05, 5.23]	H71
OLF: 1 (40); 0	1 (40)	0.67 [0.12, 3.57]	H53
Pool for similar chemotherapy[2]: 19 (1020); 5	14 (749)	0.43 [0.25, 0.75]* 28.9%	H53, H58, H65–H69, H71, H80, H85–H87, H107, H112 (H47, H103, H104, H110, H111)
XELOX: 9 (542); 1	8 (502)	0.42 [0.22, 0.78]*, 0%	H75, H76, H83, H91–H94, H109 (H114)
FOLFIRI: 3 (159); 0	3 (159)	0.51 [0.25, 1.02], 0%	H72, H88, H89
LF: 1 (60); 0	1 (60)	0.40 [0.08, 1.90]	H118
S1+oxaliplatin: 1 (66); 0	1 (66)	0.50 [0.10, 2.55]	H101
XELIRI: 2 (66); 0	2 (66)	0.47 [0.07, 2.98], 0%	H78, H79
Total pool: 35 (1913); 6	29 (1, 602)	0.48 [0.35, 0.64]*, 0%	All above

[1]Comparator was the same chemotherapy.

[2]These chemotherapy regimens all use oxaliplatin, 5-FU plus LV.

*Statistically significant.

Abbreviations: CI, confidence interval; LF, leucovorin and 5-fluorouracil; N, number; RR, risk ratio.

therapy groups (RR: 0.42 [0.22, 0.78], I^2 = 0%) but there was no significant difference in the FOLFIRI or other subgroups. The total pool of 29 studies found a significant reduction in the CHM plus chemotherapy groups, compared to the groups that used chemotherapy alone (RR: 0.48 [0.35, 0.64], I^2 = 0%).

For all grades of chemotherapy-related leukopenia (Table 5.47), there was a significant reduction in the CHM plus FOLFOX4 groups

Table 5.47 Oral Chinese Herbal Medicine plus Chemotherapy versus Chemotherapy: Chemotherapy-related Leukopenia (All Grades)

Chemotherapy Regimen[1]	N Studies (N Participants)	Effect Size (RR [95% CI]), I^2	Included Studies
FOLFOX4 (all)	13 (727)	0.72 [0.59, 0.87]*, 49.7%	H47, H65–H69, H80, H85, H104, H107, H110–H112
FOLFOX4 (adjuvant, after radical surgery)	4 (175)	0.50 [0.27, 0.92]*, 61.7%	H47, H104, H107, H110
FOLFOX6	2 (96)	0.70 [0.34, 1.44], 61.4%	H58, H86
mFOLFOX6	3 (175)	0.75 [0.57, 0.99]*, 23.1%	H87, H103, H121
FOLFOX	1 (62)	0.43 [0.19, 0.97]*	H71
OLF	1 (40)	0.44 [0.23, 0.83]*	H53
Pool for similar chemotherapy[2]	20 (1,100)	0.71 [0.61, 0.82]*, 47.9%	H47, H53, H58, H65–H69, H71, H80, H85–H87, H103, H104, H107, H110–H112, H121
XELOX (all)	9 (542)	0.73 [0.62, 0.86]*, 35.9%	H75, H76, H83, H91–H94, H109, H114
XELOX (after surgery)	1 (40)	0.44 [0.16, 1.21]	H114
XELOX (without surgery)	8 (502)	0.74 [0.63, 0.87]*, 35.8%	H75, H76, H83, H91–H94, H109
FOLFIRI	4 (203)	0.73 [0.54, 0.98]*, 55.7%	H72, H88, H89, H120
LF	1 (60)	0.65 [0.43, 0.98]*	H118
S1+oxaliplatin	1 (66)	0.72 [0.50, 1.04]	H101
XELIRI	2 (66)	0.68 [0.45, 1.01], 0%	H78, H79
HIPEC	1 (60)	0.53 [0.30, 0.94]*	H56
Total pool	38 (2,097)	0.72 [0.65, 0.78]*, 37.3%	All above

[1]Comparator was the same chemotherapy.

[2]These chemotherapy regimens all use oxaliplatin, 5-FU plus LV.

*Statistically significant.

Abbreviations: CI, confidence interval; HIPEC: hyperthermic intraperitoneal chemotherapy; LF, leucovorin and 5-fluorouracil; N, number; RR, risk ratio.

(RR: 0.72 [0.59, 0.87], I^2 = 49.7%) with moderate heterogeneity based on 13 RCTs. The result was similar in the subgroup of four studies of FOLFOX4 as adjuvant chemotherapy after radical surgery (RR: 0.50 [0.27, 0.92], I^2 = 61.7%) and in the pool of three RCTs of mFOLFOX6 (RR: 0.75 [0.57, 0.99], I^2 = 23.1%). The pooled result for 20 studies that used similar chemotherapies found a significant reduction in all grades of leukopenia in the combination therapy groups (RR: 0.71 [0.61, 0.82], I^2 = 47.9%) with moderate heterogeneity. For XELOX, the pooled result from nine RCTs showed a significant reduction in the CHM plus XELOX groups (RR: 0.73 [0.62, 0.86], I^2 = 35.9%) and the result was similar in the pool of four studies of FOLFIRI (RR: 0.73 [0.54, 0.98], I^2 = 55.7%). In the total pool of 38 RCTs there was a significant reduction in all grades of chemotherapy-related leukopenia in the combination therapy groups (RR: 0.72 [0.65, 0.78], I^2 = 37.3%) with moderate heterogeneity.

A single study used ITT analysis (H61) and the NCI-CTCAE criteria. There was no difference between groups for grade III plus IV leukopenia (RR: 0.33 [0.01, 7.93], n = 76) and the result was similar for all grades (RR: 0.47 [0.22, 1.01], n = 76). In addition, three RCTs (H46, H50, H57) did not mention which criteria were used. Each used a different chemotherapy (FOLFOX4, FOLFIRI, HIPEC, respectively). For all grades, there was no difference between groups for each study separately, but the pooled result showed a significant reduction in leukopenia in the CHM plus chemotherapy groups (RR: 0.61 [0.44, 0.85], I^2 = 0%, n = 251).

Neutrophils

Of the nine RCTs that reported data on chemotherapy-related reduced neutrophils (neutropenia) using the WHO or NCI-CTCAE criteria, eight reported on grade III plus IV of which one reported zero events in both groups, so the meta-analysis results are based on seven RCTs (Table 5.48). The pooled results showed no differences between groups for the two studies of FOLFOX4, the two studies of FOLFOX6 or the total pool of seven studies (RR: 0.67 [0.37, 1.23], I^2 = 0%).

Table 5.48 Oral Chinese Herbal Medicine plus Chemotherapy versus Chemotherapy Alone: Chemotherapy-related Neutropenia (Grade III+IV)

Chemotherapy Regimen:[1] *N* Studies (*N* Participants); *N* Studies with 0 Events in Both Groups	*N* Studies (*N* Participants) in Meta-analysis	Effect Size (RR [95% CI]), I^2	Included Studies (Studies with 0 Events in Both Groups)
FOLFOX4: 3 (294); 1	2 (160)	0.68 [0.16, 3.00], 40.1%	H70, H100 (H99)
FOLFOX6: 2 (100); 0	2 (100)	0.68 [0.12, 3.96], 0%	H44, H58
mFOLFOX6: 1 (41); 0	1 (41)	0.32 [0.01, 7.38]	H103
Pool for similar chemotherapy[2]: 6 (435); 1	5 (301)	0.63 [0.25, 1.58], 0%	H44, H58, H70, H100, H103 (H99)
XELOX: 1 (86); 0	1 (86)	1.00 [0.35, 2.86]	H76
FOLFIRI: 1 (68); 0	1 (68)	0.43 [0.12, 1.52]	H88
Total pool: 8 (629); 1	7 (455)	0.67 [0.37, 1.23], 0%	All above

[1]Comparator was the same chemotherapy.

[2]These chemotherapy regimens all use oxaliplatin, 5-FU plus LV.

*Statistically significant.

Abbreviations: CI, confidence interval; N, number; RR, risk ratio.

For all grades of chemotherapy-related neutropenia (Table 5.49), there was no difference between groups in the pooled result for three studies of FOLFOX4 (RR: 0.78 [0.54, 1.13], I^2 = 0%); however, there was a reduction in the two studies of FOLFOX6 and in the pooled result for six studies that used similar chemotherapies (RR: 0.66 [0.51, 0.86], I^2 = 0%). In the pool of two studies of XELOX, there was no difference between groups (RR: 0.67 [0.39, 1.15], I^2 = 53.6%). In the total pool of nine RCTs, there was a significant reduction in all grades of chemotherapy-related neutropenia in the CHM plus chemotherapy groups (RR: 0.70 [0.60, 0.81], I^2 = 0%).

In addition, one RCT (H62) did not mention which criteria were used. For all grades, there was a significant reduction in the CHM plus mFOLFOX6 groups (RR: 0.47 [0.22, 0.999], *n* = 68).

Table 5.49 Oral Chinese Herbal Medicine plus Chemotherapy versus Chemotherapy: Chemotherapy-related Neutropenia (All Grades)

Chemotherapy Regimen[1]	*N* Studies (*N* Participants)	Effect Size (RR [95% CI]), I^2	Included Studies
FOLFOX4	3 (294)	0.78 [0.54, 1.13], 0%	H70, H99, H100
FOLFOX6	2 (100)	0.62 [0.42, 0.90]*, 0%	H44, H58
mFOLFOX6	1 (41)	0.35 [0.13, 0.91]*	H103
Pool for similar chemotherapy[2]	6 (435)	0.66 [0.51, 0.86]*, 0%	H44, H58, H70, H99, H100, H103
XELOX	2 (148)	0.67 [0.39, 1.15], 53.6%	H76, H90
FOLFIRI	1 (68)	0.54 [0.34, 0.88]*	H88
Total pool	9 (651)	0.70 [0.60, 0.81]*, 0%	All above

[1]Comparator was the same chemotherapy.

[2]These chemotherapy regimens all use oxaliplatin, 5-FU plus LV.

*Statistically significant.

Abbreviations: CI, confidence interval; N, number; RR, risk ratio.

Red Blood Cells

Five RCTs reported on chemotherapy-related reduced red blood cells (erythropenia) using the WHO or NCI-CTCAE criteria (Table 5.50). For grade III plus IV erythropenia, there were zero events in both groups in two RCTs (H109, H111) and no significant difference between groups in the other three studies which were of FOLFOX4, FOLFOX6 or FOLFOX (RR: 0.40 [0.08, 2.06], I^2 = 0%). For all grades of erythropenia, there was no difference between groups in the pool of two studies of FOLFOX4 (RR: 0.76 [0.49, 1.18], I^2 = 0%) but there was a significant reduction in erythropenia in the pooled result for similar chemotherapies (RR: 0.67 [0.48, 0.94], I^2 = 0%) and in the total pool of five RCTs (RR: 0.68 [0.49, 0.94], I^2 = 0%) in favour of the CHM plus chemotherapy groups.

One RCT (H46) did not mention which criteria were used. For all grades of erythropenia, there was a significant reduction in the CHM plus FOLFOX4 groups (RR: 0.40 [0.18, 0.89], *n* = 60).

Table 5.50 Oral Chinese Herbal Medicine plus Chemotherapy versus Chemotherapy: Chemotherapy-related Erythropenia

Chemotherapy Regimen:[1] *N* Studies (*N* Participants); *N* Studies with 0 Events in Both Groups	*N* Studies (*N* Participants) in Meta-analysis	Effect Size (RR [95% CI]), I^2	Included Studies (Studies with 0 Events in Both Groups)
Grade III+IV			
Total pool: 5 (387); 2	3 (266)	0.40 [0.08, 2.06], 0%	H44, H71, H99 (H109, H111)
All grades			
FOLFOX4: 2 (219); 0	2 (219)	0.76 [0.49, 1.18], 0%	H99, H111
FOLFOX6: 1 (70); 0	1 (70)	0.55 [0.31, 0.97]*	H44
FOLFOX: 1 (62): 0	1 (62)	0.60 [0.16, 2.30]	H71
Pool for similar chemotherapy[2]: 4 (351); 0	4 (351)	0.67 [0.48, 0.94]*, 0%	H44, H71, H99, H111
XELOX: 1 (36); 0	1 (36)	0.80 [0.26, 2.50]	H109
Total pool: 5 (387); 0	5 (387)	0.68 [0.49, 0.94]*, 0%	All above

[1]Comparator was the same chemotherapy.

[2]These chemotherapy regimens all use oxaliplatin, 5-FU plus LV.

*Statistically significant.

Abbreviations: CI, confidence interval; N, number; RR, risk ratio.

Haemoglobin

In total, 29 RCTs reported on reduced chemotherapy-related haemoglobin levels using the WHO or NCI-CTCAE criteria, but one study (H87) had a data error in the results table and was excluded from the meta-analysis. For grade III plus IV, 14 studies reported no events in both groups (Table 5.51). In the five studies of FOLFOX4, the pooled result showed no difference between groups (RR: 0.42 [0.13, 1.34], I^2 = 0%) and there was no difference in the pool of seven studies of similar chemotherapy. For XELOX, there was no difference between groups (RR: 1.55 [0.56, 4.28], I^2 = 11.1%) based on four studies, and

Table 5.51 Oral Chinese Herbal Medicine plus Chemotherapy versus Chemotherapy: Chemotherapy-related Reduced Haemoglobin (Grade III+IV)

Chemotherapy Regimen:[1] *N* Studies (*N* Participants); *N* Studies with 0 Events in Both Groups	*N* Studies (*N* Participants) in Meta-analysis	Effect Size (RR [95% CI]), I^2	Included Studies (Studies with 0 Events in Both Groups)
FOLFOX4: 10 (570); 5	5 (343)	0.42 [0.13, 1.34], 0%	H54, H65, H70, H85, H100 (H47, H67, H107, H110, H112)
FOLFOX6: 2 (96); 1	1 (30)	0.33 [0.02, 7.58]	H58 (H86)
mFOLFOX6: 1 (41); 1	0 (0)	Both groups = 0 events	(H103)
OLF: 1 (40); 0	1 (40)	0.33 [0.01, 7.72]	H53
Pool for similar chemotherapy[2]: 14 (747); 7	7 (413)	0.40 [0.14, 1.11], 0%	H53, H54, H58, H65, H70, H85, H100 (H47, H67, H86, H103, H107, H110, H112)
XELOX: 7 (446); 3	4 (326)	1.55 [0.56, 4.28], 11.1%	H75, H76, H91, H94 (H92, H93, H114)
FOLFIRI: 2 (104); 1	1 (68)	0.33 [0.04, 3.05]	H88 (H89)
LF: 1 (60); 1	0 (0)	Both groups = 0 events	(H118)
XELIRI: 2 (66); 2	0 (0)	Both groups = 0 events	(H78, H79)
Total pool: 26 (1423); 14	12 (807)	0.87 [0.46, 1.64], 0%	All above

[1]Comparator was the same chemotherapy.

[2]These chemotherapy regimens all use oxaliplatin, 5-FU plus LV.

*Statistically significant.

Abbreviations: CI, confidence interval; N, number; RR, risk ratio.

there were no differences in any of the other subgroups or in the total pool of 12 RCTs (RR: 0.87 [0.46, 1.64], I^2 = 0%).

For all grades of reduced haemoglobin level, there was a significantly lower incidence in the ten studies of FOLFOX4 (RR: 0.69 [0.53, 0.90], I^2 = 0%), but not in the subgroup of three studies of FOLFOX4 as adjuvant chemotherapy after radical surgery (RR: 0.96 [0.53, 1.74],

Table 5.52 Oral Chinese Herbal Medicine plus Chemotherapy versus Chemotherapy: Chemotherapy-related Reduced Haemoglobin (All Grades)

Chemotherapy Regimen[1]	N Studies (N Participants)	Effect Size (RR [95% CI]), I^2	Included Studies
FOLFOX4 (all)	10 (570)	0.69 [0.53, 0.90]*, 0%	H47, H54, H65, H67, H70, H85, H100, H107, H110, H112
FOLFOX4 (adjuvant, after radical surgery)	3 (145)	0.96 [0.53, 1.74], 0%	H47, H107, H110
FOLFOX6	2 (96)	0.81 [0.42, 1.56], 0%	H58, H86
mFOLFOX6	2 (121)	0.60 [0.29, 1.22], 45.7%	H103, H121
OLF	1 (40)	0.79 [0.48, 1.28]	H53
Pool for similar chemotherapy[2]	15 (827)	0.70 [0.57, 0.86]*, 0%	H47, H53, H54, H58, H65, H67, H70, H85, H86, H100, H103, H107, H110, H112, H121
XELOX (all)	7 (446)	0.76 [0.56, 1.05], 40.7%	H75, H76, H91–H94, H114
XELOX (after surgery)	1 (40)	0.78 [0.36, 1.68]	H114
XELOX (without surgery)	6 (406)	0.75 [0.52, 1.08], 50.5%	H75, H76, H91–H94
FOLFIRI	2 (104)	0.60 [0.28, 1.30], 37.6%	H88, H89
LF	1 (60)	0.94 [0.57, 1.53]	H118
XELIRI	2 (66)	0.64 [0.35, 1.18], 0%	H78, H79
HIPEC	1 (60)	0.90 [0.43, 1.90]	H56
Total pool	28 (1,563)	0.76 [0.67, 0.87]*, 0%	All above

[1]Comparator was the same chemotherapy.

[2]These chemotherapy regimens all use oxaliplatin, 5-FU plus LV.

*Statistically significant.

Abbreviations: CI, confidence interval; HIPEC: hyperthermic intraperitoneal chemotherapy; LF, leucovorin and 5-fluorouracil; N, number; RR, risk ratio.

I^2 = 0%) or in the pools for FOLFOX6 and mFOLFOX6 (Table 5.52). The pooled result for 15 studies of similar chemotherapies showed a significantly lower incidence of reduced haemoglobin level in the CHM plus chemotherapy groups (RR: 0.70 [0.57, 0.86], I^2 = 0%). For the seven RCTs of XELOX, there was no difference between groups (RR: 0.76 [0.56, 1.05], I^2 = 40.7%) and there were similar results for the other subgroups. In the total pool of 28 studies there was a significantly lower incidence of reduced haemoglobin level (all grades) in the CHM plus chemotherapy groups (RR: 0.76 [0.67, 0.87], I^2 = 0%).

In the study that used ITT analysis (H61) and the NCI-CTCAE criteria, there was no difference between groups for grade III plus IV (RR: 0.50 [0.05, 5.29], n = 76) or for all grades of reduced haemoglobin levels (RR: 0.61 [0.34, 1.11], n = 76).

In addition, two RCTs (H50, H62) did not mention which criteria were used. Each used a different chemotherapy (mFOLFOX6 and FOLFIRI, respectively). In the pooled results of all grades of reduced haemoglobin, there was a significant reduction in the CHM plus chemotherapy groups (RR: 0.48 [0.29, 0.80], I^2 = 0%, n = 155).

Platelets

Data on chemotherapy-related reduced platelets (thrombocytopenia) were reported using the WHO or NCI-CTCAE criteria in 39 RCTs. For grade III plus IV, 22 studies reported zero events in either group, so the meta-analysis results were based on 15 RCTs (Table 5.53). In the five studies that used FOLFOX4, there was no significant difference between groups (RR: 0.83 [0.19, 3.74], I^2 = 66.6%) with substantial heterogeneity. The only subgroup that showed a significant difference between groups was XELOX (RR: 0.24 [0.07, 0.87], I^2 = 0%) based on four studies. The total pool of 15 studies showed reduced incidence of grade III plus IV thrombocytopenia in the CHM plus chemotherapy groups (RR: 0.43 [0.21, 0.91], I^2 = 27.3%).

In total, 39 studies reported on all grades of thrombocytopenia, but one study (H103) found zero events in both groups, so 38 studies were included in the meta-analysis. There was no difference between groups for FOLFOX4 (RR: 0.77 [0.59, 1.00], I^2 = 14.9%) based on 15 studies (Table 5.54). There was a significant reduction in the pool of three studies of FOLFOX6 (RR: 0.56 [0.36, 0.88], I^2 = 0%) and in the pool of 22 studies that used similar chemotherapies (RR: 0.74 [0.62, 0.89], I^2 = 0%). In the pool of all nine studies of XELOX there was a significant reduction on the combination therapy groups (RR: 0.76 [0.60, 0.97], I^2 = 0%) but there was no difference in the two

Table 5.53 Oral Chinese Herbal Medicine plus Chemotherapy versus Chemotherapy: Chemotherapy-related Thrombocytopenia (Grade III+IV)

Chemotherapy Regimen:[1] N Studies (N Participants); N Studies with 0 Events in Both Groups	N Studies (N Participants) in Meta-analysis	Effect Size (RR [95% CI]), I^2	Included Studies (Studies with 0 Events in Both Groups)
FOLFOX4: 15 (949); 10	5 (274)	0.83 [0.19, 3.74], 66.6%	H54, H66, H68, H85, H100 (H47, H65, H67, H70, H99, H104, H107, H110–H112)
FOLFOX6: 3 (166); 1	2 (100)	0.26 [0.03, 2.23], 0%	H44, H58 (H86)
mFOLFOX6: 2 (95); 1	1 (54)	0.33 [0.01, 7.84]	H87 (H103)
FOLFOX: 1 (62); 1	0 (0)	Both groups = 0 events	(H71)
OLF: 1 (40); 1	0 (0)	Both groups = 0 events	(H53)
Pool for similar chemotherapy[2]: 22 (1312); 14	8 (428)	0.63 [0.21, 1.92], 48.1%	H44, H54, H58, H66, H68, H85, H87, H100 (H47, H53, H65, H67, H70, H71, H86, H99, H103, H104, H107, H110–H112)
XELOX: 9 (512); 5	4 (246)	0.24 [0.07, 0.87]*, 0%	H75, H76, H92, H122 (H91, H93, H94, H109, H114)
FOLFIRI: 3 (159); 2	1 (68)	0.14 [0.01, 2.66]	H88 (H72, H89)
LF: 1 (60); 0	1 (60)	0.14 [0.01, 2.65]	H118
XELIRI: 2 (66); 1	1 (36)	0.37 [0.02, 8.53]	H79 (H78)
Total pool: 37 (2109); 22	15 (838)	0.43 [0.21, 0.91]*, 27.3%	All above

[1]Comparator was the same chemotherapy.

[2]These chemotherapy regimens all use oxaliplatin, 5-FU plus LV.

*Statistically significant.

Abbreviations: CI, confidence interval; LF, leucovorin and 5-fluorouracil; N, number; RR, risk ratio.

XELOX subgroups. For FOLFIRI, there was no difference between groups (RR: 0.60 [0.22, 1.60], I^2 = 45.9%) with moderate heterogeneity. The pooled result for all 38 studies showed a significant reduction in the incidence of all grades of thrombocytopenia in the CHM plus chemotherapy groups (RR: 0.73 [0.64, 0.84], I^2 = 0%).

Table 5.54 Oral Chinese Herbal Medicine plus Chemotherapy versus Chemotherapy: Chemotherapy-related Thrombocytopenia (All Grades)

Chemotherapy Regimen:[1] N Studies (N Participants); N Studies with 0 Events in Both Groups	N Studies (N Participants) in Meta-analysis	Effect Size (RR [95% CI]), I^2	Included Studies (Studies with 0 Events in Both Groups)
FOLFOX4 (all): 15 (949); 0	15 (949)	0.77 [0.59, 1.00], 14.9%	H47, H54, H65–H68, H70, H85, H99, H100, H104, H107, H110–H112
FOLFOX4 (adjuvant, after radical surgery): 5 (309); 0	5 (309)	0.74 [0.43, 1.29], 0%	H47, H99, H104, H107, H110
FOLFOX6: 3 (166); 0	3 (166)	0.56 [0.36, 0.88]*, 0%	H44, H58, H86
mFOLFOX6: 3 (175); 1	2 (134)	0.69 [0.45, 1.05], 0%	H87, H121 (H103)
FOLFOX: 1 (62); 0	1 (62)	1.00 [0.22, 4.58]	H71
OLF: 1 (40); 0	1 (40)	0.75 [0.19, 2.93]	H53
Pool for similar chemotherapy[2]: 23 (1392): 1	22 (1,351)	0.74 [0.62, 0.89]*, 0%	H44, H47, H53, H54, H58, H65–H68, H70, H71, H85–H87, H99, H100, H104, H107, H110–H112, H121 (H103)
XELOX (all): 9 (512): 0	9 (512)	0.76 [0.60, 0.97]*, 0%	H75, H76, H91–H94, H109, H114, H122
XELOX (after surgery): 2 (70): 0	2 (70)	0.79 [0.54, 1.16], 0%	H114, H122
XELOX (without surgery): 7 (442); 0	7 (442)	0.75 [0.56, 1.01], 0%	H75, H76, H91–94, H109
FOLFIRI: 3 (159): 0	3 (159)	0.60 [0.22, 1.60], 45.9%	H72, H88, H89
LF: 1 (60); 0	1 (60)	0.53 [0.28, 0.99]*	H118
XELIRI: 2 (66); 0	2 (66)	0.63 [0.27, 1.44], 0%	H78, H79
HIPEC: 1 (60); 0	1 (60)	1.17 [0.44, 3.07]	H56
Total pool: 39 (2249): 1	38 (2208)	0.73 [0.64, 0.84]*, 0%	All above

[1]Comparator was the same chemotherapy.

[2]These chemotherapy regimens all use oxaliplatin, 5-FU plus LV.

*Statistically significant.

Abbreviations: CI, confidence interval; HIPEC: hyperthermic intraperitoneal chemotherapy; LF, leucovorin and 5-fluorouracil; N, number; RR, risk ratio.

Five RCTs (H35, H46, H50, H57, H62) did not mention which criteria were used. Each used a different chemotherapy (FOLFOX4, mFOLFOX6, FOLFIRI, XELODA and HIPEC, respectively). For the subgroups, only FOLFIRI showed a significant reduction in the combination therapy group; the other subgroups showed no differences between groups. The pooled result showed a significant reduction in the CHM plus chemotherapy groups (RR: 0.62 [0.42, 0.90], I^2 = 0%, n = 409).

Myelosuppression (Type not Specified)

In eight RCTs results were reported for incidence of myelosuppression using the WHO or NCI-CTCAE criteria without specifying the groups of blood cells involved. For grade III plus IV events (Table 5.55), there were no differences between groups for the subgroups of FOLFOX4 and XELOX, however, in the single study of mFOLFOX6 in

Table 5.55 Oral Chinese Herbal Medicine plus Chemotherapy versus Chemotherapy: Chemotherapy-related Myelosuppression (Grade III+IV)

Chemotherapy Regimen:[1] *N* Studies (*N* Participants); *N* Studies with 0 Events in Both Groups	*N* Studies (*N* Participants) in Meta-analysis	Effect Size (RR [95% CI]), I^2	Included Studies (Studies with 0 Events in Both Groups)
FOLFOX4: 1 (60); 0	1 (60)	0.47 [0.05, 4.89]	H41
mFOLFOX6: 1 (75); 0	1 (75)	2.31 [1.16, 4.62]*	H63
Pool for similar chemotherapy[2]: 2 (135); 0	2 (135)	1.56 [0.40, 6.07], 39.8%	H41, H63
XELOX: 3 (160); 0	3 (160)	0.40 [0.14, 1.10], 0%	H42, H73, H105
XELIRI: 1 (55); 1	0 (0)	Both groups = 0 events	(H96)
Total pool: 6 (350); 1	5 (295)	0.65 [0.21, 2.03] 62.8%	All above

[1]Comparator was the same chemotherapy.

[2]These chemotherapy regimens all use oxaliplatin, 5-FU plus LV.

*Statistically significant.

Abbreviations: CI, confidence interval; N, number; RR, risk ratio.

advanced colon cancer there were significantly more events in the CHM plus mFOLFOX6 group after six 2-week cycles (RR: 2.31 [1.16, 4.62]). The total pool of five RCTs (RR: 0.65 [0.21, 2.03], I^2 = 62.8%) showed no difference between groups with substantial heterogeneity.

Eight studies reported data for all grades of myelosuppression (Table 5.56). There were no significant differences between groups for the single studies of FOLFOX4, mFOLFOX6, XELODA or XELIRI. The pooled result for three RCTs of XELOX showed no difference with considerable heterogeneity (RR: 0.63 [0.35, 1.13], I^2 = 79.7%), but the single study of XELOX after surgery (H105) showed a significant difference. For the total pool of eight studies, there was no significant difference between groups (RR: 0.61 [0.31, 1.22], I^2 = 96%), but the heterogeneity was considerable. This was partly due to the study of mFOLFOX6 which reported myelosuppression in all

Table 5.56 Oral Chinese Herbal Medicine plus Chemotherapy versus Chemotherapy: Chemotherapy-related Myelosuppression (All Grades)

Chemotherapy Regimen[1]	N Studies (N Participants)	Effect Size (RR [95% CI]), I^2	Included Studies
FOLFOX4	1 (60)	0.62 [0.25, 1.53]	H41
mFOLFOX6	1 (75)	1.00 [0.95, 1.05]	H63
Pool for similar chemotherapy[2]	2 (135)	0.81 [0.20, 3.20], 89%	H41, H63
XELOX (all)	3 (160)	0.63 [0.35, 1.13], 79.7%	H42, H73, H105
XELOX (after surgery)	1 (60)	0.39 [0.19, 0.79]*	H105
XELOX (without surgery)	2 (100)	0.75 [0.44, 1.30], 76.7%	H42, H73
FOLFIRI	1 (50)	0.29 [0.13, 0.62]*	H43
XELODA	1 (60)	0.50 [0.10, 2.53]	H95
XELIRI	1 (55)	0.88 [0.45, 1.72]	H96
Total pool	8 (460)	0.61 [0.31, 1.22], 96%	All above
Sensitivity	7 (385)	0.59 [0.39, 0.89]*, 65.3%	Excluding H63

[1]Comparator was the same chemotherapy.

[2]These chemotherapy regimens all use oxaliplatin, 5-FU plus LV.

*Statistically significant.

Abbreviations: CI, confidence interval; N, number; RR, risk ratio.

participants (H63). When this study was removed, the pooled result showed a significant reduction in myelosuppression in the combination therapy groups (RR: 0.59 [0.39, 0.89], I^2 = 65.3%) with reduced heterogeneity.

Chemotherapy-induced Peripheral Neurotoxicity

Forty-one RCTs reported on CIPN. Twenty-nine RCTs used the WHO criteria, five studies used Levi's modified WHO criteria,[20] four studies used the NCI-CTCAE criteria and three studies did not specify. For WHO grade III plus IV CIPN, 14 studies had zero events in both groups so 13 studies were included in the meta-analysis (Table 5.57). For the pool of seven studies of FOLFOX4, there was no difference between groups (RR: 0.41 [0.16, 1.04], I^2 = 0%). However, there was a significant reduction in the single study of mFOLFOX6 and there was a significant reduction in CIPN in the combination therapy groups in the pool of nine studies that used similar chemotherapies (RR: 0.33 [0.16, 0.70], I^2 = 0%). There was no difference between groups in the pooled result for three RCTs of XELOX, or any of the other subgroups, but the total result for 13 studies showed a significant reduction in the incidence of grade III plus IV CIPN in the CHM plus chemotherapy groups (RR: 0.41 [0.22, 0.77], I^2 = 0%).

For all grades of CIPN (WHO criteria), 29 RCTs reported data but one had zero events in both groups, so 28 studies were included in the meta-analysis (Table 5.58). There was a significant reduction in CIPN in the pooled result for all 14 studies that used FOLFOX4 (RR: 0.77 [0.66, 0.89], I^2 = 0%) but there was no significant difference between groups in the subgroup of FOLFOX4 as adjuvant chemotherapy after radical surgery. For mFOLFOX6, the pooled result for two RCTs showed no difference (RR: 0.63 [0.03, 12.41], I^2 = 99%), with considerable heterogeneity which was due to one study (H63) reporting that all participants had CIPN. In the pool of 18 studies of similar chemotherapies, there was a significant difference between groups (RR: 0.70 [0.52, 0.96], I^2 = 88%), but the heterogeneity was considerable. When the above study was removed from the pool, the heterogeneity was reduced to zero and the significant reduction in

Table 5.57 Oral Chinese Herbal Medicine plus Chemotherapy versus Chemotherapy: Chemotherapy-induced Peripheral Neurotoxicity (WHO Grade III+IV)

Chemotherapy Regimen:[1] *N* Studies (*N* Participants); *N* Studies with 0 Events in Both Groups	*N* Studies (*N* Participants) in Meta-analysis	Effect Size (RR [95% CI]), I^2	Included Studies (Studies with 0 Events in Both Groups)
FOLFOX4: 13 (836); 6	7 (532)	0.41 [0.16, 1.04], 0%	H54, H65, H67, H70, H80, H85, H99 (H47, H104, H107, H110, H111, H112)
FOLFOX6: 1 (70); 1	0 (0)	Both groups = 0 events	(H44)
mFOLFOX6: 2 (129); 1	1 (75)	0.18 [0.04, 0.75]*	H63 (H87)
FOLFOX: 1 (62); 0	1 (62)	0.50 [0.05, 5.23]	H71
Pool for similar chemotherapy[2]: 17 (1097); 8	9 (669)	0.33 [0.16, 0.70]*, 0%	H54, H63, H65, H67, H70, H71, H80, H85, H99 (H44, H47, H87, H104, H107, H110–H112)
XELOX: 7 (360); 4	3 (180)	0.66 [0.18, 2.47], 0%	H60, H74, H75 (H83, H92, H93, H114)
S1+oxaliplatin: 1 (66); 0	1 (66)	1.00 [0.07, 15.33]	H101
XELIRI: 2 (66); 2	0 (0)	Both groups = 0 events	(H78, H79)
Total pool: 27 (1589); 14	13 (915)	0.41 [0.22, 0.77]*, 0%	All above

[1]Comparator was the same chemotherapy.

[2]These chemotherapy regimens all use oxaliplatin, 5-FU plus LV.

*Statistically significant.

Abbreviations: CI, confidence interval; N, number; RR, Risk Ratio; WHO, World Health Organisation.

CIPN in the combination therapy groups remained (RR: 0.75 [0.66, 0.86], I^2 = 0%, n = 1,116). In the seven studies of XELOX the pooled result showed no difference between groups (RR: 0.93 [0.81, 1.06], I^2 = 0%) and the result was similar in the XELOX subgroups. There was no difference between groups for XELIRI. In the total pool of 28 studies, there was a significant reduction in CIPN in the CHM plus chemotherapy groups, but the heterogeneity was considerable (RR: 0.77 [0.64, 0.91], I^2 = 76%). When the study in which all participants

Table 5.58 Oral Chinese Herbal Medicine plus Chemotherapy versus Chemotherapy: Chemotherapy-induced Peripheral Neurotoxicity (WHO All Grades)

Chemotherapy Regimen:[1] *N* Studies (*N* Participants); *N* Studies with 0 Events in Both Groups	*N* Studies (*N* Participants) in Meta-analysis	Effect Size (RR [95% CI]), I^2	Included Studies (Studies with 0 Events in Both Groups)
FOLFOX4 (all): 14 (930); 0	14 (930)	0.77 [0.66, 0.89]*, 0%	H47, H54, H65, H67, H70, H80, H85, H99, H104, H107, H110–H112, H117
FOLFOX4 (adjuvant, after radical surgery): 5 (309); 0	5 (309)	0.77 [0.44, 1.33], 0%	H47, H99, H104, H107, H110
FOLFOX6: 1 (70); 0	1 (70)	0.81 [0.58, 1.13]	H44
mFOLFOX6: 2 (129); 0	2 (129)	0.63 [0.03, 12.41], 99%	H63, H87
FOLFOX: 1 (62); 0	1 (62)	0.75 [0.29, 1.91]	H71
Pool for similar chemotherapy[2]: 18 (1191): 0	18 (1191)	0.70 [0.52, 0.96]*, 88%	H44, H47, H54, H63, H65, H67, H70, H71, H80, H85, H87, H99, H104, H107, H110–H112, H117
XELOX (all): 7 (360): 0	7 (360)	0.93 [0.81, 1.06], 0%	H60, H74, H75, H83, H92, H93, H114
XELOX (after surgery): 2 (81): 0	2 (81)	0.95 [0.80, 1.13], 0%	H60, H114
XELOX (without surgery): 5 (279); 0	5 (279)	0.89 [0.72, 1.11], 0%	H74, H75, H83, H92, H93
S1+oxaliplatin: 1 (66); 0	1 (66)	0.92 [0.50, 1.71]	H101
XELODA: 1 (60): 1	0 (0)	Both groups = 0 events	(H95)
XELIRI: 2 (66); 0	2 (66)	0.57 [0.28, 1.16], 0%	H78, H79
Total pool: 29 (1743): 1	28 (1,683)	0.77 [0.64, 0.91]*, 76%	All above
Sensitivity	27 (1,608)	0.83 [0.76, 0.91]*, 0%	Excluding H63

[1]Comparator was the same chemotherapy.

[2]These chemotherapy regimens all use oxaliplatin, 5-FU plus LV.

*Statistically significant.

Abbreviations: CI, confidence interval; N, number; RR, risk ratio; WHO, World Health Organisation.

had CIPN (H63) was excluded, the result was similar without heterogeneity (RR: 0.83 [0.76, 0.91], $I^2 = 0\%$, $n = 1,608$).

Five studies used Levi's modified version of the WHO criteria[20] (Table 5.59). For grade III plus IV CIPN, the pooled result for four studies found there was a significant reduction in the combination

Table 5.59 Oral Chinese Herbal Medicine plus Chemotherapy versus Chemotherapy: Chemotherapy-induced Peripheral Neurotoxicity (Levi's Criteria)

Chemotherapy Regimen:[1] *N* Studies (*N* Participants); *N* Studies with 0 Events in Both Groups	*N* Studies (*N* Participants) in Meta-analysis	Effect Size (RR [95% CI]), I^2	Included Studies (Studies with 0 Events in Both Groups)
Grade III+IV			
FOLFOX4: 1 (60); 1	0 (0)	Both groups = 0 events	(H69)
FOLFOX6: 1 (57); 0	1 (57)	0.10 [0.01, 1.78]	H123
mFOLFOX6: 2 (219); 0	2 (219)	0.08 [0.01, 0.58]*, 0%	H124, H125
Pool for similar chemotherapy[2]: 4 (336): 1	3 (276)	0.08 [0.02, 0.44]*, 0%	H123–H125 (H69)
XELOX: 1 (53); 0	1 (53)	0.48 [0.05, 5.00]	H94
Total pool: 5 (389); 1	4 (329)	0.15 [0.04, 0.58]*, 0%	All above
All grades			
FOLFOX4: 1 (60); 0	1 (60)	0.88 [0.67, 1.15]	H69
FOLFOX6: 1 (57); 0	1 (57)	0.30 [0.13, 0.72]*	H123
mFOLFOX6: 2 (219); 0	2 (219)	0.51 [0.40, 0.65]*, 0%	H124, H125
Pool for similar chemotherapy[2]: 4 (336): 0	4 (336)	0.56 [0.37, 0.85]*, 78.2%	H69, H123–H125
XELOX: 1 (53); 0	1 (53)	0.32 [0.17, 0.62]*	H94
Total pool: 5 (389); 0	5 (389)	0.51 [0.34, 0.76]*, 78.1%	All above

[1]Comparator was the same chemotherapy.

[2]These chemotherapy regimens all use oxaliplatin, 5-FU plus LV.

*Statistically significant.

Abbreviations: CI, confidence interval; N, number; RR, risk ratio.

therapy groups (RR: 0.15 [0.04, 0.58], I^2 = 0%). For all grades, the pooled result for five studies showed a significant reduction in incidence of CIPN in the CHM plus chemotherapy groups (RR: 0.51 [0.34, 0.76], I^2 = 78.1%), but heterogeneity was considerable due mainly to the result of the single study of FOLFOX4 (H69), which found no difference between groups.

Four studies used the NCI-CTCAE criteria for CIPN (Table 5.60). Three studies reported data for grade III plus IV but there were zero events in both groups in one study, so two studies were pooled in the meta-analysis. The pooled result found no significant difference between groups (RR: 0.50 [0.09, 2.69], I^2 = 0%). For all grades, the pooled result for four RCTs showed no significant difference between the CHM plus chemotherapy groups and the chemotherapy alone groups (RR: 0.71 [0.48, 1.05], I^2 = 0%).

Table 5.60 Oral Chinese Herbal Medicine plus Chemotherapy versus Chemotherapy: Chemotherapy-induced Peripheral Neurotoxicity (NCI-CTCAE)

Chemotherapy Regimen:[1] *N* Studies (*N* Participants); *N* Studies with 0 Events in Both Groups	*N* Studies (*N* Participants) in Meta-analysis	Effect Size (RR [95% CI]), I^2	Included Studies (Studies with 0 Events in Both Groups)
Grade III+IV			
FOLFOX6: 1 (30): 0	1 (30)	0.33 [0.04, 2.85]	H58
mFOLFOX6: 1 (41); 0	1 (41)	0.95 [0.06, 14.22]	H103
XELOX: 1 (97); 1	0 (0)	Both groups = 0 events	(H91)
Total pool: 3 (138); 1	2 (71)	0.50 [0.09, 2.69], 0%	H58, H103 (H91)
All grades			
FOLFOX6: 1 (30): 0	1 (30)	0.44 [1.17, 1.13]	H58
mFOLFOX6: 1 (41); 0	1 (41)	0.64 [0.21, 1.92]	H103
XELOX: 2 (159); 0	2 (159)	0.83 [0.46, 1.50], 37.3%	H90, H91
Total pool: 4 (230); 0	4 (230)	0.71 [0.48, 1.05], 0%	All above

[1]Comparator was the same chemotherapy.

*Statistically significant.

Abbreviations: CI, confidence interval; CRC, colorectal cancer; N, number; NCI-CTCAE, National Cancer Institute-Common Terminology Criteria for Adverse Events; RR, risk ratio.

Three studies did not specify the criteria for CIPN (H57, H62, H119). For all grades of CIPN, one study of mFOLFOX6 in rectal adenocarcinoma with metastasis after radical surgery (H62) found no significant difference between groups (RR: 1.00 [0.50, 1.99], $n = 68$). One study of HIPEC for stage II/III CRC after surgery (H57) also found no significant difference (RR: 0.59 [0.34, 1.02], $n = 104$). In the pooled result for these two studies there was no significant difference in incidence of all grades of CIPN between the CHM plus chemotherapy and the chemotherapy alone groups (RR: 0.74 [0.44, 1.23], $I^2 = 28\%$, $n = 172$).

In the single study (H119) that only reported on perioral paraesthesia associated with mFOLFOX6 after radical surgery for CRC, there was a significant reduction in the CHM plus mFOLFOX6 group (RR: 0.17 [0.04, 0.68], $n = 60$).

Hand-foot Syndrome

Of the nine RCTs that reported data for chemotherapy-related hand-foot syndrome (HFS), five used the WHO criteria, three used the NCI-CTCAE criteria, and one did not specify the criteria.

For grade III plus IV (WHO) one study (H83) reported zero events in both groups (Table 5.61). There were no significant differences between groups in the other two studies and the pooled result also found no significant difference (RR: 0.42 [0.06, 2.76], $I^2 = 0\%$). For all grades, there were no significant differences between groups for the studies of FOLFOX4, mFOLFOX6 or XELOX, but there was a significant difference for HIPEC. The pooled result found no significant difference between groups (RR: 0.54 [0.12, 2.52], $I^2 = 97\%$), but the heterogeneity was considerable. This was mainly due to one study of mFOLFOX6 that reported hand-foot syndrome in all participants (H63). When this study was excluded from the meta-analysis pool, the heterogeneity was reduced and there was a significant reduction in HFS (all grades) in the CHM plus chemotherapy groups (RR: 0.56 [0.32, 0.98], $I^2 = 33.5\%$).

Three studies used the NCI-CTCAE criteria. One study (H91) reported zero grade III plus IV events in both groups (Table 5.62). In the remaining study (H94) of XELOX without surgery for stage IV

Table 5.61 Oral Chinese Herbal Medicine plus Chemotherapy versus Chemotherapy: Chemotherapy-related Hand-Foot Syndrome (WHO)

Chemotherapy Regimen:[1] *N* Studies (*N* Participants); *N* Studies with 0 Events in Both Groups	*N* Studies (*N* Participants) in Meta-analysis	Effect Size (RR [95% CI]), I^2	Included Studies (Studies with 0 Events in Both Groups)
Grade III+IV			
FOLFOX4: 1 (45): 0	1 (45)	0.32 [0.01, 7.45]	H54
mFOLFOX6: 1 (75); 0	1 (75)	0.49 [0.05, 5.14]	H63
XELOX: 1 (60); 1	0 (0)	Both groups = 0 events	(H83)
Total pool: 3 (180); 1	2 (120)	0.42 [0.06, 2.76], 0%	H54, H63 (H83)
All grades			
FOLFOX4: 1 (45): 0	1 (45)	0.82 [0.33, 2.06]	H54
mFOLFOX6: 2 (125); 0	2 (125)	0.38 [0.00, 76.97]	H43, H63
Pool for similar chemotherapy[2]: 3 (170): 0	3 (170)	0.54 [0.08, 3.83], 93%	H43, H54, H63
XELOX: 1 (60); 0	1 (60)	0.77 [0.40, 1.47]	H83
HIPEC: 1 (60); 0	1 (60)	0.38 [0.17, 0.83]*	H56
Total pool: 5 (290); 0	5 (290)	0.54 [0.12, 2.52], 97%	All above
Sensitivity	4 (215)	0.56 [0.32, 0.98]*, 33.5%	Excluding H63

[1]Comparator was the same chemotherapy

[2]These chemotherapy regimens all use oxaliplatin, 5-FU plus LV.

*Statistically significant.

Abbreviations: CI, confidence interval; N, number; RR, risk ratio; WHO, World Health Organisation.

Table 5.62 Oral Chinese Herbal Medicine plus Chemotherapy versus Chemotherapy: Chemotherapy-related Hand-Foot Syndrome (NCI-CTCAE)

Chemotherapy Regimen[1]	Cancer (*N* Participants)	Effect Size (RR [95% CI]), I^2	Included Studies
Grade III+IV			
XELOX (without surgery)	Advanced or recurrent stage IV CRC (97)	Both groups = 0 events	H91
	Stage IV CRC (53)	0.32 [0.01, 7.55]	H94
All grades			
XELOX (without surgery)	Advanced CRC (62)	0.70 [0.35, 1.43]	H90
	Advanced or recurrent stage IV CRC (97)	0.98 [0.58, 1.65]	H91
	Stage IV CRC (53)	0.41 [0.23, 0.73]*	H94
Pooled result (all grades)	3 studies (212)	0.66 [0.39, 1.13], 59.3%	All above

[1]Comparator was the same chemotherapy.

*Statistically significant.

Abbreviations: CI, confidence interval; CRC, colorectal cancer; N, number; NCI-CTCAE, National Cancer Institute-Common Terminology Criteria for Adverse Events; RR, risk ratio.

CRC, there were no significant differences between groups (RR: 0.32 [0.01, 7.55]). For all stages of HFS, all three studies used XELOX without surgery for advanced stage IV CRC. There were no differences between groups in two studies (H90, H91), but there was a difference in the other study (H94). The pooled result showed no differences between groups in incidence of all grades of HFS (RR: 0.66 [0.39, 1.13], I^2 = 59.3%) with substantial heterogeneity.

The single study (H35) that did not specify the criteria used XELODA as a maintenance treatment in stage IV CRC. There was no difference between groups in all grades of HFS (RR: 0.67 [0.12, 3.80], *n* = 90).

Fatigue

Of the four studies that reported data on chemotherapy-related fatigue, one study (H56) used the WHO criteria, one study (H61) used the NCI-CTCAE criteria and two studies (H108, H126) used the revised Piper Fatigue Scale (PFS-R). This scale includes 22 items, with higher scores indicating increased severity of fatigue.[27]

The single study that used the WHO criteria (H56) only reported data for all grades of fatigue in people with stage II/III CRC after radical surgery who received HIPEC. This study found there was a significant reduction in fatigue in the combined therapy groups (RR: 0.57 [0.35, 0.94], $n = 60$). The study that used the NCI-CTCAE criteria also reported data as ITT (H61) for FOLFOX4 (see KPS above for details). There were no differences between groups for grade III plus IV (RR: 0.14 [0.01, 2.68], $n = 76$) or all grades (RR: 0.86 [0.65, 1.15], $n = 76$) of fatigue.

In the two studies that used PFS-R, one of the studies of FOLFOX6 in people with stage III/IV advanced CRC (H108) found a significant reduction in the CHM plus FOLFOX6 group (MD: –2.40 [–3.31, –1.49], $n = 60$). The other study (H126), which used mFOLFOX6 in people with rectal cancer who had fatigue after two cycles of chemotherapy, showed no significant difference between groups (MD: –0.84 [–1.81, 0.13], $n = 52$). The pooled result for the two studies showed a significant reduction in fatigue in the CHM plus chemotherapy groups (MD: –1.63 [–3.16, –0.10], $I^2 = 81\%$, $n = 112$) with considerable heterogeneity.

Hepatotoxicity and/or Nephrotoxicity

Thirty-two RCTs reported chemotherapy-related hepatotoxicity and/or nephrotoxicity. Of these, 30 RCTs reported hepatotoxicity, 14 RCTs reported nephrotoxicity and two RCTs reported hepatotoxicity and nephrotoxicity as a single item based on the WHO criteria. These are analysed separately below.

Hepatotoxicity

Ten RCTs reported on hepatotoxicity using the WHO criteria, two RCTs used the NCI-CTCAE criteria and one study did not specify the criteria. Data on transaminases were reported by 14 RCTs using the

Table 5.63 Oral Chinese Herbal Medicine plus Chemotherapy versus Chemotherapy: Chemotherapy-related Hepatotoxicity (WHO Grade III+IV)

Chemotherapy Regimen:[1] *N* Studies (Participants); *N* Studies with 0 Events in Both Groups	*N* Studies (*N* Participants) in Meta-analysis	Effect Size (RR [95% CI]), I^2	Included Studies (Studies with 0 Events in Both Groups)
FOLFOX4: 2 (95); 1	1 (57)	1.45 [0.46, 4.59]	H80 (H67)
mFOLFOX6: 1 (54); 1	0 (0)	Both groups = 0 events	(H87)
OLF: 1 (40): 1	0 (0)	Both groups = 0 events	(H53)
XELOX: 4 (200); 2	2 (100)	0.20 [0.02, 1.65] 0%	H73, H105 (H83, H93)
XELIRI: 1 (53); 1	0 (0)	Both groups = 0 events	(H96)
Total pool: 9 (442); 6	3 (157)	0.69 [0.16, 2.88], 26.9%	All above

[1]Comparator was the same chemotherapy.

*Statistically significant.

Abbreviations: CI, confidence interval; N, number; RR, risk ratio; WHO, World Health Organisation.

WHO criteria, including four that reported alanine transaminase (ALT). Two RCTs reported on both ALT and aspartate transaminase (AST) separately using the NCI-CTCAE criteria, and one study reported ALT only but did not specify the criteria. In addition, one RCT reported on bilirubin using the WHO criteria.

In the ten studies that reported hepatotoxicity based on the WHO criteria, six reported zero events in both groups for grade III plus IV hepatotoxicity (Table 5.63). In the three studies (one of FOLFOX4 and two of XELOX) that were included in the meta-analysis, there were no significant differences between groups in the pooled result (RR: 0.69 [0.16, 2.88], I^2 = 26.9%).

For all grades of hepatotoxicity based on the WHO criteria (Table 5.64), there were no differences between groups in the two studies of FOLFOX4, or in the pool of four studies that used similar chemotherapy (RR: 0.65 [0.27, 1.58], I^2 = 58.9%). There was reduced hepatotoxicity in the combined therapy groups in the pooled result for the four studies of XELOX (RR: 0.50 [0.30, 0.83], I^2 = 0%) and in

Table 5.64 Oral Chinese Herbal Medicine plus Chemotherapy versus Chemotherapy: Chemotherapy-related Hepatotoxicity (WHO All Grades)

Chemotherapy Regimen[1]	N Studies (N Participants)	Effect Size (RR [95% CI]), I^2	Included Studies
FOLFOX4	2 (95)	1.05 [0.81, 1.35], 0%	H67, H80
mFOLFOX6	1 (54)	0.42 [0.17, 1.02]	H87
OLF	1 (40)	0.50 [0.05, 5.08]	H53
Pool for similar chemotherapy[2]	4 (189)	0.65 [0.27, 1.58], 58.9%	H53, H67, H80, H87
XELOX (all)	4 (200)	0.50 [0.30, 0.83]*, 0%	H73, H83, H93, H105
XELOX (after surgery)	1 (60)	0.40 [0.14, 1.14]	H105
XELOX (without surgery)	3 (140)	0.53 [0.30, 0.95]*, 0%	H73, H83, H93
FOLFIRI	1 (50)	0.44 [0.08, 2.43]	H43
XELIRI	1 (53)	0.80 [0.28, 2.33]	H96
Total pool	10 (492)	0.61 [0.39, 0.95]*, 48.5%	All above

[1]Comparator was the same chemotherapy.

[2]These chemotherapy regimens all use oxaliplatin, 5-FU plus LV.

*Statistically significant.

Abbreviations: CI, confidence interval; N, number; RR, risk ratio; WHO, World Health Organisation.

the subgroup of XELOX without surgery, but there were no differences between groups in the other subgroups. The pooled result for all 10 studies showed a significant reduction in hepatotoxicity in the CHM plus chemotherapy groups (RR: 0.61 [0.39, 0.95], I^2 = 48.5%) with moderate heterogeneity.

Two studies (H91, H120) used the NCI-CTCAE criteria. Only one study (I191) reported grade III plus IV hepatotoxicity and found zero events in both groups. For all grades, the study of FOLFIRI for stage IV CRC (H120) found no difference between groups (RR: 0.80 [0.25, 2.59], n = 44) and the result was similar for the study of XELOX without surgery (H91) for people with advanced or recurrent stage IV CRC (RR: 1.10 [0.65, 1.84], n = 97). The pooled result for the two studies showed no significant difference between groups (RR: 1.04 [0.65,

1.67], I^2 = 0%, n = 141). The single study of mFOLFOX6 for rectal adenocarcinoma with metastasis after radical surgery (H62) did not specify the criteria used and only reported data for all grades. This study found no significant difference between groups (RR: 0.50 [0.14, 1.84], n = 68) for chemotherapy-related hepatotoxicity.

In the 14 RCTs that reported on transaminases using the WHO criteria, ten reported zero grade III plus IV events in both groups (Table 5.65). For the three studies included in the meta-analysis, the pooled result found no significant difference between groups for elevated transaminases (RR: 0.69 [0.16, 2.94], I^2 = 0%).

For all grades of hepatotoxicity (Table 5.66) based on transaminases (WHO criteria), there were no differences between groups in the pool of five RCTs of FOLFOX4 (RR: 0.84 [0.48, 1.44], I^2 = 0%) or in the pool of six studies that used similar chemotherapies (RR: 0.85

Table 5.65 Oral Chinese Herbal Medicine plus Chemotherapy versus Chemotherapy: Chemotherapy-related Hepatotoxicity (Transaminases, WHO Grade III+IV)

Chemotherapy Regimen:[1] N Studies (N Participants); N Studies with 0 Events in Both Groups	N Studies (N Participants) in Meta-analysis	Effect Size (RR [95% CI]), I^2	Included Studies (Studies with 0 Events in Both Groups)
FOLFOX4: 5 (205); 4	1 (60)	0.50 [0.05, 5.22]	H85 (H54, H100, H104, H107)
FOLFOX6: 1 (66); 1	0 (0)	Both groups = 0 events	(H86)
XELOX: 4 (223); 3	1 (90)	0.20 [0.01, 4.05]	H75 (H92, H94, H114)
FOLFIRI: 1 (36); 1	0 (0)	Both groups = 0 events	(H89)
S1+oxaliplatin: 1 (66); 0	1 (66)	2.00 [0.19, 21.00]	H101
XELIRI: 1 (36); 1	0 (0)	Both groups = 0 events	(H78)
Total pool: 13 (632); 10	3 (216)	0.69 [0.16, 2.94], 0%	All above

[1]Comparator was the same chemotherapy.

*Statistically significant.

Abbreviations: CI, confidence interval; N, number; RR, risk ratio; WHO, World Health Organisation.

Table 5.66 Oral Chinese Herbal Medicine plus Chemotherapy versus Chemotherapy: Chemotherapy-related Hepatotoxicity (Transaminases, WHO All Grades)

Chemotherapy Regimen[1]	*N* Studies (*N* Participants)	Effect Size (RR [95% CI]), I^2	Included Studies
FOLFOX4 (all)	5 (205)	0.84 [0.48, 1.44], 0%	H54, H85, H100, H104, H107
FOLFOX4 (adjuvant, after radical surgery)	2 (60)	0.52 [0.14, 1.91], 32.6%	H104, H107
FOLFOX6	1 (66)	1.00 [0.15, 6.68]	H86
Pool for similar chemotherapy[2]	6 (271)	0.85 [0.50, 1.43], 0%	H54, H85, H86, H100, H104, H107
XELOX (all)	4 (223)	0.74 [0.43, 1.26], 0%	H75, H92, H94, H114
XELOX (after surgery)	1 (40)	0.67 [0.12, 3.57]	H114
XELOX (without surgery)	3 (183)	0.75 [0.42, 1.32], 0%	H75, H92, H94
FOLFIRI	1 (36)	0.50 [0.05, 5.04]	H89
S1+oxaliplatin	1 (66)	0.80 [0.24, 2.72]	H101
XELODA	1 (60)	0.50 [0.05, 5.22]	H95
XELIRI	1 (36)	0.45 [0.17, 1.16]	H78
Total pool	14 (692)	0.73 [0.52, 1.01], 0%	All above

[1]Comparator was the same chemotherapy.

[2]These chemotherapy regimens all use oxaliplatin, 5-FU plus LV.

*Statistically significant.

Abbreviations: CI, confidence interval; N, number; RR, risk ratio; WHO, World Health Organisation.

[0.50, 1.43], I^2 = 0%). In the four studies of XELOX there was no difference between groups (RR: 0.74 [0.43, 1.26], I^2 = 0%) and there were no differences in any of the other subgroups. In the pooled result of all 14 studies, the incidence of abnormal transaminases was not different between groups (RR: 0.73 [0.52, 1.01], I^2 = 0%).

In the two RCTs that used the NCI-CTCAE criteria for elevated ALT and AST, there were zero events in both groups for grade III plus IV events, so data suitable for meta-analysis were only available for all grades. In the study of mFOLFOX6 (H103) for people with stage III/IV CRC, there were no differences between groups for ALT or AST. In the other study (H58), which was a placebo-controlled study of FOLFOX6 for people with stage III/IV CRC, there were no significant differences between groups for ALT or AST. The pooled results for the two studies showed no differences for incidence of abnormal ALT (RR: 0.73 [0.28, 1.89], I^2 = 0%, n = 71) or abnormal AST (RR: 0.81 [0.28, 2.38], I^2 = 0%, n = 71).

In the single study that did not specify the criteria used (H50), there were no differences between groups for all grades of abnormal ALT (RR: 0.43 [0.18, 1.03], n = 87) in people with stage III/IV CRC who received FOLFIRI.

In the single RCT that reported on bilirubin (all grades, WHO) for people with stage IV CRC who received XELODA (H95), there was no difference between groups in the incidence of abnormal bilirubin levels (RR: 0.50 [0.05, 5.22], n = 60).

Nephrotoxicity

Four RCTs reported on chemotherapy-related nephrotoxicity using the WHO criteria and one study (H62) did not specify the criteria used. Five RCTs reported creatinine and one (H104) reported the ratio creatinine/blood urea nitrogen (BUN) based on the WHO criteria. Two RCTs reported creatinine based on the NCI-CTCAE criteria. One study (H50) reported creatinine and BUN but did not specify the criteria. Data were pooled for chemotherapy-related nephrotoxicity (WHO criteria) and creatinine and/or BUN (WHO criteria).

In the four studies of chemotherapy-related nephrotoxicity based on the WHO criteria, three reported zero grade III plus IV events in both groups (Table 5.67). In the remaining study (H75) there were no significant differences between groups (RR: 0.33 [0.01, 7.97]). For all grades, there were no significant differences in any of the chemotherapy subgroups and the pooled result for the four RCTs showed no significant differences between groups (RR: 0.62 [0.21, 1.80], I^2 = 0%).

Table 5.67 Oral Chinese Herbal Medicine plus Chemotherapy versus Chemotherapy: Chemotherapy-related Nephrotoxicity (WHO)

Chemotherapy Regimen:[1] *N* Studies (*N* Participants); *N* Studies with 0 Events in Both Groups	*N* Studies (*N* Participants) in Meta-analysis	Effect Size (RR [95% CI]), I^2	Included Studies (Studies with 0 Events in Both Groups)
Grade III+IV			
mFOLFOX6: 1 (54); 1	0 (0)	Both groups = 0 events	(H87)
OLF: 1 (40); 1	0 (0)	Both groups = 0 events	(H53)
XELOX: 1 (90); 0	1 (90)	0.33 [0.01, 7.97]	H75
XELIRI: 1 (55); 1	0 (0)	Both groups = 0 events	(H96)
All grades			
mFOLFOX6: 1 (54); 0	1 (54)	0.33 [0.04, 3.01]	H87
OLF: 1 (40); 0	1 (40)	0.67 [0.12, 3.57]	H53
Pool for similar chemotherapy[2]: 2 (94); 0	2 (94)	0.52 [0.14, 1.96], 0%	H53, H87
XELOX: 1 (90); 0	1 (90)	0.50 [0.10, 2.59]	H75
XELIRI: 1 (55); 0	1 (55)	0.72 [0.18, 2.93]	H96
Total pool: 4 (239); 0	4 (239)	0.62 [0.21, 1.80], 0%	All above

[1]Comparator was the same chemotherapy.

[2]These chemotherapy regimens all use oxaliplatin, 5-FU plus LV.

*Statistically significant.

Abbreviations: CI, confidence interval; N, number; RR, risk ratio; WHO, World Health Organisation.

In the study that did not specify the criteria (H62) there was no difference between groups in all grades of chemotherapy-related nephrotoxicity (RR 1.33 [0.32, 5.51], $n = 68$) in people who received mFOLFOX6 for rectal adenocarcinoma with metastasis after radical surgery.

In the six RCTs that reported creatinine or creatinine/BUN based on the WHO criteria, all reported zero grade III plus IV events in both groups. For all grades, two studies reported zero events in both

Table 5.68 Oral Chinese Herbal Medicine plus Chemotherapy versus Chemotherapy: Chemotherapy-related Abnormal Creatinine and/or Blood Urea Nitrogen (WHO All Grades)

Chemotherapy Regimen:[1] *N* Studies (*N* Participants); *N* Studies with 0 Events in Both Groups	*N* Studies (*N* Participants) in Meta-analysis	Effect Size (RR [95% CI]), I^2	Included Studies (Studies with 0 Events in Both Groups)
FOLFOX4 (all): 3 (100); 0	3 (100)	0.85 [0.30, 2.40], 0%	H100, H104, H107
FOLFOX4 (adjuvant, after radical surgery): 2 (60); 0	2 (60)	1.00 [0.20, 5.05], 0%	H104, H107
XELOX: 3 (120); 2	1 (40)	0.33 [0.01, 7.72]	H114 (H92, H93)
Total pool: 6 (220); 2	4 (140)	0.77 [0.29, 2.07], 0%	All above

[1]Comparator was the same chemotherapy.

*Statistically significant.

Abbreviations: CI, confidence interval; N, number; RR, risk ratio; WHO, World Health Organisation.

groups, so the meta-analysis included four studies (Table 5.68). There was no difference between groups in the pooled result for three RCTs of FOLFOX4 (RR: 0.85 [0.30, 2.40], I^2 = 0%) and there was no significant difference between groups in incidence of abnormal creatinine and/or BUN (RR: 0.77 [0.29, 2.07], I^2 = 0%) in the total pool.

In the two RCTs that reported creatinine based on the NCI-CTCAE criteria, both had zero grade III plus IV events. For all grades, there were no differences between groups in the study of mFOLFOX6 for stage III/IV CRC (H103) or in the study of FOLFOX6 for stage III/IV CRC (H58). The pooled result showed no significant difference in the incidence of abnormal creatinine levels (RR: 0.99 [0.22, 4.47], I^2 = 0%, *n* = 71).

In the study of FOLFIRI for stage III/IV CRC (H50) that did not specify the criteria, there were no differences between groups for all grades of abnormal creatinine levels (RR: 0.85 [0.06, 13.18], *n* = 87) or BUN (RR: 0.85 [0.06, 13.18], *n* = 87).

Hepatotoxicity and Nephrotoxicity

In the two RCTs that reported hepatotoxicity and nephrotoxicity as a single item based on the WHO criteria, there were zero grade III plus IV events in both groups. For all grades, the study of FOLFOX4 (H47) as adjuvant chemotherapy after radical surgery (n = 55) reported no events in either group. In the other study (H72) that used FOLFIRI for stage IV CRC, there were no significant differences between groups for chemotherapy-related hepatotoxicity and/or nephrotoxicity (RR: 0.72 [0.22, 2.39], n = 55).

Heart Function

Three studies reported data on heart function. In the two studies that reported heart function/cardiac toxicity based on WHO criteria, there were zero grade III plus IV events. For all grades, there were zero events in both groups in the study of FOLFOX4 (H100), and in the study of XELOX (H75), there were two events in each group (RR: 1.00 [0.15, 6.79], n = 90).

In the single study (H58) of FOLFOX6 that reported electrocardiogram (ECG) abnormalities based on the NCI-CTCAE criteria, there was one event in the combination therapy group and two events in the FOLFOX6 alone group. There was no difference between groups (RR: 0.50 [0.05, 4.94], n = 30).

Oral Mucositis

Twelve studies reported on incidence of oral mucositis. Ten used the WHO criteria, one used the NCI-CTCAE criteria and one did not specify the criteria. Of the ten studies that used the WHO criteria (Table 5.69), nine reported data for grade III plus IV events, of which five studies reported zero events in both groups. In the remaining four studies, there were no differences between groups (RR: 0.33 [0.07, 1.61], I^2 = 0%). All ten studies reported data for all grades, with one study of XELIRI (H78) reporting zero events in both groups. In the pooled results for three studies of FOLFOX4 and one study of

Table 5.69 Oral Chinese Herbal Medicine plus Chemotherapy versus Chemotherapy: Chemotherapy-related Oral Mucositis (WHO)

Chemotherapy Regimen:[1] *N* Studies (*N* Participants); *N* Studies with 0 Events in Both Groups	*N* Studies (*N* Participants) in Meta-analysis	Effect Size (RR [95% CI]), I^2	Included Studies (Studies with 0 Events in Both Groups)
Grade III+IV			
FOLFOX4: 3 (119); 2	1 (60)	0.33 [0.01, 7.87]	H85 (H54, H112)
mFOLFOX6: 1 (54); 0	1 (54)	0.33 [0.01, 7.84]	H87
Pool for similar chemotherapy[2]: 4 (173); 2	2 (114)	0.33 [0.04, 3.11], 0%	H85, H87 (H54, H112)
LF: 1 (60); 1	0 (0)	Both groups = 0 events	H118
XELOX: 2 (143); 0	2 (143)	0.33 [0.04, 3.07]	H75, H94
XELIRI: 2 (66); 2	0 (0)	Both groups = 0 events	(H78, H79)
Total pool: 9 (472); 5	4 (257)	0.33 [0.07, 1.61], 0%	All above
All grades			
FOLFOX4: 3 (119); 0	3 (119)	0.57 [0.30, 1.07], 0%	H54, H85, H112
mFOLFOX6: 1 (54); 0	1 (54)	0.58 [0.27, 1.25]	H87
Pool for similar chemotherapy[2]: 4 (173): 0	4 (173)	0.57 [0.35, 0.94]*, 0%	H54, H85, H87, H112
LF: 1 (60); 0	1 (60)	0.36 [0.15, 0.87]	H118
XELOX: 2 (143): 0	2 (143)	0.61 [0.35, 1.07], 0%	H75, H94
XELIRI: 2 (66); 1	1 (30)	3.00 [0.13, 68.26]	H79 (H78)
HIPEC: 1 (60); 0	1 (60)	0.89 [0.40, 1.99]	H56
Total pool: 10 (532); 1	9 (466)	0.60 [0.44, 0.82]*, 0%	All above

[1]Comparator was the same chemotherapy.

[2]These chemotherapy regimens all use oxaliplatin, 5-FU plus LV.

*Statistically significant.

Abbreviations: CI, confidence interval; HIPEC: hyperthermic intraperitoneal chemotherapy; N, number; RR, risk ratio; WHO, World Health Organisation.

mFOLFOX6 there was a significant reduction in the incidence of oral mucositis in the CHM plus chemotherapy groups (RR: 0.57 [0.35, 0.94], I^2 = 0%). In the pool of two studies of XELOX, there were no significant differences between groups (RR: 0.61 [0.35, 1.07], I^2 = 0%) but the total pooled result for nine studies showed a significant reduction in the combination therapy groups compared to chemotherapy alone (RR: 0.60 [0.44, 0.82], I^2 = 0%).

In the study of FOLFOX6 that used the NCI-CTCAE criteria (H58), there were zero grade III plus IV events in the combination therapy group versus one event in the FOLFOX6 alone group, which was not significant. For all grades, there were no significant differences between groups (RR: 0.29 [0.07, 1.16], $n = 30$). In the study that did not specify the criteria (H50), there was one grade III/IV event in the combination therapy group versus two in the FOLFIRI alone group, which was not a significant difference. There was no significant difference between groups for all grades of oral mucositis (RR: 0.59 [0.31, 1.11], $n = 87$).

Fever

Four studies reported on fever. Three studies (H44, H66, H68) used the WHO criteria and one study (H120) used NCI-CTCAE. Since these criteria are the same for this item, the results were combined. For grade III plus IV, there were zero events in three studies (H44, H66, H68) and the other study did not report data (H120). For all grades, there were zero events in the two studies of FOLFOX4 (H66, H68). In the two remaining studies, there were no differences between groups for FOLFOX6 (H44) or FOLFIRI (H120) and no significant differences in the pooled result (RR: 0.67 [0.33, 1.39], I^2 = 0%, $n = 114$).

Alopecia

Of the four studies that reported on chemotherapy-induced alopecia, one study (H101) used the WHO criteria, one study (H91) used

NCI-CTCAE and two studies (H50, H62) did not specify the criteria. In the study of SI plus oxaliplatin that used the WHO criteria (H101), there was one grade III plus IV event in each group and no significant difference between groups for all grades of alopecia (RR: 0.60 [0.16, 2.31], n = 66). In the study of XELOX that used the NCI-CTCAE criteria (H91), there were zero grade III plus IV events in each group, and for all grades there were no significant differences between the two groups (RR: 1.05 [0.58, 1.87], n = 97). For the two studies that did not report the criteria used (one of mFOLFOX6, one of FOLFIRI), there was no difference between groups for all grades of alopecia in either study or in the pooled result (RR 0.77 [0.41, 1.45], I^2 = 0%, n = 155).

Skin Rash

Two studies reported on chemotherapy-related skin rash. One study (H44) used the WHO criteria and the other study (H50) did not specify the criteria. For WHO grade III plus IV, there were zero events in both groups in the study of FOLFOX6 for advanced CRC and there were no differences between groups for all grades (RR: 0.50 [0.05, 5.27], n = 70). In the other study, which used FOLFIRI in stage III/IV CRC, there were no significant differences between groups for all grades of skin rash (RR: 0.43 [0.04, 4.52], n = 87).

GRADE for Oral Chinese Herbal Medicine plus Chemotherapy

Grading of Recommendations Assessment, Development and Evaluation (GRADE) assessments were according the procedures outlined in Chapter 4. Each assessment was for the integrative application of oral CHMs combined with guideline-recommended chemotherapies for CRC. The outcome measures selected were:

- Objective response rate according to the WHO criteria and the RECIST criteria;
- Chemotherapy-induced nausea and vomiting according to the WHO criteria (all grades);

- Chemotherapy-related abnormal haematological parameters (all grades) for: leukopenia, neutropenia, haemoglobin and thrombocytopenia;
- Chemotherapy-induced peripheral neurotoxicity according the WHO criteria (all grades), Levi's criteria (all grades) and NCI-CTCAE criteria (all grades).

GRADE for Objective Response Rate

For objective response rate (ORR), 25 studies provided data for 1,580 participants based on the WHO criteria and 23 studies provided data for 1,484 participants based on the RECIST criteria (Table 5.70). For both criteria the meta-analysis result indicated significantly increased tumour response rates in the groups that combined chemotherapy for

Table 5.70 GRADE for Oral Chinese Herbal Medicine plus Chemotherapy versus Chemotherapy: Objective Response Rate

Outcome (Criteria)	Absolute Effect		Relative Effect (95% CI) *N* Studies (*N* Participants)	Certainty of Evidence GRADE
	With CHM	Without CHM		
Objective response rate (WHO)	**385** per 1,000	**296** per 1,000	**RR 1.3*** (1.14 to 1.47) 25 (1,580)	⊕⊕⊕◯ MODERATE[1]
	Difference: 89 more per 1,000 patients (95% CI: 41 to 139 more)			
Objective response rate (RECIST)	**449** per 1,000	**343** per 1,000	**RR 1.31*** (1.16 to 1.48) 23 (1,484)	⊕⊕⊕◯ MODERATE[1]
	Difference: 106 more per 1,000 patients (95% CI: 55 to 165 more)			

[1]No blinding.

*Statistically significant result, random effect model.

Abbreviations: CHM, Chinese herbal medicine; CI, confidence interval; GRADE, Grading of Recommendations Assessment, Development and Evaluation; MD, mean difference; N, number; NCI-CTCAE, National Cancer Institute-Common Terminology Criteria for Adverse Events; RECIST, Response Evaluation Criteria in Solid Tumours; WHO, World Health Organisation.

Study references: Table 5.24 and Table 5.25 for included studies.

CRC with CHM compared to the same chemotherapy. There was no important statistical heterogeneity in either result. Since most of the studies were not blinded, the certainty of the evidence was rated down one grade to 'moderate' for both outcomes.

GRADE for Chemotherapy-induced Nausea and Vomiting

For chemotherapy-induced nausea and vomiting (CINV), substantial data were only available for the WHO criteria (all grades). Based on 37 studies, which provided data for 2,075 participants, there was a significant reduction in the incidence of CINV in the integrative therapy groups, which combined CHM with chemotherapy (Table 5.71). The certainty of the evidence was rated down two grades to 'low' due to lack of blinding in the majority of the studies, and substantial statistical heterogeneity (I^2 = 59.4%) in the meta-analysis pool. However, it is important to note that heterogeneity was zero in the total pool for WHO grades III plus IV (22 studies, 1,199 participants).

Table 5.71   GRADE for Oral Chinese Herbal Medicine plus Chemotherapy versus Chemotherapy: Chemotherapy-induced Nausea and Vomiting (All Grades)

Outcome (Criteria)	Absolute Effect		Relative Effect (95% CI) N studies (N participants)	Certainty of Evidence GRADE
	With CHM	Without CHM		
Chemotherapy-induced nausea and vomiting (WHO, all grades)	**391** per 1,000	**611** per 1,000	**RR 0.64*** (0.57 to 0.73) 37 (2,075)	⊕⊕◯◯ LOW[1,2]
	Difference: 220 fewer per 1,000 patients (95% CI: 165 to 263 fewer)			

[1]No blinding.

[2]Statistical heterogeneity was substantial.

*Statistically significant result, random effect model.

Abbreviations: CHM, Chinese herbal medicine; CI, confidence interval; GRADE, Grading of Recommendations Assessment, Development and Evaluation; MD, mean difference; N, number; NCI-CTCAE, National Cancer Institute-Common Terminology Criteria for Adverse Events; WHO, World Health Organisation.

Study references: see Table 5.40 for included studies.

GRADE for Chemotherapy-related Abnormal Haematological Parameters

Assessments were made for the following four categories of chemotherapy-related abnormal haematological findings: leukopenia, neutropenia, haemoglobin and thrombocytopenia. All assessments were based on incidence of all grades of these events using the WHO or NCI-CTCAE criteria (Table 5.72). For each parameter, there was a significantly reduced incidence in the CHM plus pharmacotherapy group without important heterogeneity. The number of studies included in the meta-analyses ranged from nine to 38 and the number of participants ranged from 651 to 2,208, so these results were based on substantial sample sizes. The certainty of the evidence was downgraded by one grade to 'moderate' since the majority of the studies were not blinded.

GRADE for Chemotherapy-induced Peripheral Neurotoxicity

Three measures of the incidence of all grades of CIPN were assessed: WHO criteria, Levi's modified WHO criteria and the NCI-CTCAE criteria. Most data were available for the WHO criteria with the least for the NCI-CTCAE criteria. For the WHO criteria, there was a significant reduction in the incidence of CIPN in the CHM plus pharmacotherapy groups without important heterogeneity, based on 27 studies and results for 1,608 participants (Table 5.73). The GRADE assessment was rated down one level to 'moderate' due to lack of blinding in the majority of the studies.

For Levi's criteria, data were available for 389 participants in five studies. There was a significant reduction in CIPN in the CHM plus pharmacotherapy groups, but there was considerable heterogeneity. This led to a downgrading of the certainty of the evidence by an additional level to 'low'. For the NCI-CTCAE criteria, there was no significant difference between groups without important heterogeneity based on four studies with 230 participants. It is notable that this result showed the same trend as for the other two measures. Due to the lack of blinding in most of these studies and the small overall sample size, the GRADE assessment was rated down two levels to 'low'.

Table 5.72 Oral Chinese Herbal Medicine plus Chemotherapy versus Chemotherapy: Chemotherapy-related Abnormal Haematological Parameters

Outcome (Criteria)	Absolute Effect		Relative Effect (95% CI) N Studies (N Participants)	Certainty of Evidence GRADE
	With CHM	Without CHM		
Chemotherapy-related leukopenia (WHO or NCI-CTCAE, all grades)	**485** per 1,000	**674** per 1,000	**RR 0.72*** (0.65 to 0.78) 38 (2,097)	⊕⊕⊕◯ MODERATE[1]
	Difference: 189 fewer per 1,000 patients (95% CI: 148 to 236 fewer)			
Chemotherapy-related neutropenia (WHO or NCI-CTCAE, all grades)	**358** per 1,000	**512** per 1,000	**RR 0.7*** (0.6 to 0.81) 9 (651)	⊕⊕⊕◯ MODERATE[1]
	Difference: 154 fewer per 1,000 patients (95% CI: 97 to 205 fewer)			
Chemotherapy-related reduced haemoglobin (WHO or NCI-CTCAE, all grades)	**304** per 1,000	**400** per 1,000	**RR 0.76*** (0.67 to 0.87) 28 (1,563)	⊕⊕⊕◯ MODERATE[1]
	Difference: 96 fewer per 1,000 patients (95% CI: 52 to 132 fewer)			
Chemotherapy-related thrombocytopenia (WHO or NCI-CTCAE, all grades)	**217** per 1,000	**297** per 1,000	**RR 0.73*** (0.64 to 0.84) 38 (2,208)	⊕⊕⊕◯ MODERATE[1]
	Difference: 80 fewer per 1,000 patients (95% CI: 48 to 107 fewer)			

[1]No blinding.

*Statistically significant result, random effect model.

Abbreviations: CHM, Chinese herbal medicine; CI, confidence interval; GRADE, Grading of Recommendations Assessment, Development and Evaluation; MD, mean difference; N, number; NCI-CTCAE, National Cancer Institute-Common Terminology Criteria for Adverse Events; WHO, World Health Organisation.

Study references: see Table 5.47, Table 5.49, Table 5.52 and Table 5.54 for included studies.

Table 5.73 GRADE for Oral Chinese Herbal Medicine plus Chemotherapy versus Chemotherapy: Chemotherapy-induced Peripheral Neurotoxicity

Outcome (Criteria)	Absolute Effect		Relative Effect (95% CI) N Studies (N Participants)	Certainty of Evidence GRADE
	With CHM	Without CHM		
Chemotherapy-induced peripheral neurotoxicity (WHO, all grades)	**378** per 10,00	**455** per 1,000	**RR 0.83*** (0.76 to 0.91) 27 (1,608)	⊕⊕⊕◯ MODERATE[1]
	Difference: 77 fewer per 1,000 patients (95% CI: 41 to 109 fewer)			
Chemotherapy-induced peripheral neurotoxicity (Levi, all grades)	**390** per 1,000	**764** per 1,000	**RR 0.51*** (0.34 to 0.76) 5 (389)	⊕⊕◯◯ LOW[1,2]
	Difference: 374 fewer per 1,000 patients (95% CI: 183 to 504 fewer)			
Chemotherapy-induced peripheral neurotoxicity (NCI-CTCAE, all grades)	**258** per 1,000	**363** per 1,000	**RR 0.71** (0.48 to 1.05) 4 (230)	⊕⊕◯◯ LOW[1,3]
	Difference: 105 fewer per 1,000 patients (95% CI: 189 fewer to 18 more)			

[1]No blinding.

[2]Statistical heterogeneity was considerable.

[3]Four RCTs with small sample sizes.

*Statistically significant result, random effect model.

Abbreviations: CHM, Chinese herbal medicine; CI, confidence interval; GRADE, Grading of Recommendations Assessment, Development and Evaluation; MD, mean difference; N, number; NCI-CTCAE, National Cancer Institute-Common Terminology Criteria for Adverse Events; WHO, World Health Organisation.

Study references: see Table 5.58, Table 5.59 and Table 5.60 for included studies.

Randomised Controlled Trial Evidence for Individual Oral Formulas in Conjunction with Chemotherapy

Of the 14 oral formulas used in two or more RCTs (see Table 5.21) the majority were not suitable for pooling in a meta-analysis due to differences in the comparisons and/or outcome measures. Four formulas that were combined with chemotherapy were suitable for pooling of KPS data and three of these formulas were suitable for ORR. The results are reported separately for these two outcome measures. All four formulas were named by the authors or their hospitals.

Objective Response Rate

Four of the included studies used the WHO criteria and two studies used the RECIST criteria for ORR (Table 5.74). For the two studies (H48, H49) of *Fu zheng xiao ji tang* 扶正消积汤 in colon cancer, there were no significant differences between the combined therapy group and FOLFOX4. *Qi lian fu zheng jiao nang* 芪连扶正胶囊 combined with OLF for CRC was not significantly different to OLF alone (H52, H53). *Wei tiao san hao fang* 微调 3 号方 combined with XELODA (H55) or FOLFOX (H54) for stage IV CRC with liver metastasis did not show a significant difference in ORR.

Karnofsky Performance Scale

Eight studies provided data suitable for pooling (Table 5.75). The two studies (H54, H55) of *Wei tiao san hao fang* 微调3号方 reported the

Table 5.74 Individual Oral Formulas Combined with Chemotherapy: Objective Response Rate

Formula Name (Criteria)[1]	N Studies (N Participants)	Effect Size (RR [95% CI]), I²	Included Studies
Fu zheng xiao ji tang 扶正消积汤 (RECIST)	2 (169)	1.16 [0.84, 1.61], 0%	H48, H49
Qi lian fu zheng jiao nang 芪连扶正胶囊 (WHO)	2 (89)	1.41 [0.79, 2.55], 0%	H52, H53
Wei tiao san hao fang 微调 3号方 (WHO)	2 (150)	1.46 [0.64, 3.35], 0%	H54, H55

[1]Comparator was the same chemotherapy.

*Statistically significant.

Abbreviations: CI, confidence interval; N, number; RECIST, Response Evaluation Criteria in Solid Tumours; RR, risk ratio; WHO, World Health Organisation.

Table 5.75   Individual Oral Formulas Combined with Chemotherapy: Karnofsky Performance Scale

Formula Name[1]	N Studies (N Participants)	Effect Size (RR/MD [95% CI]), I^2	Included Studies
Fu zheng xiao ji tang 扶正消积汤	2 (169)	RR 1.59 [1.18, 2.15]*, 0%	H48, H49
Qi lian fu zheng jiao nang 芪连扶正胶囊	2 (89)	RR 3.09 [1.37, 6.95]*, 0%	H52, H53
Wei tiao san hao fang 微调3号方	2 (150)	MD 5.83 [1.29, 10.36]*, 48.3%	H54, H55
Xiao liu tang 消瘤汤	2 (164)	RR 2.10 [1.42, 3.10]*, 0%	H56, H57

[1]Comparator was the same chemotherapy.

*Statistically significant.

Abbreviations: CI, confidence interval; MD, mean difference; N, number; RR, risk ratio.

KPS scores. The pooled result showed a significant improvement in KPS in the combination therapy groups. The other six studies reported the incidence of 10 points or more improvement in KPS scores. There were significant improvements in the pooled results for *Fu zheng xiao ji tang* 扶正消积汤 (H48, H49) and *Qi lian fu zheng jiao nang* 芪连扶正胶囊 (H52, H53). The same result was found for *Xiao liu tang* 消瘤汤 (H56, H57), which was combined with HIPEC for stage II/III CRC after surgery.

Frequently Reported Herbs in Meta-analyses of Oral Chinese Herbal Medicine in Conjunction with Chemotherapy Showing Favourable Effect

In the 92 RCTs that assessed oral CHMs in conjunction with chemotherapy, the most commonly used outcome measures in the meta-analyses were ORR (48 RCTs), KPS (68 RCTs), and the chemotherapy-related AEs of myelosuppression (59 RCTs) and nausea and vomiting (52 RCTs). In this section, we selected three outcomes of relevance to clinicians, researchers and patients. Objective response rate was selected since it is relevant to the selection of herbs that show potential for reducing processes associated with the growth and/or development of tumours. Nausea and vomiting were selected since these are a major source of patient distress. Myelosuppression was selected since it is a major clinical issue that may lead to discontinuation of chemotherapy; KPS was not selected since it is a less specific outcome.

In order to assess which herbs were likely to have contributed to the significant benefits found for the integrative use of oral CHMs, we selected the meta-analysis pools that showed significant differences in favour of the oral CHM plus chemotherapy test groups and calculated the frequencies of the individual herbal ingredients included in the CHM interventions. Each study was counted once only.

For ORR, the meta-analysis pools for CHM plus chemotherapy versus chemotherapy alone that used the WHO and RECIST criteria were included. In the 48 included studies, the top ten herbs were very similar to the high-frequency herbs in all 92 studies of CHM in association with chemotherapy. These included herbs typically used for anti-cancer effects such as *yi yi ren* 薏苡仁, *she she cao* 蛇舌草, *ban zhi lian* 半枝莲 and *e zhu* 莪术 (Table 5.76).

For chemotherapy-related myelosuppression, 45 RCTs were included in the five meta-analysis pools that showed significant differences in favour of the test groups for a myelosuppression outcome (all grades). The top ten herbs used in these studies (Table 5.77) were very similar to those in the previous table. The difference was in the herbs ranked number 9: *shao yao* 芍药 (including *bai shao* 白芍 and *chi shao* 赤芍) and number 10: *shan yao* 山药. For grades III/IV myelosuppression there were numerous zero events, so it was not feasible to calculate herb frequency.

For chemotherapy-induced nausea and vomiting, 39 studies were included in the meta-analyses that showed reductions in all grades of CIPN in the CHM plus chemotherapy groups (WHO criteria, all grades), compared to chemotherapy alone groups. Analysis of grade III plus IV events was not feasible. The list of herbs was very similar to the previous two tables. The included herbs were the same as for tumour response rate. Of the included herbs, *ban xia* 半夏 is a typical herb for nausea and vomiting. It is often paired with *chen pi* 陈皮 which was ranked number 11 (Table. 5.78).

Table 5.76 Frequently Reported Orally Used Herbs in Meta-analyses Showing Favourable Effect for Objective Response Rate

N Meta-analyses (N Studies)	Herbs	Scientific Name	Frequency of Use
2* (48)	*Bai zhu* 白术[1]	*Atractylodes macrocephala* Koidz.	37
	Yi yi ren 薏苡仁[2]	*Coix lacryma-jobi* L. var. *mayuen* (Roman.) Stapf	32
	Huang qi 黄芪[3]	*Astragalus membranaceus* (Fisch.) Bge.	32
	Fu ling 茯苓	*Poria cocos* (Schw.) Wolf	31
	She she cao 蛇舌草	*Hedyotis diffusa* Willd.	25
	Gan cao 甘草[4]	*Glycyrrhiza spp.*	22
	Ban zhi lian 半枝莲	*Scutellaria barbata* D. Don	19
	Dang shen 党参	*Codonopsis pilosula* (Franch.) Nannf.	17
	Ban xia 半夏[5]	*Pinellia ternata* (Thunb.) Breit.	15
	E zhu 莪术	*Curcuma phaeocaulis* Val.	15

*Objective response rate: refer to Tables 5.24 and Table 5.25.

[1]Nine RCTs used *chao bai zhu* 炒白术 and one used *jiao bai zhu* 焦白术.

[2]Nine RCTs used *sheng yi yi ren* 生薏苡仁 and one used *chao yi yi ren* 炒薏苡仁.

[3]Four RCTs used *sheng huang qi* 生黄芪 and one used *zhi huang qi* 炙黄芪.

[4]Eight RCTs used *zhi gan cao* 炙甘草 and one used *sheng gan cao* 生甘草.

[5]Five RCTs used *fa ban xia* 法半夏, two used *jiang ban xia* 姜半夏 and one used *qing ban xia* 清半夏.

Abbreviations: N, number; RCT, randomised controlled trial.

The use of some herbs may be restricted in some countries. Readers are advised to comply with relevant regulations.

Overall, the lists of the ten highest-frequency herbs used in the above three analyses were very similar to the top ten herbs for all studies (Table 5.22). The only differences were in which herbs were ranked ninth or tenth. A likely reason is most studies used multi-ingredient formulas that aimed at addressing a range of outcomes associated with CRC and chemotherapy treatment, rather than prioritising a specific outcome. In general, the high-frequency herbs

Table 5.77 Frequently Reported Orally Used Herbs in Meta-analyses Showing Favourable Effect for Myelosuppression (All Grades)

N Meta-analyses (N Studies)	Herbs	Scientific Name	Frequency of Use
5* (45)	*Bai zhu* 白术[1]	*Atractylodes macrocephala* Koidz.	35
	Huang qi 黄芪[2]	*Astragalus membranaceus* (Fisch.) Bge.	33
	Fu ling 茯苓	*Poria cocos* (Schw.) Wolf	30
	Yi yi ren 薏苡仁[3]	*Coix lacryma-jobi* L. var. *mayuen* (Roman.) Stapf	28
	Gan cao 甘草[4]	*Glycyrrhiza spp.*	21
	She she cao 蛇舌草	*Hedyotis diffusa* Willd.	21
	Ban zhi lian 半枝莲	*Scutellaria barbata* D. Don	16
	Dang shen 党参	*Codonopsis pilosula* (Franch.) Nannf.	15
	Shao yao 芍药[5]	*Dioscorea opposita* Thunb.	15
	Shan yao 山药	*Dioscorea opposita* Thunb.	13

*Myelosuppression: refer to Table 5.47, Table 5.49, Table 5.50, Table 5.52 and Table 5.54.

[1]Ten RCTs used *chao bai zhu* 炒白术 and one used *jiao bai zhu* 焦白术.

[2]Seven RCTs used *sheng huang qi* 生黄芪 and one used *zhi huang qi* 炙黄芪.

[3]Eight RCTs used *sheng yi yi ren* 生薏苡仁.

[4]Eight RCTs used *zhi gan cao* 炙甘草 and one used *sheng gan cao* 生甘草.

[5]Twelve RCTs used *bai shao* 白芍 and three used *chi shao* 赤芍.

Abbreviations: N, number; RCT, randomised controlled trial.

The use of some herbs may be restricted in some countries. Readers are advised to comply with relevant regulations.

tended to fall into the fortify the Spleen and replenish *qi* (*jian pi yi qi* 健脾益气) and resist cancer (*kang ai* 抗癌) groups.

Chinese Herbal Medicine Enema and/or Oral Chinese Herbal Medicine plus Chemotherapy versus Chemotherapy

In one RCT (H127) the participants were administered a formula called *Da huang ren shen fang* 大黄人参方 (*da huang* 大黄, *ren shen*

Table 5.78   Frequently Reported Orally Used Herbs in Meta-analyses Showing Favourable Effect for Nausea and Vomiting (All Grades)

N Meta-analyses (N Studies)	Herbs	Scientific Name	Frequency of Use
1* (39)	*Bai zhu* 白术[1]	*Atractylodes macrocephala* Koidz.	29
	Huang qi 黄芪[2]	*Astragalus membranaceus* (Fisch.) Bge.	29
	Fu ling 茯苓	*Poria cocos* (Schw.) Wolf	26
	Yi yi ren 薏苡仁[3]	*Coix lacryma-jobi* L. var. *mayuen* (Roman.) Stapf	24
	Gan cao 甘草[4]	*Glycyrrhiza spp.*	19
	She she cao 蛇舌草	*Hedyotis diffusa* Willd.	19
	Dang shen 党参	*Codonopsis pilosula* (Franch.) Nannf.	15
	Ban zhi lian 半枝莲	*Scutellaria barbata* D. Don	14
	E zhu 莪术	*Curcuma phaeocaulis* Val.	13
	Ban xia 半夏[5]	*Pinellia ternata* (Thunb.) Breit.	12

*Nausea and vomiting: refer to Table 5.40 (WHO criteria, all grades).

[1]Seven RCTs used *chao bai zhu* 炒白术 and one used *jiao bai zhu* 焦白术.

[2]Five RCTs used *sheng huang qi* 生黄芪 and one used *zhi huang qi* 炙黄芪.

[3]Seven RCTs used *sheng yi yi ren* 生薏苡仁.

[4]Nine RCTs used *zhi gan cao* 炙甘草 and one used *sheng gan cao* 生甘草.

[5]Three RCTs used *fa ban xia* 法半夏, two used *jiang ban xia* 姜半夏 and one used *qing ban xia* 清半夏.

Abbreviations: N, number; RCT, randomised controlled trial; WHO, World Health Organisation.

The use of some herbs may be restricted in some countries. Readers are advised to comply with relevant regulations.

人参, *xian he cao* 仙鹤草, *bai shao* 白芍, *yi yi ren* 薏苡仁, *ji nei jin* 鸡内金 and *gan cao* 甘草) as an oral decoction or as an enema when the person experienced vomiting. The participants ($n = 60$) were aged 41 to 70 years and all had stage IIIB/IV colon cancer and received FOLFOX4 for three cycles of two weeks each. The CHM was administered for seven days at the beginning of each cycle.

For sequence generation the RoB was judged 'unclear' due to lack of details of the method used. There was no mention of a method of allocation concealment, so the RoB was judged as 'unclear'. There was no mention of blinding of participants, personnel or outcome assessors so these domains were all judged as 'high' risk for blinding of participants and personnel and 'unclear' risk for blinding of outcome assessors. Since there were no drop-outs, the study was judged 'low' risk for incomplete outcome data. No protocol could be located but all the outcomes appear to have been reported, so the study was judged 'unclear' risk for selective outcome reporting.

For ORR (RECIST) the difference between groups was not significant (RR: 1.36 [0.76, 2.46], $n = 60$). Progression-free survival was five to nine months in the CHM plus FOLFOX4 group versus three to eight months in the FOLFOX4 alone group. For improvement in KPS of 10 points or more, the incidence was greater in the CHM plus FOLFOX4 group (RR: 1.92 [1.24, 2.98], $n = 60$).

For chemotherapy-related AEs, there was a significant reduction in WHO grade III plus IV nausea and/or vomiting, but not in any of the other grade III plus IV AEs (Table 5.79). For all grades, there were significant differences for leukopenia (RR: 0.42 [0.24, 0.71]),

Table 5.79 Chinese Herbal Medicine Enema or Oral Chinese Herbal Medicine plus FOLFOX4 versus FOLFOX4 for Chemotherapy-related Adverse Events

Chemotherapy-related Adverse Events	WHO Grade III+IV Effect Size (RR [95% CI])	WHO All Grades Effect Size (RR [95% CI])
Leukopenia	0.25 [0.06, 1.08]	0.42 [0.24, 0.71]*
Thrombocytopenia	0.33 [0.01, 7.87]	0.27 [0.08, 0.88]*
Reduced haemoglobin	0.33 [0.01, 7.87]	0.42 [0.17, 1.04]
Nausea/vomiting	0.10 [0.01, 0.73]*	0.35 [0.20, 0.61]*
Diarrhoea	0.20 [0.01, 4.00]	0.13 [0.02, 0.94]*
Abnormal liver function	0.20 [0.01, 4.00]	0.13 [0.02, 0.94]*
Abnormal kidney function	0.20 [0.01, 4.00]	0.30 [0.09, 0.98]*
CIPN	Both groups = 0	0.33 [0.01, 7.87]
Oral mucositis	0.89 [0.40, 1.99]	0.64 [0.41, 0.99]*

*Statistically significant.

Abbreviations: CI, confidence interval; CIPN, chemotherapy-induced peripheral neurotoxicity; RR, risk ratio; WHO, World Health Organisation.

thrombocytopenia (RR: 0.27 [0.08, 0.88]), nausea/vomiting (RR: 0.35 [0.20, 0.61]), diarrhoea (RR: 0.13 [0.02, 0.94]), abnormal liver function (RR: 0.13 [0.02, 0.94]), abnormal kidney function (RR: 0.30 [0.09, 0.98]) and oral mucositis (RR: 0.64 [0.41, 0.99]).

Chinese Herbal Medicine Enema plus Chemotherapy versus Chemotherapy

One RCT (H128) investigated a CHM enema (*ban zhi lian* 半枝莲, *sheng yi yi ren* 生薏苡仁, *sheng mu li* 生牡蛎, *e zhu* 莪术, *bai hua she she cao* 白花蛇舌草 and *chan su ye* 蟾酥液) combined with XELOX versus XELOX in people (*n* = 50) with stage II, III, IV CRC post-surgery. The mean age was 44 years in the CHM plus chemotherapy group and 46 years in the chemotherapy alone group). All participants had the CM syndrome *qi* deficiency with exuberant toxins (*qi xu du sheng* 气虚毒盛). The chemotherapy was for eight 3-week cycles and the enema was administered every evening for 60 days.

The RoB for sequence generation was judged 'unclear' since there were no details of the method used. There was no mention of a method of allocation concealment, so this was judged as 'unclear'. Blinding of participants or personnel was judged 'high' risk and outcome assessors was judged 'unclear' risk since the study did not mention blinding. There were no drop-outs, so the study was judged 'low' risk for incomplete outcome data. Since no protocol could be located but all the outcomes appear to have been reported, the study was judged 'unclear' risk for selective outcome reporting.

The data for KPS was reported as the number of people with increases of 10 points or more. There was no significant improvement in the CHM enema plus XELOX group (RR: 2.33 [0.68, 8.01], *n* − 50). Adverse reactions were based on the WHO criteria (all grades). In the CHM enema group, there were significant reductions in the incidence of people experiencing gastrointestinal reactions (RR: 0.43 [0.20, 0.93], *n* = 50), abnormal liver and kidney function (RR: 0.47 [0.23, 0.95], *n* = 50) and myelosuppression (RR: 0.38 [0.18, 0.80], *n* = 50). There was no difference between groups in abnormal heart function (RR: 0.33 [0.10, 1.09], $n = 50$). There was no mention of AEs associated with the enema.

Topical Chinese Herbal Medicine plus Chemotherapy versus Chemotherapy

Four RCTs (H129–H132) employed CHM hand and foot baths for CIPN and one RCT (H133) used a CHM cataplasm for myelosuppression. The results for these two groups of studies are reported separately.

Risk of Bias

Of the five RCTs of topical CHM, four were judged 'low' risk for sequence generation and one was judged 'unclear' risk, since it did not detail the method used (Table 5.80). One (H133) was judged 'low' risk for allocation concealment since a Statistics Analysis System (SAS) program was used to conceal the results of allocation. The others were 'unclear' risk for allocation concealment. Blinding of participants and personnel was judged 'low' risk in one study (H133) since it had a convincing placebo and mentioned the blinding of participants and personnel. The other studies were judged 'high' risk for blinding of participants and personnel. All studies were

Table 5.80 Risk of Bias of Randomised Controlled Trials of Topical Chinese Herbal Medicine

Risk of Bias Domain	Low Risk n (%)	Unclear Risk n (%)	High Risk n (%)
Sequence generation	4 (80)	1 (20)	0 (0)
Allocation concealment	1 (20)	4 (80)	0 (0)
Blinding of participants	1 (20)	0 (0)	4 (80)
Blinding of personnel	1 (20)	0 (0)	4 (80)
Blinding of outcome assessors	0 (0)	5 (100)	0 (0)
Incomplete outcome data	5 (100)	0 (0)	0 (0)
Selective reporting	0 (0)	5 (100)	0 (0)

judged 'unclear' risk for blinding of outcome assessors. There were no drop-outs, so all studies were judged 'low' risk for incomplete outcome data. No protocols could be located, but all the outcomes mentioned in the methods were reported so all studies were judged 'unclear' risk for selective reporting.

Chinese Herbal Medicine Hand and Foot Bath plus Chemotherapy versus Chemotherapy

Four RCTs investigated CHM decoctions used as hand and foot baths for the prevention of the symptoms of CIPN due to oxaliplatin-based chemotherapy. All used Levi's criteria.[20] The four RCTs were all conducted in mainland China and enrolled 324 participants. The age of participants ranged from 28 to 70 years, but the age range was not reported in two studies (H130, H131). Based on the reported means and standard deviations for ages, the majority of participants were aged between 35 and 63 years. There were no drop-outs and all participants completed the studies. There was no mention of syndrome differentiation.

The herbs most frequently used in the four hand and foot bath formulas were *hong hua* 红花 (*n* = 4), *huang qi* 黄芪 (*n* = 4), *tao ren* 桃仁 (*n* = 3), *di long* 地龙 (*n* = 2), *dang gui* 当归 (*n* = 2), *gui zhi* 桂枝 (*n* = 2), *fu zi* 附子 (*n* = 2) and *shao yao* 芍药 (*n* = 2) (Table 5.81).

One study (H131) involved four groups: (1) CHM plus mFOLFOX6; (2) mFOLFOX6; (3) CHM plus calcium gluconate (*pu tao tang suan gai* 葡萄糖酸钙) and magnesium sulphate (*liu suan mei* 硫酸镁) plus mFOLFOX6; and (4) calcium gluconate and magnesium sulphate plus mFOLFOX6. There were 30 people per group and this study was included as two comparisons: group 1 versus group 2 (H131.1) and group 3 versus group 4 (H131.2). The other studies all compared two groups.

The pooled incidence of people with level III or IV CIPN was not significantly different between groups (RR: 0.35 [0.10, 1.20], I^2 = 0%) but the overall incidence was very low (2 versus 9). For all grades, there was a significant reduction in the number of people developing CIPN in the CHM plus chemotherapy groups, compared to the control

Table 5.81   Frequently Used Herbs in Chinese Herbal Medicine Hand and Foot Bath Formulas in Randomised Controlled Trials

Herb Name	Scientific Name	Frequency of Use
Hong hua 红花	*Carthamus tinctorius* L.	4
Huang qi 黄芪	*Astragalus membranaceus* (Fisch.) Bge.	4
Tao ren 桃仁	*Prunus persica* (L.) Batsch	3
Di long 地龙	*Pheretima* spp.	2
Dang gui 当归[1]	*Angelica sinensis* (Oliv.) Diels	2
Gui zhi 桂枝	*Cinnamomum cassia* Presl	2
Fu zi 附子	*Aconitum carmichaelii* Debx.	2
Shao yao 芍药[2]	*Paeonia lactiflora* Pall.; *P. veitchii* Lynch	2

[1]One used *dang gui wei* 当归尾.

[2]One used *chi shao* 赤芍; one used *bai shao* 白芍.

The use of some herbs may be restricted in some countries. Readers are advised to comply with relevant regulations.

groups (RR: 0.69 [0.50, 0.95], I^2 = 66.8%) with substantial heterogeneity (Table 5.82).

Since one study included two comparisons (H131) and one of these used a complex control (calcium and magnesium plus mFOLFOX6), it was excluded in a sensitivity analysis. This did not alter the outcomes for level III + IV (RR: 0.36 [0.09, 1.34], I^2 = 0%) or for all levels (RR: 0.62 [0.39, 0.998], I^2 = 75.8%). There was no mention of any AEs associated with the CHM hand and foot baths in any study.

Chinese Herbal Medicine Cataplasm plus Chemotherapy versus Chemotherapy

One RCT (H133) enrolled people with stage III and IV CRC (*n* = 60), mean ages of 57.5 years in the CHM group and 56.1 years in the control, who were treated with FOLFIRI plus a cataplasm called *Gui lu er xian jiao ba bu ji* 龟鹿二仙胶巴布剂 (*lu jiao pian* 鹿角片, *gui ban* 龟板, *sheng shai shen* 生晒参 and *gou qi* 枸杞) or FOLFIRI (one cycle of two weeks) plus a placebo cataplasm. There was no mention of syndrome

Table 5.82   Chinese Herbal Medicine Hand and Foot Bath plus Chemotherapy versus Chemotherapy for Chemotherapy-induced Peripheral Neurotoxicity

Chemotherapy Regimen,[1] Cancer (*N* Participants)	CIPN Grade III + IV[2] Effect Size (RR [95% CI]), I^2	CIPN All Grades[2] Effect Size (RR [95% CI]), I^2	Included Studies
FOLFOX4, CRC first-time chemotherapy after surgery (120)	0.20 [0.01, 4.08]	0.59 [0.36, 0.95]*	H129
FOLFOX4, colon cancer after surgery (44)	1.00 [0.07, 15.00]	0.47 [0.26, 0.86]*	H130
Calcium and magnesium + mFOLFOX6, adjuvant chemotherapy CRC (60)	0.33 [0.01, 7.87]	0.83 [0.61, 1.14]	H131.1
mFOLFOX6, adjuvant chemotherapy CRC (60)	0.20 [0.01, 4.00]	0.96 [0.76, 1.22]	H131.2
mFOLFOX6, colon cancer after surgery (40)	0.33 [0.04, 2.94]	0.47 [0.24, 0.89]*	H132
Total pool: 4 studies, 5 comparisons (324)	0.35 [0.10, 1.20], 0%	0.69 [0.50, 0.95]*, 66.8%	All above
Sensitivity: 4 studies, 4 comparisons (264)	0.36 [0.09, 1.34], 0%	0.62 [0.39, 0.998]*, 75.8%	H129, H130, H131.2, H132

[1]Comparator was the same chemotherapy.

[2]Levi's criteria.

*Statistically significant.

Abbreviations: CI, confidence interval; CRC, colorectal cancer; N, number; RR, risk ratio.

differentiation. The cataplasm (or placebo) was applied to the acupoint RN8 *Shenque* 神阙 and changed every second day for 14 days.

The results for myelosuppression were not reported using the WHO or NCI-CTCAE criteria and were not suitable for meta-analysis. The authors reported that counts for white blood cells and neutrophils improved in the CHM group, compared to the control, while there was no change in platelets. For KPS based on an increase in 10 points or more, there was no significant difference between groups (RR: 1.86 [0.86, 4.00], *n* = 60). There was no mention of AEs.

Controlled Clinical Trials of Chinese Herbal Medicine in Conjunction with Chemotherapy

Eight non-randomised CCTs of oral CHM plus chemotherapy were identified. All were conducted in China. The studies enrolled 446 participants and no drop-outs during treatment were reported. Ages ranged from 32 to 75 years, but the age range was not reported in five studies (H134–H138). Based on the reported means and standard deviations for the ages, the majority of participants were aged between 44 and 74 years.

Syndromes

In five studies the CM syndrome was an inclusion criterion as follows:

- Spleen-stomach weakness — *pi wei xu ruo* 脾胃虚弱 (H134, H136);
- Spleen deficiency — *pi xu* 脾虚 (H139);
- Spleen *qi* deficiency — *pi qi xu* 脾气虚 (H140);
- Spleen deficiency with toxin stasis — *pi xu du yu* 脾虚毒瘀 (H138).

Formula and Herb Frequencies

Each study used a different oral CHM formula. The most common herbal ingredients in the formulas were *bai zhu* 白术, *fu ling* 茯苓, *dang shen* 党参 and *yi yi ren* 薏苡仁 (Table 5.83).

Assessable data were available for the following outcome measures: ORR (four studies), survival (one study), chemotherapy-related AEs (six studies), KPS (eight studies) and quality of life (two studies). One study (H140) was retrospective and it only reported KPS.

Objective Response Rate

All four studies used the WHO criteria (Table 5.84). All participants were stage III or IV CRC. Each study used a different chemotherapy. There were no significant differences between groups for any of the studies or in the pool of four studies (RR: 1.48 [0.97, 2.25], $I^2 = 0.9\%$).

Table 5.83   Frequently Used Herbs in Controlled Clinical Trials of Chinese Herbal Medicine in Conjunction with Chemotherapy

Herb Name	Scientific Name	Frequency of Use
Bai zhu 白术[1]	*Atractylodes macrocephala* Koidz.	7
Fu ling 茯苓	*Poria cocos* (Schw.) Wolf	7
Dang shen 党参	*Codonopsis pilosula* (Franch.) Nannf.	6
Yi yi ren 薏苡仁[2]	*Coix lacryma-jobi* L. var. *mayuen* (Roman.) Stapf	5
Gu ya 谷芽[3]	*Setaria italica* (L.) Beauv.	5
Mai ya 麦芽[4]	*Hordeum vulgare* L.	5
Gan cao 甘草[5]	*Glycyrrhiza uralensis* Fisch.	5
Huang qi 黄芪	*Astragalus membranaceus* (Fisch.) Bge.	4
Shan yao 山药	*Dioscorea opposita* Thunb.	3
Zhu ling 猪苓	*Polyporus umbellatus* (Pers.) Fires	3
Shao yao 芍药[6]	*Paeonia lactiflora* Pall.; *P. veitchii* Lynch	3
Bai bian dou 白扁豆	*Dolichos lablab* L.	2
Chen pi 陈皮	*Citrus reticulata* Blanco	2

[1]Three used *chao bai zhu* 炒白术.

[2]Two used *sheng yi yi ren* 生薏苡仁.

[3]One used *gu ya* 谷芽 and four used *chao gu ya* 炒谷芽.

[4]Two used *mai ya* 麦芽 and three used *chao mai ya* 炒麦芽.

[5]Four used *zhi gan cao* 炙甘草.

[6]One used *bai shao* 白芍, one used *chao bai shao* 炒白芍 and one used *chi shao* 赤芍.

The use of some herbs may be restricted in some countries. Readers are advised to comply with relevant regulations.

Survival Rate

One study (H141) reported on survival rates but the data were presented as percentages only. Fifty-two people with Duke's B & C rectal cancer received FOLFOX4 (four 2-week cycles) as adjuvant chemotherapy and one group of 26 people also received *Ren shen zao gan* 人参皂甙 Rg3 capsules (20 mg, twice a day for two months). This is an extract containing ginsenoside Rg3. The two-year survival rates were 79.4% in the *Ren shen zao gan* 人参皂甙 Rg3 plus FOLFOX4

Table 5.84   Controlled Clinical Trials of Oral Chinese Herbal Medicine plus Chemotherapy versus Chemotherapy: Objective Response Rate (WHO)

Chemotherapy Regimen[1]	N Studies (N Participants)	Effect Size (RR [95% CI]), I^2	Included Studies
FOLFOX4	1 (40)	3.50 [0.83, 14.83]	H134
FOLFOX	1 (60)	1.19 [0.37, 3.85]	H135
XELOX	1 (42)	2.67 [0.82, 8.69]	H138
XELODA	1 (100)	1.24 [0.75, 2.05]	H139
Total pool	4 (242)	1.48 [0.97, 2.25], 0.9%	All above

[1]Comparator was the same chemotherapy.

*Statistically significant.

Abbreviations: CI, confidence interval; N, number; RR, risk ratio; WHO, World Health Organisation.

group versus 78.2% in the FOLFOX4 alone group. The five-year survival rates were 61.4% versus 47.6%, respectively. At two years, three people were lost to follow-up and 11 people could not be followed up at five years, but the study report did not specify which groups these people were in.

Karnofsky Performance Status

In the eight studies that reported KPS, six reported scores and two studies reported improvements of ten points or more, so these data were analysed separately.

For KPS scores (Table 5.85), in the pooled result for four studies that used FOLFOX4, there was no difference between groups but there was considerable heterogeneity. Similarly, the total pool showed considerable heterogeneity. The source of this heterogeneity was the single study of rectal cancer (H141, $n = 52$). When this study was removed in the sensitivity analysis, the result for FOLFOX4 showed a significant difference between groups with no heterogeneity (MD: 4.38 [1.24, 7.51], $I^2 = 0\%$) and in the pool of five studies of CRC, there was a significant increase in KPS scores in the combination therapy groups without heterogeneity (MD: 5.86 [4.66, 7.05], $I^2 = 0\%$).

Table 5.85 Controlled Clinical Trials of Oral Chinese Herbal Medicine plus Chemotherapy versus Chemotherapy: Karnofsky Performance Status (Score)

Chemotherapy Regimen[1]	*N* Studies (*N* Participants)	Effect Size (MD [95% CI]), I[2]	Included Studies
FOLFOX4 (all)	3 (132)	10.10 [–0.56, 20.76], 93.6%	H134, H136, H141
FOLFOX	1 (60)	8.67 [3.97, 13.37]*	H135
Pooled result for similar chemotherapy[2]	4 (192)	9.72 [2.20, 17.25]*, 90.5%	H134–H136, H141
XELOX	1 (42)	7.81 [1.48, 14.14]*	H138
XELODA	1 (100)	5.81 [4.43, 7.19]*	H139
Total pool	6 (334)	8.63 [4.32, 12.95]* 86.5%	All above
Sensitivity (CRC studies only)	5 (282)	5.86 [4.66, 7.05]*, 0%	H134–H136, H138, H139

[1]Comparator was the same chemotherapy.

[2]These chemotherapy regimens all use oxaliplatin, 5-FU plus LV.

*Statistically significant.

Abbreviations: CI, confidence interval; CRC, colorectal cancer; MD, mean difference; N, number.

Of the two studies that reported KPS as a 10-point or more improvement (Table 5.86), there was a significant difference in the retrospective study of modified *Si jun zi tang* 四君子汤加减 combined with FOLFOX4 (H140). However, there was no difference in the study of FOLFIRI (H137), which used modified *Wu ling san* 五苓散加减. In the pooled result there was no significant difference between groups for the incidence of people showing a 10-point or more improvement in KPS (RR: 2.04 [0.89, 4.69], I[2] = 20.1%).

Quality of Life

Two studies reported data using the 12-item QOL scale that is frequently used in China[26] on which higher scores indicate improvement. Both studies treated people with FOLFOX4 and used similar CHMs which were made by the authors. In one study (H134) all 40 people had stage IV CRC and received FOLFOX4 (four 2-week cycles) and 20 people also received *Fu zheng gu ben fang* 扶正固本方 (*dang*

Table 5.86 Controlled Clinical Trials of Oral Chinese Herbal Medicine plus Chemotherapy versus Chemotherapy: Karnofsky Performance Status (Improvements of 10 Points or More)

Chemotherapy Regimen[1]	N Studies (N Participants)	Effect Size (RR [95% CI]), I^2	Included Studies
FOLFOX4	1 (52)	2.62 [1.23, 5.58]*	H140
FOLFIRI	1 (60)	1.00 [0.22, 4.56]	H137
Total pool	2 (112)	2.04 [0.89, 4.69], 20.1%	All above

[1]Comparator was the same chemotherapy.

*Statistically significant.

Abbreviations: CI, confidence interval; N, number; RR, risk ratio.

shen 党参, *huang qi* 黄芪, *chao bai zhu* 炒白术, *bai shao* 白芍, *fu ling* 茯苓, *sheng yi yi ren* 生薏苡仁, *bai bian dou* 白扁豆, *huang jing* 黄精, *nv zhen zi* 女贞子, *shu di huang* 熟地黄, *chuan xiong* 川芎, *ji xue teng* 鸡血藤, *gu sui bu* 骨碎补, *ji nei jin* 鸡内金, *chen pi* 陈皮, *chao gu ya* 炒谷芽, *chao mai ya* 炒麦芽 and *zhi gan cao* 炙甘草) one packet a day in two doses for eight weeks. There was a significant improvement in the combination therapy group (MD: 6.35 [2.91, 9.79], *n* = 40).

In the other study (H136), 40 people with stage II/III CRC received FOLFOX4 after radical surgery (four 2-week cycles) with 20 people also receiving *Jian pi yi qi fang* 健脾益气方 (*dang shen* 党参, *huang qi* 黄芪, *chao bai zhu* 炒白术, *chao bai shao* 炒白芍, *fu ling* 茯苓, *zhu ling* 猪苓, *sheng yi yi ren* 生薏苡仁, *shan yao* 山药, *bai bian dou* 白扁豆, *chao gu ya* 炒谷芽, *chao mai ya* 炒麦芽 and *zhi gan cao* 炙甘草) one packet a day in two doses for eight weeks. The combination therapy group showed a significantly higher QOL score than the control (MD: 6.15 [4.38, 7.92], *n* = 40). The pooled result showed a significant improvement in QOL in the CHM plus FOLFOX4 groups (MD: 6.19 [4.62, 7.77], I^2 = 0%, *n* = 80).

Chemotherapy-related Adverse Events

Four studies reported chemotherapy-related AE using the WHO criteria and two studies (H137, H141) used the NCI-CTCAE criteria. Data were available for gastrointestinal reactions (nausea and vomiting, diarrhoea, enteritis loss of appetite); myelosuppression (leukopenia, haemoglobin, thrombocytopenia); neurotoxicity; liver, kidney and heart function; and oral mucositis.

Gastrointestinal Reactions

Four studies reported on nausea and vomiting, of which three used the WI IO criteria (Table 5.87). These three studies were all of CRC. For grade III + IV nausea and vomiting, two studies (H136, H138) had zero events in both groups, and there were no differences between groups in the remaining study (H135). For all grades there were significant reductions in the FOLFOX4 or FOLFOX plus CHM groups,

Table 5.87 Controlled Clinical Trials of Oral Chinese Herbal Medicine plus Chemotherapy versus Chemotherapy: Chemotherapy-related Nausea and Vomiting (WHO)

Chemotherapy Regimen:[1] *N* Studies (*N* Participants); *N* Studies with 0 Events in Both Groups	*N* Studies (*N* Participants) in Meta-analysis	Effect Size (RR [95% CI]), I^2	Included Studies (Studies with 0 Events in Both Groups)
Grade III+IV			
FOLFOX4: 1 (40); 1	0 (0)	Both groups = 0 events	(H136)
FOLFOX: 1 (60); 0	1 (60)	0.07 [0.004, 1.12]	H135
XELOX: 1 (42); 1	0 (0)	Both groups = 0 events	(H138)
All grades			
FOLFOX4: 1 (40); 0	1 (40)	0.47 [0.24, 0.89]*	H136
FOLFOX: 1 (60); 0	1 (60)	0.58 [0.38, 0.89]*	H135
XELOX: 1 (42); 0	1 (42)	0.75 [0.48, 1.17]	H138
Total pool: 3 (142); 0	3 (142)	0.62 [0.47, 0.82]*, 0%	All above

[1]Comparator was the same chemotherapy.

*Statistically significant.

Abbreviations: CI, confidence interval; N, number; RR, risk ratio; WHO, World Health Organisation.

but not in the study of XELOX plus CHM. In the pooled result for the three studies, there were significant reductions in all grades of nausea and vomiting in the CHM plus chemotherapy groups (RR: 0.62 [0.47, 0.82], $I^2 = 0\%$). In the single study of FOLFOX4 for rectal cancer that used the NCI-CTCAE criteria (H141) there was no difference between groups (RR: 0.63 [0.35, 1.11], $n = 52$) for all grades.

Five studies reported on diarrhoea with three studies of CRC using the WHO criteria (Table 5.88) and two using the NCI-CTCAE criteria. For grade III + IV diarrhoea (WHO) two studies (H136, H138) reported zero events in both groups and there were no significant differences between groups in the remaining study (H135). For all grades, there were significant reductions in incidence of diarrhoea in the CHM plus FOLFOX4 and CHM plus FOLFOX groups. However, there was no difference for CHM plus XELOX (H138). The pooled

Table 5.88 Controlled Clinical Trials of Oral Chinese Herbal Medicine plus Chemotherapy versus Chemotherapy: Chemotherapy-related Diarrhoea (WHO)

Chemotherapy Regimen:[1] *N* Studies (*N* Participants); *N* Studies with 0 Events in Both Groups	*N* Studies (*N* Participants) in Meta-analysis	Effect Size (RR [95% CI]), I^2	Included Studies (Studies with 0 Events in Both Groups)
Grade III + IV			
FOLFOX4: 1 (40); 1	0 (0)	Both groups = 0 events	(H136)
FOLFOX: 1 (60); 0	1 (60)	0.20 [0.01, 4.00]	H135
XELOX: 1 (42); 1	0 (0)	Both groups = 0 events	(H138)
All grades			
FOLFOX4: 1 (40); 0	1 (40)	0.50 [0.28, 0.89]*	H136
FOLFOX: 1 (60); 0	1 (60)	0.38 [0.17, 0.83]*	H135
XELOX: 1 (42); 0	1 (42)	1.25 [0.39, 4.02]	H138
Total pool: 3 (142); 0	3 (142)	0.54 [0.31, 0.93]*, 29.8%	All above

[1]Comparator was the same chemotherapy.

*Statistically significant.

Abbreviations: CI, confidence interval; N, number; RR, risk ratio; WHO, World Health Organisation.

result for the three studies showed a significant improvement in diarrhoea in the CHM plus chemotherapy group (RR: 0.54 [0.31, 0.93], $I^2 = 29.8\%$).

In the study of rectal cancer that used the NCI-CTCAE criteria for diarrhoea (H141) there was no difference between groups for all grades (RR: 1.14 [0.49, 2.69], $n = 52$). In the other study that used the NCI-CTCAE criteria (H137), modified *Wu ling san* 五苓散加减 was combined with FOLFIRI. There was no difference between groups for grade III + IV diarrhoea (RR: 0.14 [0.01, 2.65], $n = 60$). For all grades there was a significant reduction in the integrative group (RR: 0.44 [0.25, 0.75], $n = 60$). However, the pooled result for all grades of diarrhoea found no significant difference between groups (RR: 0.63 [0.09, 4.36], $I^2 = 49.4\%$, $n = 112$).

One study (H141) reported on enteritis using the NCI-CTCAE criteria and found no difference between groups for all grades (RR: 1.00 [0.15, 6.57], $n = 52$).

Loss of appetite, using the WHO criteria, was reported in one study (H138) of 42 people with stage IV CRC who received XELOX (two 3-week cycles) plus an unnamed CHM (*huang qi* 黄芪, *she she cao* 蛇舌草, *yi yi ren* 薏苡仁, *ban zhi lian* 半枝莲, *teng li gen* 藤梨根, *dang shen* 党参, *fu ling* 茯苓, *bai zhu* 白术, *xian he cao* 仙鹤草, *e zhu* 莪术, *di bie chong* 地鳖虫, *chen pi* 陈皮, *shan ci gu* 山慈菇, *gu ya* 谷芽 and *mai ya* 麦芽) one packet per day in two doses for six weeks. There was no difference between groups for grade III + IV loss of appetite (RR: 0.20 [0.01, 3.93], $n = 42$). For all grades there was a significant reduction in the integrative group (RR: 0.53 [0.33, 0.84], $n = 42$).

Myelosuppression

Five studies reported on myelosuppression including leukopenia, haemoglobin and thrombocytopenia; however, the data in one study (H134) was not suitable for meta-analysis. Three of the remaining four studies used the WHO criteria and one (H141) used the NCI-CTCAE criteria. Since these criteria are the same, the data were pooled where possible.

Table 5.89   Controlled Clinical Trials of Oral Chinese Herbal Medicine plus Chemotherapy versus Chemotherapy: Chemotherapy-related Leukopenia

Chemotherapy Regimen[1]	N Studies (N Participants)	Effect Size (RR [95% CI]), I^2	Included Studies
Grade III + IV			
FOLFOX4	1 (40)	1.00 [0.16, 6.42]	H136
FOLFOX	1 (60)	0.11 [0.01, 1.98]	H135
XELOX	1 (42)	0.50 [0.05, 5.10]	H138
Total pool	3 (142)	0.52 [0.14, 1.89], 0%	All above
All grades			
FOLFOX4	2 (92)	1.03 [0.73, 1.46], 0%	H136, H142
FOLFOX	1 (60)	0.56 [0.31, 0.997]*	H135
XELOX	1 (42)	0.77 [0.52, 1.14]	H138
Total pool	4 (194)	0.83 [0.62, 1.09], 23.4%	All above

[1]Comparator was the same chemotherapy.

*Statistically significant.

Abbreviations: CI, confidence interval, N, number; RR, risk ratio.

Leukocytes

Four studies reported on leukopenia but only three reported grade III + IV (Table 5.89). There were no differences between groups in any of the three studies or in the pooled results for grade III + IV leukopenia (RR: 0.52 [0.14, 1.89], I^2 = 0%). For all grades, there was a marginally significant result for the study that used FOLFOX, but no significant differences between groups in the incidence of leukopenia in the pooled result for four studies (RR: 0.83 [0.62, 1.09], I^2 = 23.4%).

Red Blood Cells

Three studies reported incidence of reduced haemoglobin (Table 5.90). In one study there were zero grade III + IV events in both groups and the pooled result for the other studies showed no significant difference between groups (RR: 0.31 [0.05, 1.89], I^2 = 0%). For all grades,

Table 5.90 Controlled Clinical Trials of Oral Chinese Herbal Medicine plus Chemotherapy versus Chemotherapy: Chemotherapy-related Reduced Haemoglobin

Chemotherapy Regimen:[1] *N* Studies (*N* Participants); *N* Studies with 0 Events in Both Groups	*N* Studies (*N* Participants) in Meta-analysis	Effect Size (RR [95% CI]), I^2	Included Studies (Studies with 0 Events in Both Groups)
Grade III + IV			
FOLFOX4: 1 (40); 0	1 (40)	0.50 [0.05, 5.08]	H136
FOLFOX: 1 (60); 0	1 (60)	0.14 [0.01, 2.65]	H135
XELOX: 1 (42); 1	0 (0)	Both groups = 0 events	(H138)
Total pool: 3 (142); 1	2 (100)	0.31 [0.05, 1.89], 0%	All above
All grades			
FOLFOX4: 1 (40); 0	1 (40)	0.80 [0.40, 1.60]	H136
FOLFOX: 1 (60); 0	1 (60)	0.75 [0.37, 1.51]	H135
XELOX: 1 (42); 0	1 (42)	0.72 [0.50, 1.05]	H138
Total pool: 3 (142); 0	3 (142)	0.74 [0.55, 1.001], 0%	All above

[1]Comparator was the same chemotherapy.

*Statistically significant.

Abbreviations: CI, confidence interval; N, number; RR, risk ratio.

there were no differences between groups in any of the three studies or in the pooled result (RR: 0.74 [0.55, 1.001], I^2 = 0%).

Platelets

Two studies (H135, H136) reported data on thrombocytopenia. There were no grade III + IV events in either study. For all grades, there were no differences in the study of FOLFOX4 (H136) for stage II/III CRC after radical surgery (RR: 0.80 [0.25, 2.55], *n* = 40) or in the study of FOLFOX (H135) for stage III/IV CRC (RR: 0.67 [0.21, 2.13], *n* = 60). The pooled result showed no difference between groups for the incidence of all grades of thrombocytopenia (RR: 0.73 [0.32, 1.66], I^2 = 0%, *n* = 100).

Chemotherapy-induced Peripheral Neurotoxicity

Four studies provided data on CIPN. Three studies of CRC used the WHO criteria and one study of rectal cancer used the NCI-CTCAE criteria. For WHO grade III + IV there were zero events in both groups in two studies (H136, H138) and no difference between groups in the other study (Table 5.91). For all grades, there were no differences between groups for any of the three studies or in the pooled results (RR: 0.95 [0.66, 1.36], I^2 = 0%). For the single study of rectal cancer that used the NCI-CTCAE criteria (H141) there were no differences between groups in the incidence of all grades of CIPN (RR: 0.71 [0.39, 1.31], n = 52).

Table 5.91 Controlled Clinical Trials of Oral Chinese Herbal Medicine plus Chemotherapy versus Chemotherapy: Chemotherapy-induced Peripheral Neurotoxicity (WHO)

Chemotherapy Regimen:[1] *N* Studies (*N* Participants); *N* Studies with 0 Events in Both Groups	*N* Studies (*N* Participants) in Meta-analysis	Effect Size (RR [95% CI]), I^2	Included Studies (Studies with 0 Events in Both Groups)
Grade III + IV			
FOLFOX4: 1 (40); 1	0 (0)	Both groups = 0 events	(H136)
FOLFOX: 1 (60); 0	1 (60)	0.50 [0.05, 5.22]	H135
XELOX: 1 (42); 1	0 (0)	Both groups = 0 events	(H138)
All grades			
FOLFOX4: 1 (40); 0	1 (40)	1.00 [0.29, 3.45]	H136
FOLFOX: 1 (60); 0	1 (60)	0.85 [0.45, 1.58]	H135
XELOX: 1 (42); 0	1 (42)	1.00 [0.62, 1.61]	H138
Total pool: 3 (142); 0	3 (142)	0.95 [0.66, 1.36], 0%	All above

[1]Comparator was the same chemotherapy.

*Statistically significant.

Abbreviations: CI, Confidence Interval; N, number; RR, Risk Ratio; WHO, World Health Organisation.

Hepatotoxicity

Three studies of CRC reported on chemotherapy-related hepatotoxicity using the WHO criteria (Table 5.92). One study (H136) specified the measure was based on abnormal ALT/AST and the others referred to abnormal liver function. In the two studies (H136, H138) that reported grade III + IV, there were zero events in both groups. In the pool of two studies of FOLFOX4, there were no significant differences between groups with substantial heterogeneity. There was a significant reduction in the incidence of hepatotoxicity in the study of CHM plus XELOX (H138) and in the pooled results for the three studies (RR: 0.46 [0.21, 0.99], I^2 = 47.5%) with moderate heterogeneity.

Table 5.92 Controlled Clinical Trials of Oral Chinese Herbal Medicine plus Chemotherapy versus Chemotherapy: Chemotherapy-related Hepatotoxicity (WHO)

Chemotherapy Regimen:[1] N Studies (N Participants); N Studies with 0 Events in Both Groups	N Studies (N Participants) in Meta-analysis	Effect Size (RR [95% CI]), I^2	Included Studies (Studies with 0 Events in Both Groups)
Grade III + IV			
FOLFOX4: 1 (40); 1	0 (0)	Both groups = 0 events	(H136)
XELOX: 1 (42); 1	0 (0)	Both groups = 0 events	(H138)
All grades			
FOLFOX4: 2 (80); 0	2 (80)	0.54 [0.16, 1.85], 58.6%	H134, H136
XELOX: 1 (42); 0	1 (42)	0.33 [0.15, 0.75]*	H138
Total pool: 3 (122); 0	3 (122)	0.46 [0.21, 0.99]* 47.5%	All above

[1]Comparator was the same chemotherapy.

*Statistically significant.

Abbreviations: CI, confidence interval; N, number; RR, risk ratio; WHO, World Health Organisation.

Nephrotoxicity and Heart Function

Only one study (H136) reported on chemotherapy-related nephrotoxicity and abnormal heart function using the WHO criteria. In this study 40 people with stage II/III CRC received FOLFOX4 after radical surgery (see section on quality of life for details). For kidney function, abnormal creatinine was reported. There were zero grade III+IV events and no significant differences between groups for all grades (RR: 1.33 [0.34, 5.21], *n* = 40). The same study also reported that for abnormal heart function there were zero grade III + IV events and zero all grades events.

Oral Mucositis

Only one study (H141) reported on oral mucositis (see survival rate for details). This study, of FOLFOX4 in rectal cancer, used the NCI-CTCAE criteria. For all grades, there was no significant difference between groups in the incidence of oral mucositis (RR: 0.83 [0.29, 2.39], *n* = 52).

Non-controlled Clinical Trials of Chinese Herbal Medicine in Conjunction with Chemotherapy

Two case-series studies and one case report on CHM in conjunction with a guideline-recommended chemotherapy for CRC were identified. None reported a CM syndrome. All studies were conducted in mainland China. Each study used a different chemotherapy regimen and a different oral CHM, although all three CHMs included the herbs *fu ling* 茯苓, *chen pi* 陈皮 and *gan cao* 甘草.

One study (H142) included 26 people with stage IV CRC who received FOLFOX4 (six 2-week cycles) plus an oral CHM (*dang shen* 党参, *bei qi* 北芪, *fu ling* 茯苓, *yi yi ren* 薏苡仁, *chen pi* 陈皮, *fa ban xia* 法半夏, *chun sha ren* 春砂仁, *bu gu zhi* 补骨脂, *yin yang huo* 淫羊藿, *quan xie* 全蝎, *wu gong* 蜈蚣, *ban zhi lian* 半枝莲, *she she cao* 蛇舌草, *nv zhen zi* 女贞子 and *zhi gan cao* 炙甘草) once a day for three months. After treatment the response rate (WHO criteria) was 34.6%. By the end of treatment there were no grade IV AEs according to the WHO criteria, and four grade III AEs. For all grades, the main AEs were nausea and vomiting (ten people), neurotoxicity (eight people), anaemia (six people), and neutropenia (five people). The mean KPS was slightly reduced but this was less than 10 points, so it was considered 'stable'.

In another case-series study (H143), 47 people with Dukes C or D CRC, who received FOLFOX6 (four 2-week cycles), were given *Long kui he ji* 龙葵合剂 (*xian long kui guo* 鲜龙葵果, *dang shen* 党参, *bai zhu* 白术, *fu ling* 茯苓, *huai shan yao* 淮山药, *gu ya* 谷芽, *chen pi* 陈皮 and *gan cao* 甘草) one packet per day for 20 days followed by ten days' break for two months. After treatment, KPS scores increased a little but the difference was not significant. However, immune function showed significant increases in CD3+, CD4+ and the ratio CD4+/CD8+ cells.

In the case report, a 62-year-old man with stage III colon cancer (H144) received radical surgery followed by XELOX and experienced diarrhoea which did not respond to pharmaceutical treatment. He was prescribed modified *Xiang sha liu jun zi tang* 香砂六君子汤加减 (*huang qi* 黄芪, *bai zhu* 白术, *fu ling pi* 茯苓皮, *zhi gan cao* 炙甘草, *chen pi* 陈皮, *jiang ban xia* 姜半夏, *mu xiang* 木香, *sha ren* 砂仁, *dai zhe shi* 代赭石, *ze xie* 泽泻, *shi liu pi* 石榴皮, *qian shi* 芡实 and *chi shi zhi* 赤石脂) plus activated carbon. After one week the symptoms improved, so *sha ren* 砂仁 and *dai zhe shi* 代赭石 were removed. After the diarrhoea stopped, he ceased treatment.

Safety of Chinese Herbal Medicines in Conjunction with Chemotherapy

In 88 RCTs there was no specific mention of the safety of the CHMs. Five RCTs stated there were no AEs associated with the CHMs. In six studies the AEs and/or reasons for drop-outs were stated for the CHM groups. Five were of oral CHM and one was of hand and foot bath (H129). The AEs and reasons for drop-outs in the CHM and control groups are listed in Table 5.93. In two studies (H129, H118) the AEs were likely due to the CHM, but in the others it was unclear whether the AEs were due to the CHMs. Overall, there were five serious AEs, all of which were in the same study (H43), but it was not mentioned whether these deaths were related to the CHM, chemotherapy or to unrelated factors.

Table 5.93   Adverse Events and Reasons for Drop-outs in Randomised Controlled Trials of Chinese Herbal Medicines in Conjunction with Chemotherapy

Chinese Herbal Medicine plus Chemotherapy[1]	Chemotherapy	Included Studies
Myelosuppression (1 dpo)	Myelosuppression (1 dpo); diarrhoea (2 dpo); gastrointestinal bleeding (1 dpo)	H72
Allergy (1 AE)[2]	NS	H129
Allergy (1 dpo); intolerance of chemotherapy (2 dpo); no reason (2 dpo)	Intolerance of chemotherapy (3 dpo); no reason (1 dpo)	H81
Refused CHM (3 dpo)	Chemotherapy-related adverse reaction (2 dpo)	H36
Vomiting (1 AE); diarrhoea (1 AE)	NS	H118
Refused chemotherapy (2 dpo); chemotherapy-related adverse reaction (2 dpo); death (2 dpo)	Refused chemotherapy (3 dpo); chemotherapy-related adverse reaction (8 dpo); death (3 dpo)	H43

[1]Comparator was the same chemotherapy.

[2]Chinese herbal medicine was hand and foot bath.

Abbreviations: AE, adverse event but did not drop out; dpo, drop-out; NS, not specified.

In the nine CCTs, only one study (H137) mentioned the safety of the oral CHM. It stated that no AEs associated with the oral CHM were reported. None of the three non-controlled studies mentioned the safety of the oral CHMs.

In addition, the sections on chemotherapy-related AEs provide a wide range of assessments of AEs associated with the combined use of CHMs plus various chemotherapy regimens.

Section 3: Radiotherapy and Chemo-radiotherapy Combined with Chinese Herbal Medicine

Three RCTs of CHM combined with radiotherapy (H145–H147) and two RCTs of CHM combined with chemo-radiotherapy (H148, H149) were identified. No CCTs or non-controlled studies were found. All studies were conducted in mainland China and enrolled

366 participants ranging in age from 19 to 84 years. One study (H149) was of chemo-radiotherapy for CRC and the other four studies were for rectal cancer. Four studies used oral CHM and one study (H147) used a CHM enema.

No studies reported on syndrome differentiation. The CHM formulas used were different in each study and no herbal ingredients were used in multiple studies.

Risk of Bias

Two studies were judged 'low' risk for sequence generation while the others were judged 'unclear' risk. One study (H149) that used opaque envelopes was judged 'low' risk for allocation concealment. The others did not mention a method of allocation concealment and were judged 'unclear' risk. No studies mentioned the use of blinding, so all were judged 'high' risk for blinding of participants and personnel and 'unclear' risk for outcome assessors. One study (H149) had two drop-outs in the control group due to loss to follow-up, while the other studies did not report any drop-outs. The small number of drop-outs was judged unlikely to affect the outcome, so all studies were judged 'low' risk for incomplete outcome data. No protocols could be located but all studies reported on the outcomes mentioned in the method section, so all studies were judged 'unclear' risk for bias due to selective reporting (Table 5.94).

Table 5.94 Risk of Bias of Randomised Controlled Trials of Chinese Herbal Medicine plus Radiotherapy and Chemo-radiotherapy

Risk of Bias Domain	Low Risk n (%)	Unclear Risk n (%)	High Risk n (%)
Sequence generation	2 (40)	3 (60)	0 (0)
Allocation concealment	1 (20)	4 (80)	0 (0)
Blinding of participants	0 (0)	0 (0)	5 (100)
Blinding of personnel	0 (0)	0 (0)	5 (100)
Blinding of outcome assessors	0 (0)	5 (100)	0 (0)
Incomplete outcome data	5 (100)	0 (0)	0 (0)
Selective reporting	0 (0)	5 (100)	0 (0)

Oral Chinese Herbal Medicine plus Radiotherapy versus Radiotherapy

One study of 60 people, who received postoperative radiotherapy for rectal cancer (H145), were administered *Wu hong tang* 五红汤 (*hong zao* 红枣, *gou qi* 枸杞, *hong tang* 红糖, *hong pi hua sheng* 红皮花生仁 and *hong dou* 红豆) once a day from three days prior to the radiotherapy until the radiotherapy finished. Data were reported on adverse reactions to radiotherapy including leukocyte count, haemoglobin, platelets, liver function, electrocardiogram and urination/defaecation; however, the data were in terms of incidence of results meeting various thresholds so meta-analysis was not feasible. The author reported that the results were better in the CHM group for leukocyte count, haemoglobin, platelets and liver function but there were no differences for electrocardiogram and urination/defaecation. For KPS scores, there was a significant increase in the CHM group (MD: 14.37 [10.31, 18.43], *n* = 60). Data were also reported for immune function (see below).

The other RCT (H146) reported on 90 people who received radiotherapy for rectal cancer and were administered *Hua chan su jiao nang* 华蟾素胶囊, two capsules three times a day during radiotherapy. The only outcome was immune function.

Post-radiotherapy Immune Function

Both RCTs of CHM combined with radiotherapy reported data for T cells (Table 5.95). CD3+ cells were only reported in one study (H146) which found a significant increase in the CHM group after radiotherapy (MD: 4.40 [2.64, 6.16]). The pooled results showed significant increases in CD4+ cells (MD: 7.98 [5.72, 10.25], I^2 = 0%) and NK cells (MD: 6.81 [5.20, 8.42], I^2 = 39.6%), but no differences between groups for CD8+ cells (MD: –0.61 [–2.16, 0.94], I^2 = 0%) or the ratio CD4+/CD8+ (MD: 0.31 [–0.51, 1.12], I^2 = 0.2%). There was no important heterogeneity in these results.

Table 5.95   Oral Chinese Herbal Medicine plus Radiotherapy versus Radiotherapy: Immune Function

T cells	Treatment Type (*N* Participants)	Effect Size (MD [95% CI]), I^2	Included Studies
CD3+ (%)	Radiotherapy (90)	4.40 [2.64, 6.16]*	H146
CD4+ (%)	Postoperative radiotherapy (60)	9.63 [5.30, 13.96]*	H145
	Radiotherapy (90)	7.36 [4.70, 10.02]*	H146
	Pooled result (150); 2 RCTs	7.98 [5.72, 10.25]*, 0%	H146, H145
CD8+ (%)	Postoperative radiotherapy (60)	–0.73 [–4.16, 2.70]	H145
	Radiotherapy (90)	–0.58 [–2.31, 1.15]	H146
	Pooled result (150); 2 RCTs	–0.61 [–2.16, 0.94], 0%	H146, H145
CD4+/	Postoperative radiotherapy (60)	0.50 [0.14, 0.86]*	H145
CD8+	Radiotherapy (90)	–0.58 [–2.31, 1.15]	H146
	Pooled result (150); 3 RCTs	0.31 [–0.51, 1.12], 30.2%	H146, H145
NK (%)	Postoperative radiotherapy (60)	7.36 [6.19, 8.53]*	H145
	Radiotherapy (90)	5.59 [3.16, 8.02]*	H146
	Pooled result (150); 2 RCTs	6.81 [5.20, 8.42]*, 39.6%	H146, H145

[1]Comparator was the same radiotherapy.

*Statistically significant.

Abbreviations: CD, cluster of differentiation; CI, confidence interval; MD, mean difference; N, number; NK, natural killer; RCT, randomised controlled trial.

Chinese Herbal Medicine Enema plus Radiotherapy versus Radiotherapy

One study, of 68 people who had recurrent rectal cancer after surgery, received a CHM enema named *Kang fu xin ye* 康复新液 once a day after receiving radiotherapy or received radiotherapy alone (H147). The study only reported the incidence of people with radiation proctitis at severity grades 0 to IV (criteria not specified). There were no cases of grade IV in the CHM enema group and control groups. For grade III, there were no cases in the CHM enema group and four cases in the control. For the total cases (grades I–IV), there were significantly fewer cases in the CHM enema group, compared to control (RR: 0.66 [0.50, 0.87], *n* = 68).

Oral Chinese Herbal Medicine plus Chemo-radiotherapy versus Chemo-radiotherapy

Two RCTs tested oral CHMs combined with chemo-radiotherapy. In one RCT (H148), 96 people with advanced rectal cancer received a combination of XELOX chemotherapy (two 3-week cycles) and radiotherapy. One group also received an unnamed oral CHM (*shan yao* 山药, *chao bai shao* 炒白芍, *ren shen* 人参, *fu ling* 茯苓, *chao bai bian dou* 炒白扁豆, *lian zi* 莲子, *fang feng* 防风, *chen pi* 陈皮, *sha ren* 砂仁, *chao yi yi ren* 炒薏苡仁 and *zhi gan cao* 炙甘草). There was improved ORR (WHO criteria) in the CHM group (RR: 1.50 [1.09. 2.05], *n* = 96).

This study also provided data for gastrointestinal reactions, myelosuppression and radiation proctitis based on WHO grades. There were no differences between groups for grades III plus IV, but the incidence was low in both groups (Table 5.96). For all grades, there were significant reductions in the CHM group for gastrointestinal reactions (RR: 0.59 [0.40, 0.85]), myelosuppression (RR: 0.54 [0.35, 0.84]) and radiation proctitis (RR: 0.44 [0.22, 0.86]). For quality of life, based on the Chinese scale,[25] there was a significant improvement in the CHM group (MD: 6.91 [4.93, 8.89]).

Table 5.96 Oral Chinese Herbal Medicine plus Chemo-radiotherapy: Adverse Reactions to Chemo-radiotherapy

Adverse Reaction (*N* Participants), Study[1]	WHO Grade	Effect Size (RR [95% CI])
Gastrointestinal reactions (96), H148	III + IV	0.31 [0.09, 1.06]
	I to IV	0.59 [0.40, 0.85]*
Myelosuppression (96), H148	III + IV	0.15 [0.02, 1.23]
	I to IV	0.54 [0.35, 0.84]*
Radiation proctitis (96), H148	III + IV	0.23 [0.03, 1.98]
	I to IV	0.44 [0.22, 0.86]*

[1]Comparator was the same chemotherapy (XELOX) plus radiotherapy.

*Statistically significant.

Abbreviations: CI, Confidence Interval; N, number; RR, Risk Ratio; WHO, World Health Organisation.

In another RCT (H149), 52 participants with stage III CRC who had received surgery within the previous month, were treated with FOLFOX4 (12 cycles) plus radiotherapy. The CHM group also received *Xi huang jie du jiao nang* 西黄解毒胶囊 three times a day until there was tumour recurrence or metastasis. The control group received the same chemo-radiotherapy without CHM. Two people were lost to follow-up in the control group. For KPS scores at six months, there were no significant differences between groups (MD: 2.00 [–0.10, 4.10], $n = 50$). The median time to recurrence or metastasis was 21 months in the CHM group and 14 months in the control. The recurrence or metastasis rates were 15.38% for CHM versus 41.66% for control at one year; 50.00% for CHM versus 79.16% for control at two years and 57.96% for CHM versus 91.66% for control at three years.

Safety of Chinese Herbal Medicines in Conjunction with Radiotherapy or Chemo-radiotherapy

In the five studies included in this section, there was no mention of AEs associated with the CHM interventions. Two drop-outs were mentioned in one study (H149), but these were in the control group. In addition, one study (H148) reported fewer adverse reactions to chemo-radiotherapy in the integrated therapy group (see Table 5.96).

Section 4: Supportive and/or Palliative Care Incorporating Chinese Herbal Medicine

Three RCTs, no CCTs and ten non-controlled studies that studied CHMs in conjunction with various types of supportive care without current use of surgical therapies, chemotherapy, molecular targeted therapies or radiotherapy were located.

Randomised Controlled Trials of Oral Chinese Herbal Medicine

The three RCTs were conducted in mainland China and all tested different oral CHMs. They enrolled 182 participants and there were five drop-outs. Participants ranged in age from 38 to 79 years, but one study (H150) did not report the age range. In this study the mean ages were 64.09 years for the CHM group and 66.17 years for the control group.

Syndromes

One study (H151) used syndrome differentiation with all participants requiring a diagnosis of Spleen deficiency (*pi xu* 脾虚).

Formula and Herb Frequencies

Each study used a different formula. The most frequently used herbs were: *bai zhu* 白术, *fu ling* 茯苓, *xia ku cao* 夏枯草, *tai zi shen* 太子参, *hong teng* 红藤, *ye pu tao teng* 野葡萄藤 and *chen pi* 陈皮 (Table 5.97).

Risk of Bias

The RoB for sequence generation was judged 'low' in two studies since the method of randomisation was described. The other was

Table 5.97 Frequently used Herbs in Oral Formulas in Randomised Controlled Trials of Best Supportive Care

Herb Name	Scientific Name	Frequency of Use
Bai zhu 白术[1]	*Atractylodes macrocephala* Koidz.	3
Fu ling 茯苓	*Poria cocos* (Schw.) Wolf	3
Xia ku cao 夏枯草	*Prunella vulgaris* L.	2
Tai zi shen 太子参	*Pseudostellaria heterophylla* (Miq.) Pax ex Pax et Hoffm.	2
Hong teng 红藤	*Sargentodoxa cuneata* (Oliv.) Rehd. & Wils.	2
Ye pu tao teng 野葡萄藤	*Vitis quinquangularis* Rehd.	2
Chen pi 陈皮	*Citrus reticulata* Blanco	2

[1]Two studies used *chao bai zhu* 炒白术.

The use of some herbs may be restricted in some countries. Readers are advised to comply with relevant regulations.

'unclear' risk. Allocation concealment was 'low' risk in H152 and 'unclear' risk in the others. No study mentioned blinding, so all were judged 'high' risk for blinding of participants and personnel and 'unclear' risk for outcome assessors. One study (H151) had no drop-outs, one (H152) had two drop-outs and one (H150) had three drop-outs, so all were judged 'low' risk for incomplete outcome data. All studies reported the outcomes mentioned in the methods, but none had protocols, so all were judged 'unclear' risk for selective reporting. The RCTs each had different comparators and criteria, so each study is reported separately.

Oral Chinese Herbal Medicine versus Best Supportive Care

In one RCT (H152), 50 people with stage IIIB/IV advanced CRC who had received surgery were administered an oral CHM made by the author, *Yi qi fu zheng fang* 益气扶正方 (*bai zhu* 白术, *fu ling* 茯苓, *shan yao* 山药, *huang qi* 黄芪, *dang shen* 党参, *she she cao* 蛇舌草, *shan ci gu* 山慈菇, *tun li gen* 苋梨根, *wu gong* 蜈蚣 and *gan cao* 甘草), once a day for at least four weeks (mean nine weeks) combined with best supportive care, while the people in the control group received best supportive care without CHM. There were two drop-outs in the control group for unspecified reasons. There was a follow-up of two to ten months (median six months).

The ORR (WHO criteria) was zero in both groups but there was a significant increase in the incidence of stable disease in the CHM group (RR: 1.53 [0.66, 3.55], *n* = 48) and no difference between groups for progressive disease (RR: 0.81 [0.54, 1.21], *n* = 48). Median survival time was 6.5 months in the CHM group and six months in the control group. There was no mention of AEs associated with the CHM. For KPS score, there was a significant improvement in the CHM group (MD: 7.73 [1.93, 13.53], *n* = 48). There was no difference in the incidence of vomiting (WHO all grades) between the two groups (RR: 0.92 [0.14, 6.00], *n* = 48).

In another study of 48 people with advanced CRC (H150), one group received *Jian pi an chang fang* 健脾安肠方 (*tai zi shen* 太子

参, *chao bai zhu* 炒白术, *fu ling* 茯苓, *ban xia* 半夏, *qing pi* 青皮, *chen pi* 陈皮, *hong teng* 红藤, *ye pu tao teng* 野葡萄藤, *teng li gen* 藤梨根, *ba qia* 菝葜, *sheng mu li* 生牡蛎, *xia ku cao* 夏枯草, *chao gu ya* 炒谷芽 and *chao mai ya* 炒麦芽) once a day for at least eight weeks while the other group received best supportive care alone. There were three drop-outs (one in the treatment group and two in the control). The reasons for drop-outs were 'lost to follow-up' in one case (group not specified) but no reasons were given for the other two drop-outs. There was no change in ORR (RECIST criteria) in either group (both were zero). There were no significant differences for stable disease (RR; 1.91 [0.87. 4.20], *n* = 45) or progressive disease (RR: 0.60 [0.35, 1.02], *n* = 45). The median survival time was six months in the CHM group and five months in the control. For KPS there was a significant improvement in the CHM group (MD: 9.63 [3.64. 15.62], *n* = 45).

The pooled result for KPS scores in the two studies showed a significant increase in the CHM groups (MD: 8.65 [4.48, 12.82], I^2 = 0%, *n* = 93).

Oral Chinese Herbal Medicine versus Thymosin α1 for Injection

In one three-armed RCT (H151), people who had completed surgery and chemotherapy within the previous three months (*n* = 84) received an oral CHM developed by the author called *Wei chang an* 胃肠安 (*tai zi shen* 太子参, *chao bai zhu* 炒白术, *fu ling* 茯苓, *jiang ban xia* 姜半夏, *chen pi* 陈皮, *hong teng* 红藤, *ye pu tao teng* 野葡萄藤, *xia ku cao* 夏枯草, *bi hu* 壁虎 [also known as *tian long* 天龙], *bai bian dou* 白扁豆, *sheng huang qi* 生黄芪 and *dang gui* 当归) once a day separated into two doses for two months. One group received Thymosin α1 injection every second day for two months (for improving immune function), and the third group received a combination of these treatments.

There were significant reductions in regulatory T cells as a percentage of total T cells in the CHM group versus the Thymosin α1 group (MD: –5.19 [–9.35, –1.02] %, *n* = 56) and in the combined group compared to the Thymosin α1 group (MD: –5.84 [–9.29, –2.39] %, *n* = 56). The greatest reduction was in the combined group which the authors interpreted as indicating that combined therapy was more effective. For KPS, there were improvements for CHM versus Thymosin α1 (MD: 12.14 [7.45, 16.83], *n* = 56) and for combined therapy versus Thymosin α1 (MD: 13.57 [9.20, 17.94], *n* = 56). There was no mention of any AEs.

Non-controlled Studies of Chinese Herbal Medicine in Conjunction with Supportive Care

Of the ten non-controlled studies, seven were case-series studies (H153–H159) and three were case reports (H160–H162. The case-series and case reports are discussed separately.

Case-series Studies

Of the case-series studies, four tested oral CHMs, two combined oral CHM with an enema (H153, H156), and one used an enema alone (H155). Two were of advanced rectal cancer (H153, H155), two were of CRC (H156, H157), and three studies were of advanced CRC (H154, H158, H159). One study was conducted in Singapore (H159) and the others were in mainland China. None of the studies specified syndrome differentiation.

The oral formulas in the case-series studies were all different. The main herbs in the oral formulas were *hong teng* 红藤, *yi yi ren* 薏苡仁 and *bai hua she she cao* 白花蛇舌草. The three enema formulas were different. The main herbs were *bai hua she she cao* 白花蛇舌草, *tu fu ling* 土茯苓, *bi hu* 壁虎, *ku shen* 苦参 and *yi yi ren* 薏苡仁 (Table 5.98).

Survival Rate

Four case-series studies reported survival at one to ten years. All used oral formulas and two combined an oral formula with an enema for rectal cancer (H153) or CRC (H156). In H154, 24 people with

Table 5.98   Frequently Used Herbs in Case-series Studies

Herb Name in Chinese	Scientific Name	Frequency of Use
Oral Chinese Herbal Medicine		
Hong teng 红藤	*Sargentodoxa cuneata* (Oliv.) Rehd. & Wils.	3
Yi yi ren 薏苡仁	*Coix lacryma-jobi* L. var. *mayuen* (Roman.) Stapf	3
Bai hua she she cao 白花蛇舌草	*Hedyotis diffusa* Willd.	3
Dang shen 党参	*Codonopsis pilosula* (Franch.) Nannf.	2
Ban zhi lian 半枝莲	*Scutellaria barbata* D. Don	2
Mu xiang 木香	*Aucklandia lappa* Decne.	2
Ma chi xian 马齿苋	*Portulaca oleracea* L.	2
Chinese Herbal Medicine Enema		
Bai hua she she cao 白花蛇舌草	*Hedyotis diffusa* Willd.	3
Tu fu ling 土茯苓	*Smilax glabra* Roxb.	2
Bi hu 壁虎	*Gekko* spp.	2
Ku shen 苦参	*Sophora flavescens* Ait.	2
Yi yi ren 薏苡仁	*Coix lacryma-jobi* L. var. *mayuen* (Roman.) Stapf	2

The use of some herbs may be restricted in some countries. Readers are advised to comply with relevant regulations.

advanced CRC were treated with *Chang ji xiao fang* 肠积消方 once a day (in three doses) for at least three months. The authors reported the CHM improved symptoms and there was 8.3% survival at three years. In H158, 44 advanced CRC patients took *Zhao shi wei tiao san hao* 赵氏微调三号 (*dang shen* 党参, *chao bai zhu* 炒白术, *fu ling* 茯苓, *yi ren* 苡仁, *zhi pi pa ye* 灸枇杷叶, *zhi ban xia* 制半夏, *chen pi* 陈皮 and *zhu ling* 猪苓) as an oral liquid (30 ml/1–3 times a day) for 60 days. After treatment, KPS improved and survival at two years was 45.45%.

In H153, 18 people with advanced rectal cancer (mainly C1, C2 — modified Dukes) took *Chang ai fang* 肠癌方 once a day for at

Table 5.99   Survival Rates in Case-series Studies

Study, Intervention (*N* Participants)	1 Year (%)[3]	2 Year (%)[3]	3 Year (%)[3]	5 Year (%)[3]	10 Year (%)[3]
H154, *Chang ji xiao fang* 肠积消方 oral (24)[1]	10/24 (41.7)	6/24 (25.0)	2/24 (8.3)	na	na
H158, *Zhao shi wei tiao san hao* 赵氏微调三号 oral (44)[1]	32/44 (72.7)	20/44 (45.5)	na	na	na
H153, *Chang ai fang* 肠癌方 oral plus enema (18)[2]	(100)	na	(66.7)	(38.9)	na
H156, *Qing chang xiao zhong tang* 清肠消肿汤, oral plus enema (50)	40/50 (80.0)	20/46 (43.5)	13/41 (31.7)	7/35 (20.0)	1/11 (9.1)

[1]Advanced colon rectal cancer.

[2]Advanced rectal cancer.

[3]Survivors/total (% survival).

Abbreviations: na, not available.

least three months plus an enema composed of *huai hua* 槐花, *ya dan zi* 鸦胆子, *bai jiang cao* 败酱草, *tu fu ling* 土茯苓, *bai hua she she cao* 白花蛇舌草, *hua rui shi* 花蕊石, *xue xie* 血竭 and *zao jiao ci* 皂角刺 once a day. The authors reported symptom improvement and 38.9% survival at five years. In H156, 50 people with cancer of the rectum or sigmoid colon (stage unspecified) received *Qing chang xiao zhong tang* 清肠消肿汤 orally and as an enema once or twice a day for at least three months. The five-year survival was 20% and the ten-year survival was 9.1%. However, at the time of writing, data were not yet available for all time periods, hence the different baseline numbers (Table 5.99).

Immune Function

Two studies reported on immune function. In H155, 32 people with advanced rectal cancer were administered an enema of *Hua yan tang* 化岩汤 once a day for more than one hour for ten days as a cycle, followed by a one-day break, and then a further two cycles. The authors reported that symptoms and immune function improved.

In H159, 47 people with advanced CRC took *ling zhi* 灵芝 *Ganoderma lucidum*, 5.4 g/day for 12 weeks. The authors reported increases in CD3+, CD4+, CD8+ and CD56+ lymphocyte counts, and increased plasma concentrations of interleukin (IL)-2, IL-6, interferon (IFN)-gamma and NK activity, combined with decreased plasma concentrations of IL-1 and tumour necrosis factor (TNF)-alpha which suggests an immune-modulatory effect. There were six drop-outs, including one death, but these were not related to the CHM.

Tumour Response and KPS

In H157, 20 CRC patients (stage unclear) received *Chang fu kang jiao nang* 肠复康胶囊 two capsules, three times a day for 30 days. The authors reported there was 45% partial tumour response and KPS improved in ten participants.

Case Reports

The three case reports were all from mainland China. One case was of an 83-year-old woman with sigmoid colon cancer (H160) who had received oral chemotherapy for one week (she refused surgery and further chemotherapy). She sought treatment for diarrhoea and bleeding, abdominal pain, weight loss and other symptoms. She was diagnosed with the syndrome Liver depression and Spleen deficiency (*gan yu pi xu* 肝郁脾虚) and received modified *Gu chang zhi xie wan* 固肠止泻丸 (*wu mei* 乌梅, *huang lian* 黄连, *gan jiang* 干姜, *mu xiang* 木香, *ying su ke* 罂粟壳, *yuan hu* 元胡, *huang hua cai* 黄花菜, *hei mu er* 黑木耳 and *xue yu tan* 血余炭) for two weeks. The symptoms reduced and the bleeding stopped. At five-year follow-up, she had continued treatment and there was no evidence of metastasis or AEs associated with the CHM.

In another case (H161), a 40-year-old woman with rectal cancer sought treatment for diarrhoea with bleeding and abdominal pain. She was treated with *Bai tou weng tang jia jian* 白头翁汤加减

(*bai tou weng* 白头翁, *huang lian* 黄连, *huang bai* 黄柏, *mu xiang* 木香, *di yu* 地榆, *he zi* 诃子, *zhi ke* 枳壳, *jiao shan zha* 焦山楂, and *san qi fen* 三七粉) combined with *Yun nan bai yao* 云南白药 plus an enema of *huang lian* 黄连, *huang bai* 黄柏 and *peng sha* 硼砂. A colonoscopy identified rectal cancer. Seventeen days later her symptoms had improved. The oral CHM was modified with the addition of *bing lang* 槟榔 and was continued for two months, by which time the symptoms had resolved. She was referred for surgery.

In the third case (H162), a woman aged 74 who had colon cancer with metastases of the lung, liver and lymph nodes refused chemotherapy. She had abdominal distension, abdominal pain, loose stool and intestinal bleeding. She was treated with *sheng huang qi* 生黄芪, *chao bai zhu* 炒白术, *chao bai shao* 炒白芍, *teng li gen* 藤梨根, *chao dang shen* 炒党参, *fu ling* 茯苓, *chao dang gui* 炒当归, *zhi ke* 枳壳, *fo shou* 佛手, *jiang ban xia* 姜半夏, *chen pi* 陈皮, *chai hu* 柴胡, *yu jin* 郁金, *bai hua she she cao* 白花蛇舌草, *xian he cao* 仙鹤草, *di yu tan* 地榆炭 and *huai hua tan* 槐花炭 for two weeks. The bleeding stopped and the symptoms improved. The formula was modified by removing *di yu tan* 地榆炭 and *huai hua tan* 槐花炭 and adding *yuan hu* 元胡, *da zao* 大枣 and *zhi gan cao* 炙甘草 which was consumed for 15 days. The distension and pain disappeared, and defaecation became normal. The woman continued to take this formula for more than one year. After 16 months, the computerized tomography scan showed the tumour to be stable.

Safety of Chinese Herbal Medicine in Supportive and/or Palliative Care

There were five drop-outs in two of the three RCTs (one in CHMs, four in controls) which did not appear to be due to the CHMs causing AEs. None of the RCTs mentioned AEs associated with the CHMs, although one study found no difference in vomiting between groups. In the non-controlled case-series studies, one reported six drop-outs

(H159), and one serious AE (death), but these were reported as not related to the CHM.

Evidence for Chinese Herbal Medicine Treatments Commonly Used in Clinical Practice

Of the formulas included in textbooks and guidelines in Chapter 2, 12 were also tested in one or more of the clinical studies in Chapter 5. In some studies, the formulas were modified or combined with other formulas, so these have been grouped. In two studies (H36, H40) multiple formulas were used according to syndrome differentiation.

Formulas Based on Syndrome Differentiation

In one RCT (H36) of CHM versus XELODA as maintenance treatment for stage IV CRC, eight different formulas were prescribed according to the syndrome, including four that appear in Chapter 2: *Si jun zi tang* 四君子汤, *Si wu tang* 四物汤, *Tao hong si wu tang* 桃红四物汤 and *Zhi bai di huang tang* 知柏地黄汤. However, there was no data on which formulas were more commonly prescribed. There was a significant increase in incidence of a 10-point or more improvement in KPS in the CHM group compared to the XELODA group (Table 5.100). For T cells, the percentage of NK cells was significantly higher in the CHM group and the ratio CD4+/CD8+ was significantly increased. For PFS, the mPFS in the CHM group was 5.4 months versus two months in the XELODA group. In the CHM group, PFS was 1.7–18 months versus 1.5–12 months in the XELODA group. There were three drop-outs in the CHM group (all refused CHM) versus two in the XELODA group due to chemotherapy-related AEs, which may have affected the PFS results.

In another multi-formula RCT (H40) of CHM plus XELODA versus XELODA alone as maintenance therapy for advanced CRC (*n* = 150), 11 different formulas were prescribed according to syndrome. The following six are in Chapter 2: *Si jun zi tang* 四君子汤, *Si wu*

Table 5.100 Multi-formula Randomised Controlled Trial of Chinese Herbal Medicine versus XELODA: Results

Outcome	Comparison[1] (Cancer)	Effect Size (RR or MD [95% CI]), Participants	Included Study, Type
KPS (increase of 10 points or more)	Chinese herbal formula based on syndrome versus XELODA (stage IV CRC)	RR 1.85 [1.04, 3.27]*, $n = 120$	H36, RCT
NK cells (%)		MD 7.10 [4.22, 9.98]*, $n = 120$	
CD4+/CD8+ (ratio)		MD 0.59 [0.36, 0.82]*, $n = 120$	
mPFS (months)		5.4 versus 2	
PFS (months)		1.7–18 versus 1.5–12	

[1]Comparator was the same chemotherapy.

*Statistically significant.

Abbreviations: CD, cluster of differentiation; CI, confidence interval; CRC, colorectal cancer; MD, mean difference; n, number; NK, natural killer; RCT, randomised controlled trial; RR, risk ratio.

tang 四物汤, *Ge xia zu yu tang* 膈下逐瘀汤, *Tao hong si wu tang* 桃红四物汤, *Zhi bai di huang tang* 知柏地黄汤 and *Bai tou weng tang* 白头翁汤. There was an improvement in immune function in the CHM plus XELODA group in terms of NK cells and the ratio of CD4+/CD8+ cells. Time to progression (TTP) was longer in the integrative therapy group at 2–12 months (median six months) compared to 2–10 months (median three months) in the XELODA alone group; however, eight participants dropped out during follow-up (treatment:5 / control:3) which may have influenced the TPP result (Table 5.101).

Liu jun zi tang

The formula most frequently investigated in single-formula studies was *Liu jun zi tang* 六君子汤 (including modified versions) which was an intervention in five RCTs and one non-controlled study (H144). In the pooled results for two RCTs (H15, H17) of postoperative recovery, there were significant reductions in time to first flatus and defaecation but no significant changes in immunoglobulins

Table 5.101 Multi-formula Randomised Controlled Trial of Chinese Herbal Medicine plus XELODA versus XELODA: Results

Outcome	Comparison[1] (Cancer)	Effect Size (MD [95% CI]), Participants	Included Study, Type
NK cells (%)	Chinese herbal formula based on syndrome plus XELODA versus XELODA (advanced CRC)	5.10 [2.50, 7.70]*, $n = 150$	H40, RCT
CD4+/CD8+ (ratio)		0.51 [0.27, 0.75]*, $n = 150$	
mTTP (months)		6 versus 3	
TTP (months)		2–12 versus 2–10	

[1]Comparator was the same chemotherapy.

*Statistically significant.

Abbreviations: CD, cluster of differentiation; CI, confidence interval; CRC, colorectal cancer; MD, mean difference; mTTP, median time to progression; n, number; NK, natural killer; RCT, randomised controlled trial; TTP, time to progression.

(Table 5.11). When combined with XELOX chemotherapy (H45), ORR (RECIST) was not significantly improved and a similar result was found in combination with FOLIRI (H43) (Table 5.102). Combination with XELOX did not significantly change KPS scores (H45). For improvements of 10 points or more on KPS, the pooled result for two RCTs (H43, H42) showed no significant difference. One study provided data for T cells (H45) and found significant increases in CD3+, CD4+ and CD8+ cells but no change in the ratio CD4+/CD8+. For chemotherapy-related AEs, one RCT (H43) found significant improvements in all grades (WHO) of nausea and vomiting, diarrhoea and myelosuppression, but not in hand-foot syndrome or hepatotoxicity. In the other RCT (H42), which used NCI-CTCAE criteria, there were no significant differences for nausea and vomiting, diarrhoea or myelosuppression. The single non-controlled study (H144) reported an improvement in chemotherapy-related diarrhoea. In the study of *Jia wei xiang sha liu jun zi tang* 加味香砂六君子汤 plus FOLIRI (H43), there were six drop-outs in the integrative therapy group versus 14 in the FOLIRI alone group for the following reasons: refused chemotherapy (2 versus 3), chemotherapy-related adverse reaction (2 versus 8), and death (2 versus 3).

Table 5.102 *Liu Jun Zi Tang* **(Including Modified Versions): Additional Results**

Outcome (Criteria, Unit)	Comparison[1]	Effect Size (RR, MD [95% CI]) or T/C, I^2, Participants	Included Study, Type
ORR (WHO)	CHM plus XELOX (no surgery)	RR 1.27 [0.69, 2.33], $n = 60$	H45, RCT
ORR (RECIST)	CHM plus FOLFIRI	RR 1.07 [0.62, 1.85], $n = 50$	H43, RCT
1-year survival T/C	CHM plus XELOX (no surgery)	T/C 25/17 (83.3%/56.7%), $n = 60$	H45, RCT
KPS score	CHM plus XELOX (no surgery)	MD −0.67 [−4.04, 2.70], $n = 60$	H45, RCT
KPS (increase of 10 points or more)	CHM plus FOLFIRI	RR 1.60 [0.67, 3.84], $n = 50$	H43, RCT
	CHM plus XELOX (no surgery)	RR 4.50 [1.06, 19.11]*, $n = 60$	H42, RCT
KPS Pooled Result	CHM plus chemo	RR 2.29 [0.85, 6.12], 33.3%, $n = 110$	H43, H42
CD3+ (%)	CHM plus XELOX (no surgery)	MD 7.87 [5.39, 10.35]*, $n = 60$	H45, RCT
CD4+ (%)		MD 5.17 [3.27, 7.07]*, $n = 60$	
CD8+ (%)		MD −1.96 [−3.45, −0.47]*, $n = 60$	
CD4+/CD8+ (ratio)		MD 0.26 [−0.01, 0.53], $n = 60$	
Chemotherapy-related Adverse Events			
Nausea and vomiting (NCI-CTCAE)	CHM plus XELOX (no surgery)	Grades III+IV: RR 0.25 [0.06, 1.08]; All grades: RR 0.93 [0.81, 1.07], $n = 60$	H42, RCT
Nausea and vomiting (WHO)	CHM plus FOLFIRI	All grades: RR 0.25 [0.12, 0.53]*, $n = 50$	H43, RCT
Diarrhoea (NCI-CTCAE)	CHM plus XELOX (no surgery)	Grades III+IV: RR 0.17 [0.02, 1.30]; All grades: RR 0.65 [0.37, 1.14], $n = 60$	H42, RCT

(*Continued*)

Table 5.102   (*Continued*)

Outcome (Criteria, Unit)	Comparison[1]	Effect Size (RR, MD [95% CI]) or T/C, I^2, Participants	Included Study, Type
Diarrhoea (WHO)	CHM plus FOLFIRI	All grades: RR 0.29 [0.15, 0.58]*, $n = 50$	H43, RCT
Diarrhoea (NS) due to XELOX	CHM plus XELOX	Improved, $n = 1$	H144, NCS
Myelosuppression (NCI-CTCAE)	CHM plus XELOX (no surgery)	Grades III + IV: RR 0.75 [0.18, 3.07]; All grades: RR 0.96 [0.73, 1.25], $n = 60$	H42, RCT
Myelosuppression (WHO)	CHM plus FOLFIRI	All grades: RR 0.29 [0.13, 0.62]*, $n = 50$	H43, RCT
Hand-foot syndrome		All grades: RR 0.13 [0.02, 1.06], $n = 50$	
Hepatotoxicity		All grades: RR 0.44 [0.08, 2.43], $n = 50$	

[1]Versus the same chemotherapy.

*Statistically significant.

Abbreviations: C, control group; CHM, Chinese herbal medicine; CI, confidence interval; KPS, Karnofsky Performance Status; MD, mean difference; n, number; NCI-CTCAE, National Cancer Institute-Common Terminology Criteria for Adverse Events; NCS: non-controlled study; ORR, objective response rate; RCT, randomised controlled trial; RECIST, Response Evaluation Criteria in Solid Tumours; RR, risk ratio; T, treatment group; WHO, World Health Organisation.

Specific formulas: *Xiang sha liu jun wan* 香砂六君丸 (H42), *Jia wei xiang sha liu jun zi tang* 加味香砂六君子汤 (H43), *Gui qi liu jun tang* 归芪六君汤 (H45) and modified *Xiang sha liu jun zi tang* 香砂六君子汤加减 (H144).

Si jun zi tang

The formula *Si jun zi tang* 四君子汤 was included in each of the multi-formula RCTs discussed above (H36, H40), and in a further two RCTs and two CCTs. For recovery after surgery, one RCT (H12) of *Si jun zi tang jia wei* 四君子汤加味 plus FTP found non-significant reductions in time to measures of gastrointestinal recovery after laparoscopic surgery (Table 5.103). For measures of postoperative

Table 5.103 *Si Jun Zi Tang* (Including Modified Versions): Additional Results

Outcome (Criteria)	Comparison	Effect Size (MD or RR [95% CI]), Participants	Included Study, Type
Time to first flatus	CHM plus FTP versus FTP (laparoscopy, CRC)	MD –2.50 [–13.44, 8.44], $n = 61$	H12, RCT
Time to food intake		MD –1.60 [–4.68, 1.48], $n = 61$	
Postoperative immune function	CHM plus PEN versus saline plus PEN (colon cancer)	See Table 5.19 for results for T cells and immunoglobulins, $n = 84$	H27, CCT
ORR (RECIST)	CHM plus FOLFOX6[1]	RR 1.56 [0.78, 3.11], $n = 70$	H44, RCT
KPS score		MD 9.89 [7.07, 12.71]*, $n = 70$	
KPS (increase of 10 points or more)	CHM plus FOLFOX4[1,2]	RR 2.62 [1.23, 5.58]*, $n = 52$	H140, CCT[2]
Chemotherapy-related AEs (WHO Criteria)			
Nausea and vomiting	CHM plus FOLFOX6[1] Participants = 70	Grade III + IV: RR 0.25 [0.03, 2.13]; all grades: RR 0.57 [0.34, 0.97]*	H44, RCT
Diarrhoea		Grade III + IV: RR 1.00 [0.07, 15.36]; all grades: RR 0.80 [0.37, 1.79]	
Neutropenia		Grade III + IV: RR 0.50 [0.05, 5.27]; all grades: RR 0.64 [0.42, 0.97]*	
Erythropenia		Grade III + IV: RR 0.33 [0.01, 7.91]; all grades: RR 0.55 [0.31, 0.97]*	
Thrombocytopenia		Grade III + IV: RR 0.20 [0.01, 4.02]; all grades: RR 0.59 [0.36, 0.98]*	
CIPN		all grades: RR 0.81 [0.58, 1.13]	
Fever		all grades: RR 1.00 [0.22, 4.62]	
Skin rash		all grades: RR 0.50 [0.05, 5.27]	

[1]Versus the same chemotherapy.

[2]The syndrome *pi qi xu* 脾气虚 was an inclusion criterion.

*Statistically significant.

Abbreviations: C, control group; CCT, controlled clinical trial; CHM, Chinese herbal medicine; CI, confidence interval; CIPN, chemotherapy-induced peripheral neuropathy; CRC, colorectal cancer; FTP, Fast Track Programme; KPS, Karnofsky Performance Status; MD, mean difference; n, number; NCS: non-controlled study; ORR, objective response rate; PEN, postoperative enteral nutrition; RCT, randomised controlled trial; RECIST, Response Evaluation Criteria in Solid Tumours; RR, risk ratio; T, treatment group; WHO, World Health Organisation.

immune function, one CCT (H27) of CHM plus PEN versus saline plus PEN found significant improvements in the CHM group for counts of CD3+, CD4+ and NK cells, but not for CD8+ cells or the ratio CD4+/CD8+, and higher levels of immunoglobulins IgG, IgA and IgM (see Table 5.19). When *Jia wei si jun zi tang* 加味四君子汤 was combined with FOLFOX6 in one RCT (H44), there was no significant difference in ORR and a significant improvement in KPS score. Of the chemotherapy-related AEs, there were improvements in nausea and vomiting, thrombocytopenia, erythropenia and neutropenia (Table 5.103). In a retrospective CCT (H140) of *Si jun zi tang jia jian* 四君子汤加减 plus FOLFOX4 in people with the syndrome Spleen *qi* deficiency (*pi qi xu* 脾气虚), there was an increased incidence of improvements in KPS of 10 points or more.

Bu zhong yi qi tang/wan

Bu zhong yi qi tang/wan 补中益气汤/丸 (Table 5.104) was used for postoperative diarrhoea after surgery in two RCTs (H9, H19) and one non-controlled study which specified that all participants had the syndrome sunken middle *qi* (*zhong qi xia xian* 中气下陷) (H33). There was no significant difference between groups in either RCT for incidence of complete recovery. The non-controlled study reported improvement in diarrhoea and a range of other symptoms. Adverse events were not reported.

Table 5.104 ***Bu Zhong Yi Qi Tang/Wan*** **for Postoperative Diarrhoea**

Cancer Type	Comparison	Effect Size (RR [95% CI]), Participants	Included Study, Type
Colorectal cancer	CHM plus LOP vs LOP	1.83 [0.78. 4.32], *n* = 60	H19, RCT
Rectal cancer	CHM plus LOP plus MON vs LOP plus MON	1.09 [0.62, 1.92], *n* = 48	H9, RCT
Rectal cancer	Single group	Improvements, *n* = 73	H33, NCS

*Statistically significant.

Abbreviations: CHM, Chinese herbal medicine; CI, confidence interval; LOP, loperamide; MON, montmorillonite; NCS: non-controlled study; RCT, randomised controlled trial; RR, risk ratio.

Table 5.105 ***Shen Ling Bai Zhu San* (Including Modified Versions): Results**

Outcome	Comparison[1]	Effect Size (RR [95% CI]), Participants	Included Study, Type
Postoperative diarrhoea	CHM plus usual care for CRC	RR 4.00 [1.51, 10.57]*, $n = 60$	H8, RCT
Chemotherapy-related Adverse Events (NCI-CTCAE Criteria: All Grades)			
Leukopenia	CHM plus mFOLFOX6	RR 0.83 [0.56, 1.24], $n = 80$	H121, RCT
Reduced haemoglobin		RR 0.41 [0.19, 0.88]*, $n = 80$	
Thrombocytopenia		RR 0.74 [0.43, 1.26], $n = 80$	

[1]Versus the same chemotherapy/usual care.

*Statistically significant.

Abbreviations: CHM, Chinese herbal medicine; CI, confidence interval; CRC, colorectal cancer; n, number; NCI-CTCAE, National Cancer Institute-Common Terminology Criteria for Adverse Events; RCT, randomised controlled trial; RR, risk ratio.

Shen ling bai zhu san

Shen ling bai zhu san 参苓白术散 (modified) was used for diarrhoea following surgery for CRC in one RCT (H8) which reported a significant improvement in incidence of complete recovery, compared to usual care alone (Table 5.105). In another RCT (H121) of *Shen ling bai zhu san* plus *Gui pi tang* 参苓白术散合归脾汤加减 combined with mFOLFOX6, there was a significant improvement in incidence of reduced haemoglobin level in the integrative therapy group, but no significant differences for leukopenia or thrombocytopenia.

Bai tou weng tang

Bai tou weng tang 白头翁汤 (including modified versions) was used in one of the two multi-syndrome RCTs described above (H40), a single RCT (H81) and a case study (H161). The RCT (H81) used *Si miao san* plus *Bai tou weng tang* 四妙散和白头翁汤 combined with FOLFOX4 in people with stage III/IV colon cancer. There were no significant differences between groups for ORR or KPS score

Table 5.106 ***Bai Tou Weng Tang*** **(Including Modified Versions): Additional Results**

Outcome	Comparison	Effect Size (RR or MD [95% CI]), Participants	Included Study, Type
ORR (RECIST)	CHM plus FOLFOX4[1] (colon cancer)	RR 1.04 [0.60, 1.79], $n = 41$	H81, RCT
KPS score		MD 5.47 [–0.96, 11.90], $n = 41$	
Diarrhoea with bleeding and abdominal pain	Oral CHM plus CHM enema (rectal cancer)	Symptoms improved prior to surgery, $n = 1$	H161, NCS

[1]Versus the same chemotherapy.

*Statistically significant.

Abbreviations: CHM, Chinese herbal medicine; CI, confidence interval; KPS, Karnofsky Performance Status; MD, mean difference; NCS, non-controlled study; ORR, objective response rate; RCT, randomised controlled trial; RECIST, Response Evaluation Criteria in Solid Tumours; RR, risk ratio.

(Table 5.106). Of the five drop-outs in the CHM plus FOLFOX4 group, one was due to allergy, two were due to intolerance of chemotherapy and no reason was given for the other two ($n = 5$). In the FOLFOX4 group there were three drop-outs due to intolerance of chemotherapy and no reason was given for one drop-out ($n = 4$). In the case study (H161), a 40-year-old woman with rectal cancer was treated with *Bai tou weng tang jia jian* 白头翁汤加减 combined with *Yun nan bai yao* 云南白药 plus an enema of *huang lian* 黄连, *huang bai* 黄柏 and *peng sha* 硼砂 for diarrhoea with bleeding and abdominal pain associated with rectal cancer. After the symptoms had resolved, she was referred for surgery.

Ba zhen tang

Ba zhen tang 八珍汤 (including modified versions) was investigated in two RCTs. In one study (H47) *Ba zhen tang jia jian* 八珍汤加减 was combined with FOLFOX4 as adjuvant chemotherapy after radical surgery for colon cancer. There were significant improvements in KPS scores, T cell subsets, and in the levels of IgG and IgM, but not IgA or IgE (Table 5.107). For chemotherapy-related AEs, in the

Table 5.107 *Ba Zhen Tang* (Including Modified Versions): Results

Outcome (Unit)	Comparison[1]	Effect Size (MD or RR [95% CI]), Participants	Included Study, Type
KPS score	CHM plus FOLFOX4 (adjuvant, after radical surgery)	MD 6.44 [2.60, 10.28]*, $n = 55$	H47, RCT
KPS (increase of 10 points or more)		RR 1.67 [1.13, 2.47]*, $n = 60$	H46, RCT
1-year recurrence T/C (%)		2/4 (6.7/13.3)	
1-year metastasis T/C (%)		1/4 (3.3/13.3)	
T Cell Subsets			
CD3+ (%)	CHM plus FOLFOX4 (adjuvant, after radical surgery for colon cancer)	MD 3.99 [1.15, 6.83]*, $n = 55$	H47, RCT
CD4+ (%)		MD 6.56 [3.93, 9.19]*, $n = 55$	
CD8+ (%)		MD –3.17 [–5.16, –1.18]*, $n = 55$	
CD4+/CD8+ (ratio)		MD 0.42 [0.25, 0.59]*, $n = 55$	
NK cells (%)		MD 10.70 [9.20, 12.20]*, $n = 55$	
Immunoglobulins			
IgA (g/L)	CHM plus FOLFOX4 (adjuvant, after radical surgery for colon cancer)	MD –0.12 [–0.37, 0.13], $n = 55$	H47, RCT
IgG (g/L)		MD 2.46 [0.97, 3.95]*, $n = 55$	
IgM (g/L)		MD 0.59 [0.26, 0.92]* $n = 55$	
IgE (mg/L)		MD 0.03 [–0.08, 0.14], $n = 55$	
Chemotherapy-related Adverse Events (WHO Criteria)			
Nausea and vomiting	CHM plus FOLFOX4 (adjuvant, after radical surgery for colon cancer) Participants = 55	Grade III + IV: RR 0.96 [0.06, 14.65]; all grades: RR 0.35 [0.13, 0.97]*	H47, RCT
Diarrhoea		All grades: RR 0.32 [0.12, 0.87]*	
Constipation		All grades: RR 0.48 [0.13, 1.74]	
Leukopenia		All grades: RR 0.48 [0.25, 0.94]*	
Thrombocytopenia		All grades: RR 0.24 [0.06, 1.03]	
Reduced haemoglobin		All grades: RR 1.21 [0.36, 4.02]	
CIPN		All grades: RR 0.64 [0.12, 3.55]	

(Continued)

Table 5.107   (*Continued*)

Outcome (Unit)	Comparison[1]	Effect Size (MD or RR [95% CI]), Participants	Included Study, Type
Chemotherapy-related Adverse Events (Criteria Not Specified: All Grades)			
Nausea and vomiting	CHM plus FOLFOX4 (adjuvant, after radical surgery for CRC)	RR 0.56 [0.31, 1.00], $n = 60$	H46, RCT
Diarrhoea		RR 0.67 [0.21, 2.13], $n = 60$	
Leukopenia		RR 0.57 [0.28, 1.16], $n = 60$	
Thrombocytopenia		RR 0.67 [0.27, 1.64], $n = 60$	
Erythropenia		RR 0.40 [0.18, 0.89]*, $n = 60$	

[1]Versus the same chemotherapy.

*Statistically significant.

Abbreviations: C, control group; CHM, Chinese herbal medicine; CD, cluster of differentiation; CI, confidence interval; CIPN, chemotherapy-induced peripheral neurotoxicity; CRC, colorectal cancer; Ig, immunoglobulin; KPS, Karnofsky Performance Status; MD, mean difference; n, number; NK, natural killer; RCT, randomised controlled trial; RR, risk ratio; T, treatment group; WHO, World Health Organisation.

integrative groups there were significant reductions for all grades of nausea and vomiting, diarrhoea and leukopenia, but not for the other AEs. In the other RCT (H46), *Ba zhen tang* 八珍汤 was used with adjuvant FOLFOX4 chemotherapy following radical surgery for CRC. The incidence of improvements in KPS of 10 points or more was significantly increased in the integrative therapy group. For chemotherapy-related AEs the criteria used were not specified, so results were not pooled. There was a significant reduction in erythropenia, but not in the other AEs. One-year recurrence and one-year metastasis rates were lower in the integrative therapy group.

Fu fang ban mao jiao nang

Fu fang ban mao jiao nang 复方斑蝥胶囊 was mentioned in Chapter 2 as a manufactured medicine for CRC and was investigated in two RCTs (Table 5.108). In one RCT (H51), *Fu fang ban mao jiao nang* 复方斑蝥胶囊 was combined with FOLFOX4 for CRC, but there was no significant increase in ORR. In the other RCT (H50) *Fu fang ban mao jiao nang* 复方斑蝥胶囊 was

Table 5.108   *Fu Fang Ban Mao Jiao Nang*: **Results**

Outcome (Criteria, Units)	Comparison[1] (Cancer)	Effect Size (RR [95% CI]), Participants	Included Study, Type
ORR (RECIST)	CHM plus FOLFOX4 (CRC)	RR 1.18 [0.75, 1.86], $n = 107$	H51, RCT
ORR (WHO)	CHM plus FOLFIRI (stage III/IV CRC)	RR 1.31 [0.75, 2.28], $n = 87$	H50, RCT
KPS (increase of 10 points or more)		RR 1.65 [1.07, 2.54]*, $n = 87$	
Chemotherapy-related Adverse Events (Criteria Not Specified: All Grades)			
Nausea and vomiting	CHM plus FOLFIRI (stage III/IV CRC)	RR 0.66 [0.44, 0.98]*, $n = 87$	H50, RCT
Diarrhoea		RR 0.67 [0.40, 1.14], $n = 87$	
Leukopenia		RR 0.58 [0.37, 0.91]*, $n = 87$	
Reduced haemoglobin		RR 0.49 [0.23, 1.04], $n = 87$	
Thrombocytopenia		RR 0.57 [0.35, 0.91]*, $n = 87$	
ALT		RR 0.43 [0.18, 1.03], $n = 87$	
BUN		RR 0.85 [0.06, 13.18], $n = 87$	
Creatinine level		RR 0.85 [0.06, 13.18], $n = 87$	
Oral mucositis		RR 0.59 [0.31, 1.11], $n = 87$	
Alopecia		RR 0.78 [0.39, 1.57], $n = 87$	
Skin rash		RR 0.43 [0.04, 4.52], $n = 87$	
Survival			
1-year survival T/C (%)	CHM plus FOLFIRI (stage III/IV CRC)	25/16 (53.2/40)	H50, RCT
Overall survival T/C (months)		7–38/5–31	
MST T/C (months)		12.5/10.8	

[1]Versus the same chemotherapy.

*Statistically significant.

Abbreviations: ALT, alanine transaminase; BUN, blood urea nitrogen; C, control group; CHM, Chinese herbal medicine; CI, confidence interval; CRC, colorectal cancer; KPS, Karnofsky Performance Status; MST, mean survival time; n, number; ORR, objective response rate; RECIST, Response Evaluation Criteria in Solid Tumours; RCT, randomised controlled trial; RR, risk ratio; T, treatment group; WHO, World Health Organisation.

combined with FOLFIRI for stage III/IV CRC that had recurred after surgery or was not suitable for surgery. The ORR showed no significant improvement, but there was a significant increase in the incidence of improvement in KPS of 10 points or more. For chemotherapy-related AEs, there were significant reductions in all grades of nausea and vomiting, and thrombocytopenia but not in the other AEs. Measures of liver and kidney function were not significantly different in the integrative therapy group. One-year survival, overall survival and MST were all improved in the *Fu fang ban mao jiao nang* 复方斑蝥胶囊 plus FOLFIRI group.

Hua chan su pian/jiao nang

Hua chan su pian 华蟾素片 (tablets) is another manufactured medicine mentioned in Chapter 2. *Hua chan su jiao nang* 华蟾素胶囊 (capsules) was investigated in one RCT (H146) for people who were receiving radiotherapy for rectal cancer for its effect on immune function. The combination therapy showed significant increases in CD3+, CD4+ and NK cells but there were no significant differences between groups for CD8+ cells or the ratio CD4+/CD8+. Adverse events were not reported (Table 5.109).

Table 5.109 *Hua Chan Su Jiao Nang*: **Results**

Outcome	Comparison (Cancer)	Effect Size (MD [95% CI]), Participants	Included Study, Type
T Cell Subsets			
CD3+ (%)	CHM plus radiotherapy versus radiotherapy (rectal cancer)	4.40 [2.64, 6.16]*, $n = 90$	H146, RCT
CD4+ (%)		7.36 [4.70, 10.02]*, $n = 90$	
CD8+ (%)		−0.58 [−2.31, 1.15], $n = 90$	
CD4+/CD8+ (ratio)		−0.58 [−2.31, 1.15], $n = 90$	
NK cells (%)		5.59 [3.16, 8.02]*, $n = 90$	

*Statistically significant.

Abbreviations: CD, cluster of differentiation; CHM, Chinese herbal medicine; CI, confidence interval; MD, mean difference; n, number; NK, natural killer; RCT, randomised controlled trial.

Safety of Chinese Herbal Medicines

Of 19 RCTs of oral CHM for postoperative recovery, six reported on safety (31.6%), five reported no AEs associated with the CHM and one reported a drop-out who had vomiting. There was no data for the RCTs of topical CHM.

For orally administered CHMs in conjunction with chemotherapy, safety reporting was focused on the chemotherapy aspect. Only ten studies (10.9%) specifically reported on the safety of the CHMs. Five RCTs had no AEs and five reported specific AEs and/or reasons for drop-out (Table 5.93). In addition, 32 studies reported on hepatotoxicity and nephrotoxicity, and the meta-analysis results did not show any elevated incidences in the groups that took oral CHMs. For incidence of skin rash, there were no significant differences between groups. In the five RCTs that used topical CHM there was no mention of AEs in three hand and foot bath studies and the single study of a CHM cataplasm. In one hand and foot bath study there was one case of probable allergy to the CHM (Table 5.93). None of the five RCTs of CHMs, in conjunction with radio-therapy, chemo-radiotherapy or the three RCTs of supportive and/or palliative care mentioned AEs associated with the CHMs. Overall, the reporting of AEs associated with the CHM was inadequate and there was insufficient data for a complete statistical assessment.

Summary of the Clinical Evidence for Chinese Herbal Medicine

The database searches identified a substantial volume of data from clinical trials of CHM for CRC. Most studies were of orally administered CHM to assist in recovery after CRC surgery or of oral CHM combined with chemotherapy. The majority of these studies were RCTs so there were opportunities to pool data from multiple studies. For the topical CHMs and the other comparisons, data analyses were based on only a few studies, so it is difficult to draw strong conclusions.

Overall, the results of the RCTs suggest that oral CHM reduced the time to postoperative recovery of gastrointestinal function and improved KPS, with weaker evidence for no improvement in diarrhoea, reduced incidence of abdominal distension, and reduced nausea and vomiting. However, most studies were not investigator-blind so there was potential for bias. This factor, combined with statistical heterogeneity and small samples sizes, reduced the grades of evidence from 'low' to 'very low' (Table 5.9).

For oral CHM combined with chemotherapy, the evidence was also based mainly on unblinded studies. Combining CHM with chemotherapy appeared to increase ORR. The grade of evidence was 'moderate' (Table 5.70). Similar results were reported in previous meta-analyses.[9,10,15] While there appeared to be improvements in survival outcomes, longer-term data were few and it was unclear whether the reported differences reflected a bias towards positive results. Nevertheless, improved survival with CHM use has been reported in other systematic reviews[15,5,6] and in longitudinal studies.[28,29]

Although results were reported for a large number of chemotherapy-associated AEs, most data were available for nausea and vomiting (CINV), abnormal haematological parameters and peripheral neurotoxicity (CIPN). All of these showed a reduction in incidence of AEs in the integrative CHM groups, with 'low' to 'moderate' grades of evidence (Table 5.71, Table 5.72, Table 5.73). These results were broadly consistent with previous meta-analyses.[7–9,11–13]

Overall, the available evidence suggests that CHM has a role to play in the integrative management of CRC, but further well-controlled studies are needed to provide better estimates of effect sizes and identify which CHMs show the most promise.

Summary of Results of Randomised Controlled Trials for Main Clinical Outcomes

Overall, 133 RCTs, 11 CCTs, and 18 non-controlled studies contributed to the data analyses which were organised under the following four main sections:

1. CHM used during postoperative recovery;
2. CHM used in association with chemotherapies;

3. CHM used in association with radiotherapy or chemo-radiotherapy;
4. CHM used for supportive and/or palliative care.

In this summary we have focused on the main meta-analyses results for RCTs and on the larger pools (where available). For complete data see the corresponding sections.

Section 1: Chinese Herbal Medicine Used during Postoperative Recovery

This section included 19 RCTs of oral CHM, six RCTs of topical CHM, and one RCT of CHM inhalation.

Oral Chinese Herbal Medicine

Orally administered CHMs were tested in 19 RCTs. Only four mentioned syndrome differentiation (21%), with three of these syndromes relating to *qi* deficiency (*qi xu* 气虚). However, the high-frequency herbs tended to be those for tonifying *qi* (*bai zhu* 白术, *huang qi* 黄芪, *dang shen* 党参, etc.) so it is likely that in many of the studies that made no mention of syndromes, the formulas were focused on this aspect. Sequence generation was considered 'low' risk in 57.9% of studies. A total of 26.3% of studies used a procedure intended to blind participants but the effectiveness of this blinding was judged 'unclear'. Also, it was likely that personnel were aware of group allocation in all studies so they were judged 'high' risk.

Most studies tested measures of recovery of gastrointestinal function. Meta-analyses of oral CHM combined with usual postoperative care versus usual postoperative care found reductions in time to the following events:

- First bowel sounds (three RCTs): reduced by 6.09 hours;
- First flatus (six RCTs): reduced by 24.42 hours;
- First defaecation (five RCTs): reduced by 32.41 hours (Table 5.3).

These differences were all statistically significant, but the statistical heterogeneity was considerable.

The formulas *Si mo tang* 四磨汤 and modified *Liu jun zi tang* 六君子汤 were compared with usual care in two RCTs each. For time to first flatus and defaecation the first formula showed non-significant reductions (Table 5.10), whereas the second formula showed significant reductions (Table 5.11). However, there was substantial to considerable heterogeneity in all pools.

When oral CHM was combined with Fast Track Programme (FTP) versus FTP alone, the results were as follows:

- First bowel sounds (three RCTs): reduced by 3.09 hours;
- First flatus (five RCTs): reduced by 11.57 hours;
- First defaecation (three RCTs): reduced by 19.44 hours (Table 5.4).

In this group, there were significant reductions in time to first flatus and defaecation. The magnitudes of the reductions in time were less than when oral CHM was compared to usual postoperative care alone. Statistical heterogeneity was reduced for these outcomes but remained substantial.

For oral CHM combined with postoperative enteral nutrition (PET) versus postoperative enteral nutrition, data were only available for two of the above outcomes:

- First flatus (four RCTs): reduced by 10.13 hours;
- First defaecation (four RCTs): reduced by 9.42 hours (Table 5.5).

Both these reductions were statistically significant, but the heterogeneity was substantial to considerable.

These results suggest that the use of oral CHM, in conjunction with postoperative care, reduced time to recovery. The magnitudes of the reductions were less when patients were also receiving additional care such as FTP and PEN. The likely reason is these conventional therapies also improved recovery time, so the additional benefits of the CHMs were proportionally less. Although heterogeneity was substantial to considerable, all the studies showed a reduction in recovery time in the group that received CHM. The different magnitudes of the effects generated the heterogeneity.

Postoperative diarrhoea was assessed for two groups of two studies. For incidence of complete recovery:

- CHM plus usual care versus usual care (two RCTs): no significant difference;
- *Bu zhong yi qi wan/tang* 补中益气丸/汤 plus anti-diarrhoea medicines versus anti-diarrhoea medicines (two RCTs): No significant difference.

In both cases the CHMs appeared to have a beneficial effect, but this was too small to make a significant difference. It should be noted that usual care is likely to have involved anti-diarrhoea medicines which are effective in most cases.

Postoperative abdominal distension (two RCTs) was significantly reduced in CHM groups compared to usual care. There was no heterogeneity in the result, but the overall incidences were low.

Postoperative nausea and vomiting (three RCTs) showed a significant reduction in all grades without heterogeneity.

KPS, based on incidence of a 10-point or more increase in scores, showed a significant improvement in the oral CHM groups (four RCTs), compared to usual care, without heterogeneity (Table 5.6).

Postoperative immune function was assessed in five RCTs that combined CHM with FTP or enteral nutrition. For immunoglobulins:

- IgG, IgA and IgM levels significantly improved (one RCT of CHM plus FTP);
- IgA levels significantly improved, but IgG and IgM levels showed no difference (four RCTs of CHM plus PET) (Table 5.7).

Overall, the meta-analysis results for the RCTs indicated that the time to recovery of the three main measures of gastrointestinal function significantly improved in the groups that received oral CHM, and this effect was evident in the various subgroup analyses as well as in the two CCTs.

The GRADE assessments downgraded the certainty of the effect size estimates based on lack of blinding, statistical heterogeneity and small sample size. However, the heterogeneity mainly reflected the variability between studies in the magnitudes of the improvements, rather than disagreement between studies regarding whether the CHM groups improved or not relative to the controls that received usual care alone. Such heterogeneity was likely when the results of studies of different kinds of surgery and diverse patient groups were pooled. Regarding sample sizes, these were not large since we divided the studies into three main groups based on the type of usual care. Had all three groups been pooled together, the GRADE for time to first defaecation would have increased from 'very low' to 'low' due to the larger number of participants in the pool, but the GRADE for time to first bowel sounds would have remained 'very low'.

Topical Chinese Herbal Medicine

For topical CHM, six RCTs, and no CCTs or non-controlled studies provided data for postoperative recovery. Sequence generation was judged as 'low' risk in 33.3% of RCTs. One used a method for blinding participants, but it was not clear whether this was successful. All studies were judged 'high' risk for blinding of personnel.

Recovery of gastrointestinal function was assessed for topical CHM fomentation combined with usual postoperative care versus usual postoperative care alone for:

- First bowel sounds (three RCTs): reduced by 1.43 hours;
- First flatus (three RCTs): reduced by 6.33 hours;
- First defaecation (two RCTs): reduced by 4.74 hours (Table 5.16).

These differences were only statistically significant for time to first flatus, but heterogeneity was considerable.

For two RCTs of topical CHM cataplasm combined with usual postoperative care versus usual postoperative care alone, the meta-analysis results were as follows:

- First bowel sounds (two RCTs): reduced by 10.68 hours;
- First flatus (two RCTs): reduced by 11.19 hours;
- First defaecation (one RCT): reduced by 14.88 hours (Table 5.17).

All of these showed significant reductions, but heterogeneity was substantial for time to first flatus. Overall, the results of the RCTs suggested that topical CHM improved postoperative recovery, but the evidence was based on only a few unblinded studies.

Section 2: Chinese Herbal Medicine Used in Association with Chemotherapies

This section included 92 RCTs of oral CHM, two RCTs of CHM enema and five RCTs of topical CHM.

Oral Chinese Herbal Medicine

In 92 RCTs, orally administered CHMs were used in conjunction with chemotherapies. Two RCTs compared CHM with chemotherapy in advanced CRC, and three were of post-chemotherapy AEs. In addition, 88 RCTs combined oral CHM with chemotherapy. Of these, 38 RCTs used syndrome differentiation (43%). Most syndromes referred to *qi* deficiency (*qi xu* 气虚), mainly Spleen deficiency (*pi xu* 脾虚), followed by stasis (*yu* 瘀) and dampness (*shi* 湿). The most frequently used formulas were *Si jun zi tang* 四君子汤 and modified *Liu jun zi tang* 六君子汤. The more commonly used herbs tended to focus on *qi* deficiency (*bai zhu* 白术, *huang qi* 黄芪, *dang shen* 党参, etc.) but anti-cancer herbs (*yi yi ren* 薏苡仁, *she she cao* 蛇舌草, *ban zhi lian* 半枝莲, *e zhu* 莪术, etc.) were also frequently used. The RoB for sequence generation was judged 'low' in 40.2% of studies but only 1.1% were judged 'low' risk for blinding of participants, so the meta-analysis data are based mainly on open-label studies.

Only four RCTs were comparisons with chemotherapy. The only poolable result was for KPS, which showed an improvement in the oral CHM groups based on two studies. Another 88 RCTs compared oral CHM plus chemotherapy versus the same chemotherapy alone, so this summary focuses on these RCTs of integrative therapy.

Objective response rate (ORR) was significantly improved when assessed using the WHO criteria (25 RCTs) and the RECIST criteria (23 RCTs) without heterogeneity.

Survival rate and median survival time (MST) were not amenable to meta-analysis. In the integrative therapy groups, one-year survival was generally higher (six RCTs), MST was longer (three RCTs), median progression-free survival (mPFS) was longer (four RCTs), time to progression was longer (one RCT) and recurrence/metastasis rates were lower (three RCTs).

Quality of life data suitable for meta-analysis were available for ten RCTs. Significant improvements in the integrative groups were found for FACT-C (two RCTs), EORTC QLQ-C30 (two RCTs) and the Chinese QOL scale (six RCTs). KPS scores were significantly improved in the integrative groups (30 RCTs) and there was a greater incidence of improvements of 10 points or more on the KPS (37 RCTs).

Immune function (T cells and/or immunoglobulins) data suitable for meta-analysis were available in 28 RCTs. For T cells, there were significant increases in the integrative groups for CD3+ (18 RCTs), CD4+ (22 RCTs), CD4+/CD8+ (19 RCTS) and NK cells (17 RCTS), but no difference in CD8+ (19 RCTS). However, heterogeneity was considerable. For immunoglobulins, there were no differences in IgA (two RCTs), IgG (two RCTs) or IgE (one RCT), but there was a significant increase in IgM (two RCTs).

Chemotherapy-related AE data suitable for meta-analysis were reported by 71 RCTs. Of the 14 AEs reported, most data were for the following six AEs.

Results for all grades tended to favour the integrative medicine groups so the grade III + IV results are the focus in this summary:

- Nausea/vomiting showed significant reductions in the integrative groups based on WHO criteria (two RCTs) and NCI-CTCAE criteria (three RCTs);
- Diarrhoea was significantly reduced based on WHO criteria (19 RCTs), but not NCI-CTCAE criteria (four RCTs);
- Myelosuppression outcomes showed significant improvements for leukocytes (29 RCTs) and platelets (12 RCTs), but not for neutrophils (seven RCTs), red blood cells (seven RCTs) or haemoglobin (12 RCTs);

- Chemotherapy-induced peripheral neurotoxicity (CIPN) was significantly reduced based on WHO (13 RCTs) and Levi's criteria (four RCTs), but not NCI-CTCAE criteria (two RCTs);
- Hepatotoxicity was not different between groups for WHO criteria (three RCTs), nor was transaminases based on WHO criteria (three RCTs) or NCI-CTCAE criteria (two RCTs);
- Oral mucositis was not different between groups for WHO criteria (four RCTs) or NCI-CTCAE criteria (one RCT).

Overall, the clinical studies suggested that the integrative application of oral CHM improved outcomes for people receiving chemotherapy for CRC.

For the main outcomes the GRADE assessments were:

- Objective response rate: 'moderate' for both WHO and RECIST criteria;
- Chemotherapy-related nausea and vomiting: 'low' for WHO criteria (all grades);
- Chemotherapy-related abnormal haematological parameters: 'moderate' for all grades of leukopenia, neutropenia, haemoglobin and thrombocytopenia;
- Chemotherapy-induced peripheral neurotoxicity: 'moderate' for WHO criteria (all grades), 'low' for Levi's criteria (all grades) and 'low' for NCI-CTCAE criteria (all grades).

Each of the GRADE assessments was downgraded based on lack of blinding, with some being further downgraded based on statistical heterogeneity or small sample size.

Topical Chinese Herbal Medicine

Meta-analysis results were available for four RCTs of CHM hand and foot baths plus chemotherapy for CIPN. There were no differences between groups for level III + IV neurotoxicity (four RCTs), but for all levels there was a reduction in the integrative groups (four RCTs). While these studies of CHM hand and foot baths suggest these treatments alleviated the symptoms of CIPN, there were too few studies for any strong conclusions.

In the single study of a CHM cataplasm plus FOLFIRI versus a placebo cataplasm plus FOLFIRI (H133), the authors reported improvements in white blood cells and neutrophils with no change in platelets, but these data could not be analysed. Meta-analysis showed no change in KPS.

Section 3: Chinese Herbal Medicine Used in Association with Radiotherapy or Chemo-radiotherapy

For CHM combined with radiotherapy versus radiotherapy, two RCTs were of oral CHM and one was of CHM enema. None mentioned syndrome differentiation. Two were judged 'low' risk for sequence generation but none were blinded.

Post-radiotherapy immune function was reported in both RCTs of oral CHM. The pooled results showed significant increases in CD4+ and NK cells, but no differences in CD8+ cells or the ratio CD4+/CD8+.

The single enema study reported significantly reduced incidence of radiation proctitis (all grades) in the CHM enema group.

For CHM combined with chemo-radiotherapy, there were two RCTs of oral CHM but they reported different outcomes. One RCT reported improved tumour response rate, improved QOL, reductions in grade I to IV gastrointestinal reactions, myelosuppression and radiation proctitis in the oral CHM group, but no differences for grade III plus IV. The other RCT reported no significant difference between groups for KPS scores, but longer median times to recurrence or metastasis in the oral CHM group.

Overall, the available studies suggested some benefits for combining CHM with radiotherapy or chemo-radiotherapy, but there were too few studies for any strong conclusions.

Section 4: Chinese Herbal Medicine Used for Supportive and/or Palliative Care

Oral CHMs were tested in three RCTs, but there were no studies of topical CHM. One mentioned syndrome differentiation. Two were judged 'low' risk for sequence generation and none were blinded. In the two studies of CHM compared to best supportive care alone in advanced CRC, differences in criteria precluded pooling for most outcomes. The main results were as follows:

- For objective response rate, there were no responses in any of the groups (2 RCTs);
- For incidence of stable disease, there was a significant increase in one study after nine weeks, but no difference in the other study after eight weeks of treatment;
- For progressive disease there was no significant difference between groups in either study;
- Median survival was slightly longer in the CHM groups in both studies;
- For KPS, both studies showed improvements in the CHM groups, and the pooled result was significant;
- One of the studies reported no difference in the incidence of vomiting between groups, suggesting that the CHM was not causing this symptom.

In one study of CHM combined with thymosin $\alpha1$ injection (for improving immune function) there was:

- A significant reduction in regulatory T cells (%) in the combination group;
- A significant improvement in KPS scores.

References

1. Jiangsu New Medical Academy, ed. (1986) *Zhong Yao Da Ci Dian* 中药大辞典 [*Great Compendium of Chinese Medicines.*] Shanghai Scientific and Technical Publishers, Shanghai.
2. Chinese Pharmacopoeia Commission. (2015) *Zhong Hua Ren Min Gong He Guo Yao Dian* [*Pharmacopoeia of the People's Republic of China.*] China Medical Science Press, Beijing.
3. Bensky D, Clavey S, Stöger E. (2004) *Chinese Herbal Medicine: Materia Medica*, 3rd ed. Eastland Press, Seattle.

4. Zhong LLD, Chen HY, Cho WCS, *et al.* (2012) The efficacy of Chinese herbal medicine as an adjunctive therapy for colorectal cancer: A systematic review and meta-analysis. *Complement Ther Med* **20(4):** 240–252.

5. 黎春华, 符国长, 杨雨, 陈轶劼, 靖林林. (2012) 中西医结合治疗对中晚期结直肠癌生存期影响的荟萃分析. 数理医学杂志 **25(5):** 520–525.

6. 戚益铭, 吴霜霜, 沈敏鹤, *et al.* (2014) 扶正中药联合化疗对 III–IV 期结直肠癌患者生存期影响的 meta 分析. 中华中医药学刊 **32(12):** 2835–2838.

7. 王丽芬, 曹蕊芸, 李方平, 诸孟娟. (2014) 中草药联合化疗治疗晚期大肠癌疗效分析. 辽宁中医药大学学报 **16(12):** 130–133.

8. 张美霞, 徐细明, 余婷婷, 胡毅, 韩娜娜. (2015) 大肠癌术后患者行化疗联合中药治疗的 meta 分析. 中国医药导报 **12(23):** 92–96.

9. Chen M, May BH, Zhou IW, *et al.* (2014) FOLFOX 4 combined with herbal medicine for advanced colorectal cancer: A systematic review. *Phytother Res* **28(7):** 976–991.

10. Chen M, May BH, Zhou IW, *et al.* (2016) Meta-analysis of oxaliplatin-based chemotherapy combined with traditional medicines for colorectal cancer: Contributions of specific plants to tumor response. *Integr Cancer Ther* **15(1):** 40–59.

11. Chen MH, May BH, Zhou IW, *et al.* (2016) Integrative medicine for relief of nausea and vomiting in the treatment of colorectal cancer using oxaliplatin-based chemotherapy: A systematic review and meta-analysis. *Phytother Res* **30(5):** 741–753.

12. Chen M, May BH, Zhou IW, *et al.* (2016) Oxaliplatin-based chemotherapy combined with traditional medicines for neutropenia in colorectal cancer: A meta-analysis of the contributions of specific plants. *Crit Rev Oncol Hematol* **105:** 18–34.

13. 刘静, 朱琦. (2009) 健脾中药减少大肠癌患者化疗后不良反应的系统评价. 中国循证医学杂志 **9(7):** 802–808.

14. 刘静, 朱琦. (2009) 健脾中药联合化疗改善大肠癌患者免疫功能的系统评价. 中国中医药信息杂志 **16(12):** 104–106.

15. 陈琴, 杨向东, 巫加, 曹暂剑. (2015) 健脾方联合化疗治疗晚期大肠癌患者近期疗效及生存质量的 meta 分析. 中国肛肠病杂志 **35(5):** 7–9.

16. 李泓佳, 石齐, 李文, 刘珊珊, 宗绍其, 侯风刚. (2016) 健脾除湿,祛瘀解毒中药联合化疗对晚期大肠癌的疗效及安全性评估. 肿瘤研究与临床 **28(4):** 256–261.

17. 陈文婷, 任建琳, 侯风刚, 李琦. (2015) 健脾补肾复方联合化疗治疗大肠癌患者疗效指标的系统评价. 辽宁中医杂志 **42(7):** 1162–1166.

18. 李悠然, 谷云飞, 陈邑岐, 王浩. (2016) 四君子汤加减联合化疗对结直肠癌患者的 meta 分析. 中国实验方剂学杂志 **22(6):** 204–209.

19. Peng HR, ed. (1994) *Zhong Yi Fang Ji Da Ci Dian* 中医方剂大辞典 [*Great Compendium of Chinese Medical Formulae.*] People's Medical Publishing House, Beijing.

20. Levi F, Misset JL, Brienza S, *et al.* (1992) A chronopharmacologic phase-II clinical-trial with 5-fluorouracil, folinic acid, and oxaliplatin using an ambulatory multichannel programmable pump: High antitumor effectiveness against metastatic colorectal-cancer. *Cancer* **69(4):** 893–900.

21. Miller AB, Hoogstraten B, Staquet M, Winkler A. (1981) Reporting results of cancer treatment. *Cancer* **47(1):** 207–214.

22 Schwartz LH, Litiere S, de Vries E, *et al.* (2016) Recist 1.1-update and clarification: From the recist committee. *Eur J Cancer* **62:** 132–137.

23. Wong CK, Lam CL, Law WL, *et al.* (2012) Validity and reliability study on traditional Chinese FACT-C in Chinese patients with colorectal neoplasm. *J Eval Clin Pract* **18(6):** 1186–1195.

24. Ward WL, Hahn EA, Mo F, *et al.* (1999) Reliability and validity of the Functional assessment of cancer therapy-colorectal (FACT-C) quality of life instrument. *Qual Life Res* **8(3):** 181–195.

25. Aaronson NK, Ahmedzai S, Bergman B, *et al.* (1993) The European-Organization-for-Research-and-Treatment-of-Cancer QLQ-C30: A quality-of-life instrument for use in international clinical-trials in oncology. *J Natl Cancer Inst* **85(5):** 365–376.

26. 孙燕. (2001) 内科肿瘤学. 北京: 人民卫生出版社, pp. 996–997.

27. Piper BF, Dibble SL, Dodd MJ, *et al.* (1998) The revised Piper Fatigue Scale: Psychometric evaluation in women with breast cancer. *Oncol Nurs Forum* **25(4):** 677–684.

28. McCulloch M, Broffman M, van der Laan M, *et al.* (2011) Colon cancer survival with herbal medicine and vitamins combined with standard therapy in a whole-systems approach: Ten-year follow-up data analyzed with marginal structural models and propensity score methods. *Integr Cancer Ther* **10(3):** 240–259.

29. Xu Y, Mao JJ, Sun L, *et al.* (2017) Association between use of traditional Chinese medicine herbal therapy and survival outcomes in patients with stage II and III colorectal cancer: A multicenter prospective cohort study. *J Natl Cancer Inst Monogr* **2017(52):** 19–25.

List of Clinical Studies Included in Chapter 5

Study Number	References
H1	杨满菊. (2012) 益气健脾方治疗结肠癌外科术后的临床疗效观察. 中国实验方剂学杂志 **18(13):** 262–265.
H2	于边芳, 李师, 姚力. (2012) 四磨汤对腹腔镜直肠癌术后胃肠道反应疗效观察. 辽宁中医药大学学报 **14(7):** 234–235.
H3	张喆, 刘瑜, 张挽澜, 王微, 王文跃, 符思. (2013) 加味三香颗粒治疗结肠癌术后胃肠功能障碍 32 例. 中医杂志 **54(11):** 966–967.
H4	郑子洲, 徐巍. (2013) 益气健脾方治疗结肠癌外科术后 66 例. 陕西中医 **34(10):** 1322–1323.
H5	张双燕, 杜业勤. (2011) 温针灸对肠癌术后患者胃肠功能及免疫功能的影响. 中国针灸 **31(6):** 513–517.
H6	邱剑锋, 李国栋, 舒涛, 寇玉明. (2009) 加味大承气汤对直肠癌术后胃肠功能恢复的影响. 中国中医药信息杂志 **16(6):** 78.
H7	侯庆, 马原驰, 姚德蛟. (2015) 益气固摄升提方治疗直肠癌术后腹泻25例疗效观察. 国医论坛 **30(4):** 32–33.
H8	刘晓. (2011) 益气健脾渗湿法治疗大肠癌术后腹泻的临床研究. 学位论文. 山东中医药大学, pp. 1–10.
H9	张艳玲, 刘丽, 叶桦. (2014) 补中益气汤联合西药治疗直肠癌术后腹泻随机平行对照研究. 实用中医内科杂志 **28(1):** 121–122.
H10	何国伟. (2014) 太根饮在胃肠外科快速康复方案中的应用价值. 中国实用医刊 **41(8):** 24–25.
H11	田昭春. (2011) 通里扶正法促进结直肠癌术后快速康复的临床研究. 学位论文. 山东中医药大学, pp. 1–9.
H12	邹瞭南, 刁德昌, 万进. (2013) 中医健脾通腑法联合快速康复外科在腹腔镜结直肠癌围手术期中的应用. 广东医学 **34(14):** 2256–2258.
H13	杨双. (2015) 加味枳术汤促进腹腔镜下结直肠癌术后快速康复的研究. 学位论文. 广州中医药大学, pp. 13–25.
H14	周康. (2011) 结直肠癌快速康复外科中加味厚朴三物汤促胃肠功能恢复的临床观察. 学位论文. 南京中医药大学, pp. 10–21.
H15	陈念. (2013) 早期肠内营养配合柴芍六君子汤对大肠癌术后恢复影响的临床研究. 学位论文. 湖南中医药大学, pp. 1–21.
H16	彭章艳. (2015) 济川养生驻颜不老药酒联合肠内营养液促进直肠癌术后康复的随机、对照临床研究. 学位论文. 成都中医药大学, pp. 4–19.

(Continued)

(*Continued*)

Study Number	References
H17	肖兵, 孙月梅, 郭宏珺. (2015) 肠内营养联合香砂六君子汤对结肠癌患者术后营养状态及免疫功能的影响. 河南中医 **35(12):** 3030–3032.
H18	陆军, 童宗培, 潘龙, 颜成杰. (2016) 益气通里中药煎剂对结、直肠癌术后早期免疫功能及胃肠功能的影响. 现代中西医结合杂志 **25(3):** 297–298, 303.
H19	尹涛, 黄岩. (2015) 补中益气丸联合盐酸洛哌丁胺胶囊治疗大肠癌术后腹泻疗效观察. 中国继续医学教育 **7(23):** 171–172.
H20	郑军营. (2011) 以吴茱萸热熨为主的中医外治法对结直肠癌术后胃肠功能恢复的影响. 学位论文. 广州中医药大学 pp. 12–20.
H21	杨东亮, 赵翠苗. (2016) 枳术散热敷腹部治疗结肠癌术后胃肠功能紊乱临床观察. 中医临床研究 **8(5):** 73–74.
H22	郑燕生, 罗立杰, 王伟, 万进, 陈志强. (2013) 吴茱萸热敷在腹腔镜结直肠癌外科快速康复中的应用. 广东医学 **34(9):** 1442–1444.
H23	陈玲, 田永明, 印义琼, 文曰. (2012) 超声电导透皮给药对结肠癌患者术后肠功能恢复的影响研究. 华西医学 **27(12):** 1893–1894.
H24	杨茜湄. (2015) 四黄水蜜方联合芒硝冰片散对结肠癌患者术后胃肠功能恢复的影响. 中医临床研究 **7(16):** 101–103.
H25	张莉莉, 李云飞, 卢丹, 曹波. (2014) 神阙穴经吴茱萸贴敷促进直肠癌术后胃肠功能恢复的临床观察. 新教育时代电子杂志（教师版）**12:** 297.
H26	严伟华, 严孟瑜, 黄进林, 伍志辉. (2013) 雾化吸人加味枳术煎对乙直肠癌术后肠道功能的影响. 广州中医药大学学报 **30(3):** 323–325.
H27	王少言, 初巍巍. (2015) 肠内营养联合四君子汤对结肠癌患者术后营养状态及免疫功能的影响. 解放军医药杂志 **27(5):** 49–52.
H28	Suehiro T, Matsumata T, Shikada Y, Sugimachi K. (2005) The effect of the herbal medicines dai-kenchu-to and keishi-bukuryo-gan on bowel movement after colorectal surgery. *Hepatogastroenterology* **52(61):** 97–100.
H29	Yoshikawa K, Shimada M, Nishioka M, *et al.* (2012) The effects of the Kampo medicine (Japanese herbal medicine) 'Daikenchuto' on the surgical inflammatory response following laparoscopic colorectal resection. *Surg Today* **42(7):** 646–651.

(Continued)

(Continued)

Study Number	References
H30	陈武进, 夏传宝, 欧阳观峰, 任丽萍, 陈江田, 余养生. (2013) 益气解毒方合微波消融治疗结直肠癌肝转移 42 例临床观察. 福建中医药大学学报 **23(5):** 5–7.
H31	李敏贤, 周醒华, 杨关根, 沈忠, 金夏兰. (2003) 葱白醋炒外敷合加味大承气汤内服治疗大肠癌术后早期炎性肠梗阻 56 例观察. 浙江中医杂志, pp. 10–11.
H32	王文海, 周荣耀, 邹菁. (2000) 肠益煎治疗大肠癌术后 50 例临床观察. 浙江中西医结合杂志 **10(6):** 325–326.
H33	张倩. (2015) 补中益气汤在治疗直肠癌 Dixon 术后早期腹泻相关症状中的应用. 学位论文. 山东中医药大学, pp. 2–14.
H34	Schnell, N. (2012) Case study: Herbal treatment of recurrent colon polyps in a colon cancer patient. *Journal of the American Herbalists Guild* **11(1):** 31–39.
H35	焦士洁, 范春琦, 安广宇, 权红, 严冬. (2016) 滋补汤联合卡培他滨维持治疗一线化疗后气血两虚证晚期结直肠癌的研究. 现代中西医结合杂志 **25(12):** 1258–1260, 1317.
H36	李辰慧, 赵文硕, 冯利, 胡凤山, 杨国旺, 唐武军, 等. (2014) 中医辨证维持治疗晚期结直肠癌的临床研究. 北京中医药 **33(2):** 93–96.
H37	李静. (2010) 中西医结合治疗大肠癌化疗相关性腹泻的临床研究. 学位论文. 成都中医药大学, pp. 6–22.
H38	唐建清, 邓天好. (2015) 痛泄 I 号方干预大肠癌 mFOLFOX6 方案化疗后腹泻 66 例临床观察. 湖南中医杂志 **31(8):** 47–49.
H39	徐晓卿, 齐元富. (2014) 益气和血法治疗大肠癌患者化疗所致神经毒性疗效分析. 世界中西医结合杂志 **9(10):** 1087–1089.
H40	杨为伟. (2014) 晚期结直肠癌维持期中药治疗疗效观察. 学位论文. 北京中医药大学, pp. 27–34.
H41	张华堂, 方灿途, 黄振炎, 刘立文. (2008) 中医辨证配合化疗治疗晚期大肠癌 31 例近期疗效观察. 新中医 **40(7):** 22–23.
H42	沈建明, 胡学文, 杜伟. (2012) 香砂六君丸联合奥沙利铂和卡培他滨方案对大肠癌患者不良反应和生活质量的影响. 中成药 **34(12):** 2302–2304.
H43	徐川, 于小伟, 李敏. (2012) 加味香砂六君子汤联合 FOLFIRI 方案治疗晚期结肠癌. 中国临床医学 **19(1):** 36–37.

(Continued)

(*Continued*)

Study Number	References
H44	蒋志明, 胡黎清, 蒋思思. (2014) 加味四君子汤联合 FOLFOX6 方案治疗晚期结直肠癌临床观察. 浙江临床医学 **16(8)**: 1296–1298.
H45	肖卫云. (2013) 益气健脾法联合 XELOX 方案治疗晚期大肠癌的临床观察. 实用癌症杂志 **28(3)**: 305–306.
H46	魏海梁, 闫曙光, 李京涛. (2015) 八珍汤联合 FOLFOX4 方案治疗结肠癌术后患者 30 例. 陕西中医 **36(10)**: 1347–1348.
H47	高小明. (2015) 八珍汤加减对结肠癌术后气血两虚型患者辅助化疗减毒作用的临床研究. 学位论文. 福建中医药大学, pp. 3–11.
H48	王辉, 邓晓明. (2014) 中西医结合治疗晚期结肠癌 78 例临床观察. 河南医学研究 **23(3)**: 123–124.
H49	曾琛, 邓晓明, 杜纪英, 崔伟锋. (2013) 中西医结合治疗中晚期结肠癌 61 例. 中国实验方剂学杂志 **19(8)**: 335–337.
H50	林燕, 陆明. (2011) 复方斑蝥胶囊联合 CPT-11+CF+5Fu 治疗晚期大肠癌的临床观察. 西部医学 **23(9)**: 1650–1652, 1655.
H51	赵文英, 程宜福. (2010) 复方斑蝥胶囊联合化学治疗对转移性结直肠癌的疗效观察. 中华消化杂志 **30(7)**: 452–455.
H52	王志鹏. (2010)芪连扶正胶囊联合化疗治疗大肠癌的临床研究. 学位论文. 山东中医药大学, pp. 2–8.
H53	于慧敏. (2011) 芪连扶正胶囊联合 OLF 方案治疗晚期大肠癌的临床研究. 学位论文. 山东中医药大学, pp. 2–9.
H54	浦琼华. (2012) 微调三号方对大肠癌肝转移 VEGF, nm23-H1 和 CK20 的影响的实验研究及其联合 FOLFOX4 方案的临床研究. 学位论文. 南京中医药大学, 31–41.
H55	薛青, 尤建良, 王旺胜, 龚时夏. (2015) 中药微调3号方治疗大肠癌肝转移的临床分析. 内蒙古中医药 **34(12)**: 1–2.
H56	谢威. (2010) 消瘤汤对结直肠癌VEGF抑制作用的临床研究. 学位论文. 广西中医学院, 6–14.
H57	曾家耀, 赫军, 王清坚, 傅汉琨, 谢威. (2010) 消瘤汤联合热灌注化疗对进展期结直肠癌术后免疫功能和血清血管内皮生长因子水平的影响. 广西医科大学学报 **27(3)**: 415–416.
H58	刘姝晨. (2011) 益气养阴中药配合 FOLFOX6 方案化疗治疗中晚期大肠癌的临床观察. 学位论文. 北京中医药大学, 26–35.

(*Continued*)

(Continued)

Study Number	References
H59	张娟. (2015) 清热化湿解毒汤联合 XELOX 方案治疗湿热蕴毒型晚期结直肠癌的临床疗效观察. 学位论文. 黑龙江中医药大学, pp. 15–25.
H60	侯中博. (2014) 半夏泻心汤加减对结直肠癌术后的临床疗效及相关血清肿瘤标志物的影响. 学位论文. 贵阳中医学院, pp. 7–21.
H61	肖春霞. (2011) 芫菁膏对脾虚湿盛型大肠癌 FOLFOX4 化疗减毒作用的临床观察. 学位论文. 新疆医科大学, pp. 6–15.
H62	王桦. (2008) 益气活血补肠汤合化疗治疗直肠癌术后患者的疗效观察. 辽宁中医药大学学报 **10(5):** 81–82.
H63	王全玉, 何炜, 蔺强, 李莉蕊. (2015) 中药联合化疗治疗晚期结肠癌的临床疗效观察. 现代消化及介入诊疗 **20(4):** 387–389.
H64	周鏊, 张建平, 苏立, 孙贵银, 黄大春, 付敏, 等. (2007) 十济汤联合化疗治疗结直肠癌临床研究. 中国中医急症 **16(9):** 1068–1069, 1106.
H65	胡凤山, 张青, 王笑民, 杨国旺, 赵文硕. (2007) 固本消瘤胶囊联合 FOLFOX4 方案治疗晚期大肠癌的临床研究. 中国中医药信息杂志 **14(7):** 13–14.
H66	赖景春, 彭卫卫, 邓江华, 汪琛. (2012) "健脾益气, 解毒祛瘀法" 联合 FOLFOX4 方案治疗晚期大肠癌的临床研究. 辽宁中医杂志 **39(5):** 849–851.
H67	李毅俊, 陈劲智, 黄伟贤, 李晓峰. (2007) 温肾健脾方联合化疗治疗老年进展期大肠癌的临床观察. 福建中医药 **38(4):** 13–14.
H68	吴文通, 方军, 平进. (2015) 自拟中药方联合化疗治疗晚期大肠癌的临床观察. 中国中医药科技 **22(3):** 293–294.
H69	曾纪权, 黎治平, 王晓. (2008) 中医辨证施治配合化疗治疗晚期大肠癌 30 例. 江西中医学院学报 **20(6):** 39–41.
H70	张青, 王笑民, 杨国旺, 胡凤山, 赵文硕, 唐武军, 等. (2010) 固本消瘤胶囊联合 FOLFOX4 化疗方案治疗晚期大肠癌的临床研究. 北京中医药 **29(4):** 255–257.
H71	方志红, 李雁, 陈晏, 陈东林. (2009) 健脾抗癌方配合化疗治疗晚期大肠癌 31 例. 上海中医药杂志 **43(3):** 29–31.
H72	戴玲玲. (2013) 健脾祛浊消积方联合 FOLFIRI 方案治疗晚期大肠癌临床研究. 山东中医杂志 **32(7):** 476–478.
H73	丁志佳. (2011) 健脾益气解毒散结方联合 XELOX 方案治疗晚期大肠癌的临床研究. 学位论文. 南京中医药大学, pp. 11–20.

(Continued)

(*Continued*)

Study Number	References
H74	盖领, 施兵, 张秀兵. (2010) 参一胶囊联合 XELOX 方案与单纯 XELOX 方案治疗晚期直肠癌的临床观察. 现代中西医结合杂志 **19(9):** 1066–1067.
H75	束家和, 周荣耀, 钟薏, 吴丽英. (2011)益气解毒汤联合 CapeOX 方案治疗晚期大肠癌 45 例. 上海中医药杂志 **45(5):** 33–35, 45.
H76	许炜茹, 张青, 富琦, 徐咏梅, 于洁, 杨国旺, 等. (2015) 升血汤对转移性结直肠癌化疗患者骨髓抑制及免疫功能的影响. 中华中医药杂志 **30(6):** 2230–2232.
H77	殷晓聆, 赵凡尘, 蔡淦, 李雁. (2011) 健脾中药配合化疗治疗晚期大肠癌临床观察. 上海中医药杂志 **45(7):** 43–44.
H78	陈小娟. (2010) 健脾化湿祛瘀方联合化疗治疗晚期大肠癌的临床研究. 学位论文. 南京中医药大学, pp. 14–20.
H79	李黎. (2007) 健脾化湿祛瘀方联合Caplri方案化疗治疗晚期大肠癌的临床研究. 学位论文. 南京中医药大学, pp. 11–20.
H80	贺佳蓓, 屈景辉. (2013) 固本解毒法联合 FOLFOX4 方案化疗治疗晚期或复发性直肠癌的临床. 四川中医 **31(12):** 76–78.
H81	黄丽. (2015) 清热燥湿法联合化疗治疗晚期湿热型结肠癌的临床观察. 学位论文. 成都中医药大学, pp. 9–22.
H82	欧阳郴生, 杨振江, 古宏晖, 杨丽娜, 陈钟, 汪桃利. (2012) 髓清丸联合 FOLFOX 方案治疗晚期结肠癌50例疗效观察. 中国肿瘤临床与康复 **19(5):** 460–462.
H83	黄伶, 郭俊华. (2014) 益气化痰散结方联合 XELOX 化疗方案治疗晚期复发性结肠癌的临床研究. 中华中医药学刊 **32(3):** 670–672.
H84	孙波, 王志敏, 沈静, 余资笔, 郑坚. (2015) 健脾益气法联合化疗治疗晚期大肠癌临床观察. 辽宁中医杂志 **42(3):** 518–521.
H85	王建中, 柯友辉, 刘鹏程, 吴春迎, 陈浩波. (2011) 宜肠宁方联合 FOLFOX-4 方案治疗晚期结直肠癌30例临床研究. 福建中医药 **42(5):** 23–24.
H86	廖振华, 左文娟, 刘丽. (2015) 平瘤康胶囊联合 FOLFOX6 治疗晚期结直肠癌33例临床观察. 湖南中医杂志 **31(1):** 51–52.
H87	朱方勇, 王斌, 艾岩, 周晓, 邱文斌, 周焱冰, 等.(2016) 健脾益气解毒方联合化疗治疗晚期大肠癌临床研究. 现代中西医结合杂志 **25(3):** 261–263.

(*Continued*)

(Continued)

Study Number	References
H88	王容容, 王其美, 蒋益兰, 阳鹏. (2016) 健脾消癌方联合化疗治疗晚期转移性结直肠癌的临床研究. 中华中医药杂志 **31(5)**: 1732–1736.
H89	支晟. (2010) 肠癌转移Ⅰ号方联合 FOLFIRI 方案治疗晚期结直肠癌的临床疗效观察. 学位论文. 南京中医药大学, pp. 13–22.
H90	胡兵, 李刚, 安红梅, 杜琴, 沈克平, 许玲, 等. (2015) 藤龙补中汤联合化疗治疗晚期大肠癌临床研究. 中华中医药学刊 **33(1)**: 37–39.
H91	柯诗文, 黄国栋, 赵俊. (2015) 抗癌抑瘤方联合 CapeOx 方案治疗晚期结直肠癌. 中成药 **37(1)**: 49–54.
H92	李京. (2011) 扶正化瘀解毒散结配合化疗治疗晚期大肠癌的临床观察及机理研究. 学位论文. 南京中医药大学, pp. 12–24.
H93	王舒雯. (2012) 通泰合剂联合 XELOX 方案化疗治疗晚期大肠癌疗效临床观察. 学位论文. 南京中医药大学, pp. 14–23.
H94	胡清清. (2013) 中药三步周期疗法联合改良 XELOX 方案治疗Ⅳ期大肠癌的临床研究. 学位论文. 南京中医药大学, pp. 15–28.
H95	张微微, 陈洁, 谢国群, 贺天临, 郭晓冬, 张学民, 等. (2013) 健脾解毒方结合卡培他滨片治疗晚期大肠癌临床研究. 上海中医药大学学报 **27(4)**: 31–34.
H96	陈歆妮. (2011) 克瘤丸治疗晚期大肠癌的临床观察及其对血清 VEGF 的影响. 学位论文. 南京中医药大学, pp. 15–24.
H97	唐智军, 谭世平, 李实忠. (2007) 莲花解毒抗癌汤抗大肠癌复发转移的临床研究. 中国医药论坛 **5(5)**: 33.
H98	曾柏荣, 刘华, 何欣. (2008) 抗癌防移片预防Ⅲ期结肠癌术后复发转移的临床观察. 中华中医药杂志 **23(7)**: 654–655.
H99	茅伟达, 蒋立新, 周锦仪, 蒋红妹. (2011) 中药加化疗对大肠癌术后复发转移的影响研究. 中外健康文摘 **8(39)**: 70–72.
H100	陈娟. (2009) 健脾益气养血方联合 FOLFOX4 方案对大肠癌术后患者免疫功能影响的临床研究. 学位论文. 南京中医药大学, pp. 19–33.
H101	钟妙文, 叶慧青, 黎群足, 唐荣德, 曾黎明. (2016) 芪附龙葵汤联合化疗对转移性结直肠癌患者生存质量的影响. 现代中西医结合杂志 **25(18)**: 1980–1982.
H102	崔虎军. (2011) 健脾祛瘀方联合卡培他滨、伊立替康治疗晚期大肠癌 20 例. 实用中医内科杂志 **25(8)**: 48–50.

(Continued)

(*Continued*)

Study Number	References
H103	秦春艳. (2014) 健脾益肾治法防治中晚期结直肠癌化疗毒副反应的临床观察. 学位论文. 北京中医药大学, pp. 25–35.
H104	李灵常. (2009) 复方肠泰治疗大肠癌的临床和实验研究. 学位论文. 南京中医药大学, pp. 7–12.
H105	杨海淦. (2015) 健脾渗湿抑瘤法联合XELOX化疗治疗结肠癌根治术后疗效研究. 学位论文. 广州中医药大学, pp. 7–18.
H106	白凤桐. (2011) 直肠癌1号方联合 FOLFOX-4 治疗直肠癌术后患者 21 例. 中国中西医结合外科杂志 **17(1):** 80–81.
H107	何正飞. (2006) 益气健脾、化瘀解毒方合 FOLFOX 方案化疗治疗术后大肠癌的临床研究. 学位论文. 南京中医药大学, pp. 8–17.
H108	李志明. (2015) 健脾益肾法对行 FOLFOX6 化疗的晚期大肠癌患者癌因性疲乏和证候积分及生存状态的影响. 中国全科医学 **18(36):** 4492–4495.
H109	邓德厚, 沈小珩. (2010) 益气消积方配合化疗治疗晚期大肠癌 18 例临床观察. 福建中医药 **41(3):** 13–14.
H110	包益洁, 邱艳艳, 胡送娇, 石晓静, 于卉, 邹瑜, 等. (2014) 健脾补肾方对大肠癌术后辅助治疗的疗效. 上海医学 **37(11):** 984–986.
H111	曹波. (2011) 益气健脾汤联合 FOLFOX4 方案治疗结直肠癌术后患者的临床疗效. 肿瘤防治研究 **38(7):** 820–822.
H112	陈诚刚. (2005) 健脾益肾、化瘀解毒法联合 FOLFOX-4 方案治疗中、晚期大肠癌的临床研究. 学位论文. 南京中医药大学, pp. 20–31.
H113	海艳洁, 卢林, 丁艳波. (2010) 健脾渗湿汤对晚期大肠癌患者肠道微生态的影响. 中国药师 **13(11):** 1545–1547.
H114	李诺. (2012) 健脾益肾法治疗术后大肠癌的临床研究. 学位论文. 南京中医药大学, pp. 10–18.
H115	胡兵, 李刚, 安红梅, 杜琴, 沈克平, 许玲, 等. (2014) 藤龙补中汤对晚期大肠癌患者Th1型免疫反应作用. 中国中西医结合消化杂志 **22(8):** 434–435, 439.
H116	任秋生, 乔天渊, 贺天临, 张微微. (2014) 自拟扶本固元汤对患者行直肠癌根治术后化学治疗的胃肠道反应和免疫力的影响. 上海医学 **37(5):** 423–425.
H117	刘平, 刘剑辉, 朱道奇, 马进安, 胡春宏. (2007) 博尔宁胶囊联合 FOLFOX4 方案治疗结肠癌的临床观察. 中国肿瘤临床 **34(2):** 89–91.

(*Continued*)

(Continued)

Study Number	References
H118	彭南勇. (2007) 固本抑瘤法对大肠癌化疗减毒增效作用的临床研究. 学位论文. 云南中医学院, pp. 6–16.
H119	张超, 韩振国. (2015) 化疗联合中药治疗在结直肠癌术后的临床效果观察. 中国当代医药 **22(14):** 135–138, 141.
H120	任延毅, 徐阳, 刘兆酷, 郑振东, 谢晓冬. (2013) 黄芩汤预防含伊立替康方案化疗后腹泻的临床研究. 辽宁中医杂志 **40(11):** 2264–2266.
H121	张康梅. (2012) 参苓白术散合归脾汤加减对结直肠癌术后辅助化疗相关毒副反应的影响. 健康必读杂志 **10:** 345–346.
H122	张继峰, 周学鲁, 胡灏. (2013) 六味地黄丸防治化疗后血小板减少的临床观察. 中医临床研究 **5(4):** 17–18.
H123	赖义勤, 陈乃杰, 吴丹红, 陈云莺. (2009) 健脾益肾法预防奥沙利铂周围神经毒性 27 例. 福建中医药 **40(5):** 22–23.
H124	梁学书, 颜玲玲, 林琪. (2015) 理血祛风汤防治大肠癌术后奥沙利铂所致外周神经毒性反应74例. 浙江中医杂志 **50(7):** 522–523.
H125	梁学书, 陈明聪, 陈德连, 林琪. (2012) 益气理血愈风汤防治奥沙利铂所致外周神经毒性反应46例. 中国中医药科技 **19(1):** 94.
H126	刘青. (2015) 中药干预直肠癌化疗后疲乏 26 例. 江西中医药 **5:** 37–38.
H127	胡志强, 韩轶超, 彭晔, 张旭刚, 姜瑞博, 李炳茂. (2015) 大黄人参方联合 FOLFOX4 方案治疗晚期结肠癌疗效观察. 现代中西医结合杂志 **24(33):** 3649–3651, 3654.
H128	刘平贤. (2014) 结直肠癌术后中医药联合化疗临床疗效分析. 学位论文. 新乡医学院, pp. 6–16.
H129	高军, 闫绍辉, 李大鹏, 徐强松, 温博. (2015) 中药泡洗预防奥沙利铂所致神经毒性的疗效观察. 河北中医 **37(7):** 994–996.
H130	杨春娣. (2015) 中药熏洗治疗奥沙利铂所致周围神经毒性的临床观察. 中国临床护理 **7(3):** 234–235.
H131	王强. (2015) 黄芪桂枝五物汤手足浴联合钙镁合剂防治奥沙利铂神经毒性的临床观察. 现代中西医结合杂志 **24(3):** 318–320.
H132	冯娅清. (2011) 中药外洗防治奥沙利铂神经毒性的护理观察. 海峡药学 **23(12):** 203–204.
H133	王珏, 魏澹宁, 张卫平, 冉冉, 徐凯, 高聚伟, 等. (2014) 龟鹿二仙胶巴布剂辅助治疗大肠癌患者化疗后骨髓抑制的临床观察. 中国中西医结合杂志 **34(8):** 947–951.

(Continued)

(*Continued*)

Study Number	References
H134	符常军. (2011) 扶正固本方加减联合 FOLFOX4 方案治疗中晚期大肠癌的临床研究. 学位论文. 南京中医药大, pp. 11–19.
H135	龚时夏. (2008) 中药微调三号方治疗中晚期大肠癌的临床及实验研究. 学位论文. 南京中医药大学 pp. 16–27.
H136	胡虞睿. (2015) 健脾益气方联合 FOLFOX 方案治疗大肠癌术后患者的临床研究. 学位论文. 南京中医药大学, pp. 8–14.
H137	黄丹云. (2014) 五苓散加减防治结（直）肠癌 FOLFIRI 方案化疗相关性腹泻的临床研究. 学位论文. 广州中医药大学, pp. 8–18.
H138	姚成, 任函承. (2014) 中西医结合治疗晚期大肠癌 21 例疗效观察. 新中医**46(12)**: 161–163.
H139	候东东. (2014) 益气健脾中医疗法联合化疗对于中晚期大肠癌患者的效果分析. 中医临床研究 **6(33)**: 147–148.
H140	王彩虹. (2010) 四君子汤加减对脾气虚型肠癌术后患者生命质量改善的临床研究. 学位论文. 辽宁中医药大学, pp. 11–16.
H141	陈大富, 庄永敬, 黄建强. (2013) 人参皂甙 Rg3 联合 FOLFOX4 方案治疗直肠癌的疗效观察. 临床肿瘤学杂志 **18(2)**: 163–165.
H142	李柳宁, 刘丽荣, 潘宗奇, 刘译红, 邓华, 白建平, 等. (2009) 健脾补肾祛瘀解毒法联合化疗治疗晚期结直肠癌的疗效观察. 辽宁中医杂志 **36(5)**: 772–774.
H143	黄东彬, 管静. (2012) 龙葵合剂联合化疗对 47 例中晚期大肠癌患者生活质量和免疫功能的影响. 亚太传统医药 **8(10)**: 37–38.
H144	赖小平. (2008) 中西医结合治疗希罗达导致严重腹泻1例. 中国中西医结合杂志 **28(2)**: 164.
H145	陈金鸣, 魏霞, 姚伟荣. (2015) 五红汤减轻直肠癌术后放疗反应提高患者免疫功能. 江西医药 **50(7)**: 664–666, 672.
H146	马海锋. (2014) 华蟾素胶囊对直肠癌放疗后气阴两虚证患者的疗效及对免疫功能的影响. 中国中西医结合消化杂志**22(4)**: 185–188.
H147	严布谷, 姜照林. (2014) 康复新液保留灌肠预防放射性直肠炎的效果观察. 中国临床护理 **6(2)**: 153–154.
H148	蔡卫东, 陶德友, 张艳, 王微. (2015) 中医自拟方联合同步放化疗治疗晚期直肠癌临床疗效. 辽宁中医杂志 **42(1)**: 102–104.
H149	刘浩, 关念波, 王辉. (2013) 西黄解毒胶囊控制大肠癌术后复发转移临床研究. 中华中医药学刊 **31(1)**: 72–73.

(*Continued*)

(*Continued*)

Study Number	References
H150	石惠燕, 田义洲, 黄立萍, 张凌燕, 余达, 邵莉莉, 等. (2016) 健脾安肠方治疗晚期结直肠癌疗效观察. 浙江中医杂志 **51(2)**: 122–123.
H151	顾贤, 何宝仪, 沈克平, 朱凌宇. (2011) 胃肠安对大肠癌术后化疗后患者调节性T细胞及生存质量的影响. 上海中医药杂志 **45(11)**: 54–56.
H152	张毅, 胡兴寿. (2010) 自拟益气扶正方治疗晚期结直肠癌研究. 现代中西医结合杂志**19(27)**: 3424–3426.
H153	陈培丰. (1995) 单纯中医药治疗晚期直肠癌18例. 陕西中医 **16(1)**: 12.
H154	冯晓飞. (2007) 胡志敏教授中药治疗晚期大肠癌24例经验总结. 实用中医内科杂志**21(7)**: 19–20.
H155	郭小培, 曹一敏. (2004) 化岩汤灌肠对晚期直肠癌患者T淋巴细胞免疫活性的影响. 中国肛肠病杂志 **24(12)**: 19–20.
H156	刘嘉湘. (1981) 中医中药治疗大肠癌50例疗效观察. 中医杂志 **(12)**: 33–36.
H157	吴雪梅, 姚德蛟. (2001) 肠复康胶囊治疗原发性中晚期大肠癌近期临床疗效观察. 成都中医药大学学报 **24(2)**: 12, 19.
H158	周留勇, 单珍珠, 尤建良. (2008) 赵氏微调三号治疗晚期大肠癌患者44例. 陕西中医 **29(9)**: 1151–1152.
H159	Chen X, Hu ZP, Yang XX, *et al.* (2006) Monitoring of immune responses to a herbal immuno-modulator in patients with advanced colorectal cancer. *Int Immunopharmacol* **6(3)**: 499–508.
H160	蔡舜金. (2012) 固肠止泻丸治疗老年结肠癌1例报告. 中国社区医师·医学专业 **14(7)**: 293.
H161	丁明星, 许咏, 唐兴广. (2010) 大肠癌的中医辨证与治疗. 中国煤炭工业医学杂志 **13(4)**: 605.
H162	卢晓峰, 黄海燕, 张谈. (2015) 升清降浊法治疗大肠癌临证应用初探. 浙江中医杂志 **50(3)**: 219.

6

Pharmacological Actions of the Common Herbs

OVERVIEW

This section reviews the available experimental evidence for the ten Chinese herbs most frequently used in the formulas tested in the randomised clinical trials included in Chapter 5 that showed evidence of tumour response in order to identify their biological activities relevant to colorectal cancer.

Introduction

Chinese herbal formulas exert their actions via the multiple constituent compounds contained in the herbs that are ingested. While clinical trials assess the efficacy and safety of formulas and herbs, investigation of the mechanisms of action of the herbs and their constituent compounds mainly depends on experimental studies using *in vitro* and/or *in vivo* models that are relevant to the physiological processes involved in the development of colorectal cancer (CRC), its prevention and its management.

In Chapter 5, the meta-analyses results of randomised controlled trials (RCTs) found that the addition of Chinese herbal medicine (CHM) to conventional chemotherapy for CRC resulted in increases in the objective response rate (ORR), suggesting that CHM assisted in reducing tumour growth. In order to identify the actions and potential mechanisms of action of the herbs included in these clinical studies, this chapter reviews evidence from animal models, cell lines and other experimental studies of the herbs most frequently included in the CHM interventions in the RCTs. The ten most commonly used herbs (see table 5.76) were *bai zhu* 白术, *yi yi ren* 薏苡仁, *huang qi* 黄芪, *fu ling* 茯苓, *she she cao* 蛇舌草, *gan cao* 甘草, *ban zhi lian* 半枝莲, *dang shen* 党参, *ban xia* 半夏 and *e zhu* 莪术. The included studies investigated either an extract of one or more of these herbs, and/or at least one of their known constituent compounds, and reported their (1) actions on cancer cell proliferation, migration, invasion and/or metastasis; (2) effects on inflammation, the immune system and oxidative stress; and (3) actions when combined with conventional anti-cancer drugs.

The included studies were identified by searches of PubMed using the botanical names of the plants from which the herbs are sourced and the names of major compounds as search terms. In general, studies of plant extracts are presented first, followed by studies of major compounds.

Experimental Studies on *Bai Zhu* 白术

The official source of the Chinese herb *bai zhu* 白术 is the rhizomes of *Atractylodes macrocephala* Koidz.[1] A large number of compounds from this herb have been identified. The main classes are sesquiterpenoids, triterpenoids, polyacetylenes, coumarins, phenylpropanoids (including phenolic acids), flavonoids and flavonoid glycosides, steroids, benzoquinones and polysaccharides. Most of the research attention has focused on the sesquiterpenoid lactones: atractylenolide I, atractylenolide II, atractylenolide III (also known as codonolactone), atractylenolide IV, atractylon (also known as atractylone) and biatractylolide, and the polysaccharide fraction which mainly contains inulin-type polysaccharides.[2-5] A number of these compounds are also found in other *Atractylodes* species and other plants. *Bai zhu* 白术 is a commonly used herb for gastrointestinal disorders. An assay of embryonic stem cells indicated that an extract of *A. macrocephala* had negligible embryotoxicity.[6] *Bai zhu* 白术 is often used in its processed form (*chao bai zhu* 炒白术) which involves stir-frying the herb with wheat bran; this reduces the proportion of volatile compounds found in the oils.[7,8]

A few studies of *A. macrocephala* and its constituent compounds in models of CRC were located. However, there were numerous studies in other cancers. These studies have shown effects relevant to CRC including induction of apoptosis, immunomodulation, anti-inflammatory effects and free-radical scavenging.

Effects in Cancer

The formula *Shen ling bai zhu san* 参苓白术散 (SBS), of which *bai zhu* 白术, *fu ling* 茯苓and *gan cao* 甘草 are major ingredients, was investigated in mice with dextran sodium sulfate (DSS)-induced colitis which produced pre-neoplastic and neoplastic lesions. Administration of SBS improved body weight and survival time, and reduced the number and size of colonic neoplasms. When the human CRC cell lines SW-480 and HCT-116 were treated with SBS, atractylenolide-1 and ginsenoside Rc, there was a time- and dose-dependent decrease in viability for SBS and atractylenolide-1, but not for ginsenoside Rc. Also, SBS reduced expression of proliferating cell nuclear antigen (PCNA), β-catenin and p53 in both cell lines.[9]

Atractylenolide I and II

The effects of atractylenolide I on CRC were explored in mice with a mutated adenomatous polyposis coli (APC) gene, which develop intestinal adenomatous polyps that progress to carcinomas. Treatment with atractylenolide I reduced the number of intestinal adenomas in the mice and down-regulated the expression of the tumorigenic proteins β-catenin, PCNA and cyclooxygenase-2 (COX-2). Further, atractylenolide I promoted autophagy in mouse tissues, and in the HCT-116 human colon cancer cell line. Autophagy is an important process that enables the immune elimination of transformed cells.[10] A clinical trial of atractylenolide I for people with cachexia associated with gastric cancer, reported improvements in appetite but there was no significant weight gain. Serological tests indicated upregulation of tumour necrosis factor (TNF) and downregulation of interleukin (IL)-1, and urine analysis showed a decrease in the proteolysis-inducing factor (PIF) positive rate.[11]

Atractylenolide II was found to inhibit proliferation in the human gastric cancer HGC-27, and in AGS cell lines to inhibit cell motility and induce apoptosis. The expression level of pro-apoptotic protein Bax was upregulated, B-cell lymphoma 2 (Bcl-2) was downregulated, and there was downregulation of phosphorylated protein kinase B (Akt) and phosphorylated extracellular signal-regulated kinases (ERK), suggesting modulation of the Akt/ERK signalling pathway.[12] In B16 melanoma cells, atractylenolide II induced apoptosis, downregulated phosphorylated Akt and ERK, increased the expression of phosphorylated-p38 and p53, and activated caspase-8, -9 and -3.[13] In nude mice with A549 human lung carcinoma transplants, atractylenolide II suppressed tumour growth, upregulated caspase-3, caspase-9 and Bax, and downregulated Bcl-2 and Bcl-XL.[14]

Codonolactone

Codonolactone (also known as atractylenolide III) was reported to induce apoptosis in human lung carcinoma A-549 cells. It increased active caspase-3 and caspase-9, and cleaved the nuclear protein poly-(ADP)-ribose polymerase (PARP). It also increased release of cytochrome-c into the cytosol, upregulated the expression of Bax and induced the translocation of apoptosis-inducing factor (AIF) to the nucleus. This result suggests apoptosis may involve a caspase-independent pathway. In a separate assay in human umbilical vein endothelial cells (HUVEC), codonolactone inhibited cell proliferation and capillary tube formation, indicating potential anti-angiogenic effects.[15] In a subsequent study in HUVECs and the EA.hy926 human umbilical vein cell line, codonolactone inhibited tube formation in both cell lines. In rat thoracic aortas, it dose-dependently decreased the number of micro vessels formed from explants, and reduced the development of blood vessels in breast cancer MDA-MB-231 tissue samples. Furthermore, codonolactone dose-dependently reduced vascular endothelial growth factor (VEGF) expression in HUVECs at both the RNA and protein levels, and reduced the phosphorylation of VEGFR-2, suggesting a likely mechanism of action.[16]

Codonolactone was one of a number of compounds investigated in a screen of beta-tubulin inhibitors. It showed significant binding with beta-tubulin and inhibitory activity against the polymerization of tubulin. The pharmacological mechanism was the same as for paclitaxel, suggesting codonolactone as a potential lead compound for developing antineoplastic agents.[17]

Atractylochromene

Using a TOPFlash assay to screen for inhibitors of Wnt/β-catenin signalling, atractylochromene was identified and isolated from *A. macrocephala* extracts. In the human colorectal adenocarcinoma SW-480 cell line, atractylochromene suppressed cell proliferation and decreased the nuclear level of β-catenin and cyclin D1, suggesting it is a potential lead compound for the down-modulation of Wnt/β-catenin signalling.[18]

Polysaccharides

In glioma C6 cells, a model of brain tumours, the polysaccharide fraction of *A. macrocephala* was found to induce apoptosis and increase expression of activated caspase-3 and caspase-9, and cleaved PARP, suggesting that apoptosis occurs via a mitochondria-dependent pathway.[19]

Anti-inflammatory Effects

The anti-inflammatory activity of four fractions of *A. macrocephala* were investigated in rabbits and mice to determine the most effective fraction, from which the compounds atractylenolide I and 14-acetoxy-12-senecioyloxytetradeca-2E, 8E, 10E-trien4,6-diyn-1-ol were identified.[20] In peritoneal macrophages treated with lipopolysaccharide (LPS) to induce inflammation, atractylenolide I and atractylenolide III, at concentrations that did not induce cytotoxicity, reduced the LPS-induced production of TNF-alpha and nitric oxide (NO), and attenuated the synthesis of inducible nitric oxide synthase (iNOS) in dose-dependent manners. Atractylenolide I showed greater inhibition than atractylenolide III.[21] In a mouse air-pouch model of inflamma-tion-induced angiogenesis, atractylenolide I reduced the numbers of granulocytes and macrophages, and reduced the levels of TNF-alpha, IL-1beta, IL-6, VEGF, placenta growth factor (PlGF), basic fibroblast growth factor (bFGF) and NO.[22]

In a mouse model of inflammatory bowel disease (IBD) induced by dextran sulfate sodium (DSS), pre-treatment with an extract of *A. macrocephala* was protective against DSS-induced rectal bleeding, diarrhoea and poor oral intake. Colon sections showed reduced inflammation and ulceration which was associated with reduced COX-2, iNOS, IL-1beta and TNF-alpha.[23]

Immunoregulatory Effects

A study of the effects of the polysaccharides of *A. macrocephala* on RAW 264.7 macrophages found dose-dependent enhancement of phagocytosis. There was an increased production of TNF-alpha, interferon (IFN)-gamma and NO. Inhibition of nuclear factor-kap-paB (NF-κB) reduced the induction of TNF-alpha and NO, suggesting the immunomodulatory activity of the polysaccharides were via the NF-κB pathway.[24] The effects of polysaccharide fractions derived from *A. macrocephala* on proliferation of peripheral lymphocytes showed considerable variation between fractions, with the total polysaccharide fraction and one of the four partial fractions showing significant increases in CD4+ and CD8+ T-lymphocytes, suggesting enhancement of immune function.[25] Furthermore, in geese treated with cyclophosphamide (CTX) to induce immunosuppression, poly-saccharides of *A. macrocephala* improved spleen morphology and tended to normalise the proportions of leukocytes and spleen lym-phocytes, indicating that the polysaccharides attenuated the immunosuppressive effects of CTX.[26]

Antioxidant Effects

A study of the antioxidant activity of *A. macrocephala* rhizomes reported that the fractions of total phenolics and total flavonoids showed higher activity compared to total sugars and total saponins. In addition, the antioxidant actions of the phenolic acids (notably caffeic acid, ferulic acid and protocatechuic acid) were higher for free-radical scavenging, while the flavonoids showed higher activity in metal-chelating assays.[27]

Experimental Studies on *Yi Yi Ren* 薏苡仁

The official source of *yi yi ren* 薏苡仁 is the seeds of *Coix lacryma-jobi* L. var. *mayuen* (Roman.) Stapf.[1] It is also called 'Job's tears' or 'adlay' and is widely used as a grain in east and south Asia. The whole grain of *Coix* contains a large number of compounds including coixenolide, coixans A-C, a-monolinolein, fatty acids (such as palmitic, stearic, oleic and linoleic acids), phenolics (chlorogenic acid, vanillic acid, vanillin, caffeic acid, p-coumaric acid, ferulic acid, syringic acid, quercetin, narigenin, sinapaldehyde, apigenin and rutin), lactams (such as coixlactam and coixspirolactams A-C), coixol, oils, proteins (such as the coixins) and amino acids (notably glutamine).[28–33]

Kanglaite is an injectable adjuvant anti-cancer drug developed in China. It is composed of a purified oil from *Coix* that contains coixenolide. It has been tested in clinical trials and is used in treatment for multiple cancers in China including CRC. Its mechanisms included induction of apoptosis and halting tumour cell progression in the G2/M phase.[34] Kanglaite is not reviewed in this section.

Effects in Cancer

Aberrant crypt foci (ACF) and mucin-depleted foci (MDF) are pre-neoplastic lesions of CRC in rodents and humans. F344 rats were randomly divided into five groups with the experimental groups being fed a diet that included different proportions of dehulled *Coix* seed. After one week they were injected once a week with the carcinogen azoxymethane (AOM). After five or 52 weeks their colons were assessed for ACF. There was a reduction in ACF in the distal colons at five weeks, and at 52 weeks there was a small decrease in the number of tumours and a decrease in COX-2 protein expression in tumours, but no effect on tumour volume.[35]

In an experimental model of CRC development in rats injected with the colon-specific carcinogen 1,2-dimethylhydrazine (DMH), the animals were tube-fed an ethyl acetate fraction for nine weeks. The medium dose of the extract reduced MDF formation in rat colons; the oncogenes RAS and ETS2 were significantly downregulated; and the protein expression of COX-2 was significantly suppressed. The extract contained a number of phenolic compounds, of which the authors suggested ferulic acid contributed to the extract's activity.[36] *Coix* bran is high in bioactive phytochemicals. An ethanol extract of the bran, and the residue of the extract, were each fed to rats as part of their diet. After one week, rats were injected weekly with the carcinogen DMH. The bran and its ethanolic extract suppressed small ACFs (one, two or three crypts) and ACFs in the distal colon, while the residue of the extract suppressed large ACFs (four or more crypts), suggesting *Coix* has potential as a chemo-preventive cereal product.[37]

The whole seeds of five cultivars of *Coix* were processed by different methods and extracted with different solvents to produce 330 extracts which were investigated for anti-proliferative activity on human colon adenocarcinoma HT-29 cells. The hull of the Thai Black Loei variety was found to have the highest anti-proliferative and free-radical scavenging activity.[38] A methanol extract of Thai Black Loei *Coix* was further fractionated with ethyl acetate to make a semi-purified extract and formed into liposomes using supercritical carbon dioxide. Mice with HT-29 human colon adenocarcinoma cell xenografts that were administered the liposomes showed dose-dependent reductions in tumour volumes.[39] An aqueous extract of *Coix* sprouts reduced viability of HCT-116 cells but not normal cells. It reduced their migratory potency, invasion and adhesion under hypoxic conditions, and down-regulated the hypoxia-induced activation of ERK1/2 and AKT.[40]

Anti-inflammatory Effects

In RAW-264.7 macrophages activated by LPS and INF-gamma, a methanol extract of *Coix* seeds inhibited NO production in a dose-dependent manner and suppressed the mRNA expression of iNOS. Pre-treatment with the extract reduced superoxide production.[41] An ethanolic extract, that was further fractionated by column chromatography, was tested for radical scavenging capacity, antioxidative effects and anti-inflammatory activities. In LPS-stimulated RAW-264.7 macrophages, four fractions inhibited NO production and three fractions down-regulated the expression of iNOS and COX-2. Four fractions showed 2,2-diphenyl-1-picrylhydrazyl (DPPH)-scavenging capacity. Further isolation of compounds found the anti-inflammatory and antioxidant activities were mainly due to chlorogenic acid, caffeic acid and ferulic acid.[29]

When hulled and unhulled *Coix* seeds were compared in terms of their anti-inflammatory effects, the ethyl acetate extract of unhulled seeds was found to reduce NO production in LPS-activated RAW-264.7 macrophages. In comparison, the extract of the hulled seeds showed little effect. The extract of unhulled seeds also suppressed the protein expression of iNOS and COX-2 in a concentration-dependent manner.[42]

Antioxidant Effects

Three varieties of *yi yi ren* 薏苡仁, which were rich in free and bound phenolics, were shown to have high antioxidant activity and inhibited proliferation of HepG2 liver cancer cells. It was considered likely that release of bound phytochemicals by colonic bacteria may contribute to the protective effect of *Coix* against CRC.[43] Defatted *Coix* seed, which is left over after the removal of oil and is rich in phenolics, was fractionated and investigated in three antioxidant assays: the oxygen radical absorbance capacity (ORAC) assay, the peroxyl radical scavenging capacity (PSC) assay and the cellular anti-oxidant activity (CAA) assay. The subfraction that had the highest total phenolic content also possessed the highest antioxidant activity. In this subfraction, the most abundant phenolic acid was ferulic acid, while its predominant flavonoid was rutin. The highest ORAC values were for p-coumaric acid and vanillin, followed by vanillic acid, ferulic acid, quercetin and rutin. The PSC values were highest for quercetin and vanillic acid, and CAA values were highest for quercetin, rutin, ferulic acid and vanillic acid. These differences reflected differences between methods. Overall, the antioxidant activity of the extracts was positively correlated with the phenolic content.[32]

Experimental Studies on *Huang Qi* 黄芪

The official botanical sources of *huang qi* 黄芪 are the roots of *Astragalus membranaceus* (Fisch.) Bge. or *A. membranaceus* (Fisch.) Bge. var. *mongholicus* (Bge.) Hsiao.[1] The plant *Hedysarum polybotrys* Hand.-Mazz. is also used as *huang qi* 黄芪 but is more properly called *hong qi* 红芪.[44] It is not considered an official source of *huang qi* 黄芪 so it is not reviewed here. The roots of *huang qi* 黄芪 contain saponins (such as astragalosides I-IV), flavonoids (such as calycosin, calycosin-7-O-β-d-glucoside, ononin and formononetin), polysaccharides and amino acids.[44,45]

Effects in Cancer

An extract of *Astragalus* saponins was found to inhibit proliferation in HT-29 human colon cancer cells, induce apoptosis via caspase-3 activation and PARP cleavage, and induce cell cycle arrest. In HT-29 cell xenografts in nude mice, the extract reduced tumour volume without decreasing body weight and immunohistochemical analysis showed increased apoptotic cell numbers in tumour tissues. An extract of *Astragalus* polysaccharides was not found to inhibit HT-29 cell proliferation.[46] In a subsequent study of the same extract in HT-29 cells, cell cycle arrest was induced by modulation of both the mTOR and ERK signalling pathways.[47]

In HCT-116 human colon cancer cells, the extract of total saponins reduced the protein expression of the two angiogenic factors bFGF and VEGF. In HCT-116 cells treated with cobalt chloride (II) to mimic hypoxia and upregulate hypoxia inducible factor 1 alpha (HIF-1a), the extract abolished the cobalt chloride-induced protein expression of both HIF-1a and VEGF. In HT-29 cells which express COX-2, the extract reduced COX-2 protein expression under normoxic conditions and showed a similar effect in HCT-116 cells with cobalt chloride-induced hypoxia. In HCT-116 mouse xenografts, the extract reduced tumour size, downregulated the protein expression of VEGF and its receptors VEGFR1 and VEGFR2, and inhibited COX-2 expression.[48] When the same extract was combined with vinblastine and studied in human colorectal carcinoma HCT-116 cells and metastatic colorectal adenocarcinoma LoVo cells, the combination showed greater reductions in angiogenic factors and numbers of invaded cells, compared to the two treatments separately. In mice with HCT-116 xenografts, serum VEGF levels were reduced by both the extract and vinblastine. There were further reductions when both treatments were combined together, and there were reductions in the neutropenic and anaemic effects of vinblastine.[49]

Formononetin

The isoflavonoid, formononetin, was found to inhibit the viability of HCT-116 cells and induce apoptosis, as indicated by activation of caspase-3 and caspase-9 and downregulation of the anti-apoptotic proteins Bcl-2 and Bcl-x(L).[47] In HCT-116 cells, formononetin time-dependently downregulated the protein expression of bFGF, VEGF and the matrix metalloproteinases MMP2 and MMP9, and both the gene and protein expression of VEGF. In LoVo human colorectal adenocarcinoma cells from metastatic sites, formononetin significantly decreased the number of invaded cells. In nude mice with HCT-116 xenografts, tumour volume was reduced in the formononetin-treated group and serum VEGF levels were reduced, as was VEGF staining in tumour samples. Immunohistochemical assessment showed reduced cell proliferation in tumour tissues.[50]

In SW-1116 and HCT-116 cells, formononetin inhibited proliferation and cell invasion, induced cell-cycle arrest, and inhibited expression of MMP2 and MMP9. It upregulated microRNA (miR)-149 and downregulated the mRNA expression of EphB3 (the direct target of miR-149) in both cancer cell lines, but not in normal colon cells. In addition, it suppressed phosphorylation of AKT/PI3K and signal transducer and activator of transcription (STAT)3 in both SW-1116 and HCT-116 cells. In HCT-116 cell xenografts, formononetin reduced tumour volume.[51]

Astragaloside IV

Astragaloside IV has received considerable research attention in multiple diseases and has been shown to inhibit oxidative stress injury via scavenging reactive oxygen species (ROS), inhibit the expression of pro-inflammatory cytokines, and inhibit cell proliferation in multiple cancers.[52] In two CRC cell lines, HCT-116 and SW-480, astragaloside IV reduced cell viability but did not significantly inhibit normal colonic epithelial cells. When cells were incubated with cisplatin plus astragaloside IV, the sensitivity to cisplatin was increased. Compared with cisplatin, the combination downregulated the protein level and mRNA expression of NOTCH3, which is increased in some primary and metastatic colon cancers.[53]

The effects of astragaloside IV on epithelial to mesenchymal transition (EMT), which is involved in the initiation of metastasis, was investigated in SW-480 CRC cells. Astragaloside IV suppressed cell proliferation in a dose and time-dependent manner. In addition, it inhibited SW-480 CRC cell migration and invasion. Astragaloside IV increased the protein level of E-cadherin and decreased the protein levels of N-cadherin, Snail (Zinc finger protein SNAI1) and vimentin, which indicated it had an inhibitory effect on EMT signalling. It induced expression of miR-134 and downregulated the CREB1 signalling pathway. This pathway is involved in cancer cell proliferation, survival and differentiation. In addition, astragaloside IV increased the sensitivity of SW-480 cells to oxaliplatin.[54]

In SW-620 and HCT-116 CRC cell lines, astragaloside IV dose-dependently reduced cell growth without affecting the proliferation of normal cells. It induced cell cycle arrest at the G0/G1 checkpoint. Moreover, it decreased the mRNA expression level of the immune checkpoint molecule B7-H3 which regulates the immune response,[55] is overexpressed in a number of cancers, and is associated with poor survival via upregulation of miR-29c.[56]

Anti-inflammatory Effects

Using *in-vitro* bioassay-guided fractionation in LPS-stimulated mouse RAW-264.7 macrophages, aqueous extracts were tested for inhibition of NO release. Two major active fractions were identified, and formononetin was found to have the greatest anti-inflammatory effects.[57] In LPS-stimulated RAW-264.7 cells, an aqueous extract reduced NO production by downregulating iNOS expression in a concentration-dependent manner. It reduced the release of IL-1beta, IL-6 and TNF-alpha, inhibited prostaglandin E2 (PGE2) production and decreased expression of COX-2. Reductions in the phosphorylated forms of ERK, c-Jun N-terminal kinase (JNK) and p38 suggested that the anti-inflammatory effects were mediated by the mitogen-activated protein kinase (MAPK) signalling pathway.[58]

In mice treated with LPS, astragaloside IV inhibited increases in serum levels of monocyte chemoattractant protein 1 (MCP-1) and TNF-alpha, but not vascular cell adhesion molecule 1 (VCAM-1) and intercellular adhesion molecule 1 (ICAM-1). It had no effect on body weight. Pre-treatment with astragaloside IV reduced LPS-induced increases in the mRNA levels of the adhesion molecules VCAM-1, ICAM-1, E-selectin and P-selectin, as well as in the proinflammatory mediators MCP-1, TNF-alpha, IL-6 and toll-like receptor 4 (TLR4) in the lung, heart, aorta, kidney and liver of the mice, indicating that astragaloside IV could reduce acute inflammatory responses *in-vivo*.[59]

In LPS-stimulated RAW-264.7 cells, an extract of total flavonoids of *Astragalus* dose-dependently inhibited the mRNA levels of TNF-alpha, IL-1beta, IL-6, iNOS and COX-2, and increased the mRNA level of IL-10. Further analyses indicated its actions were mediated via the MAPK and NF-κB signalling pathways.[60]

Immunoregulatory Effects

A fraction derived from *A. membranaceus* roots, which contained polysaccharides and proteins, increased the proliferation of mouse splenocytes and restored depressed immune functions in tumour-bearing mice. In addition, murine macrophages pre-treated with the fraction showed increased cytostatic activities towards tumour cells *in-vitro* and *in-vivo*. These studies suggest the anti-cancer effects involve modulation of host immune mechanisms.[61,62]

A comparison of the immunoregulatory effects of *Astragalus membranaceus* var. *mongholicus*, *A. membranaceus* and *Hedysarum polybotrys* found the polysaccharide extracts all increased the spleen and thymus index in mice, and the phagocytosis indices of mouse macrophages. Serum hemolysin level, an indicator of humoral immunity, was also increased by the polysaccharide extracts of all three plants — even though there were distinct differences between the *Astragalus* species and *Hedysarum* in their polysaccharides. The extracts of flavonoids, saponins and amino acids showed less effect than the polysaccharides in all three species.[44]

Experimental Studies on *Fu Ling* 茯苓

The official source of *fu ling* 茯苓 is the fungus *Poria cocos* (Schw.) Wolf, which is also called *Wolfiporia cocos* (F.A.Wolf) Ryvarden & Gilb.[1] It contains a number of bioactive triterpenoids including pachymic acid, dehydropachymic acid, poricoic acid A, polyporenic acid C, dehydrotumulosic acid, dehydrotrametenolic acid, dehydroe-buricoic acid, poricotriol A and multiple polysaccharides.[63–67]

Effects in Cancer

When triterpenoids from *fu ling* 茯苓 were tested in 60 human tumour cell lines, poricoic acid A was found to show significant cytotoxic effects in leukemia HL-60 cells, and moderate cytotoxicity in lung, colon, renal, ovarian and brain cancer, melanoma, and other leukaemia cell lines.[68] The effects of lanostane-type triterpenes in cancer have been reviewed in detail, and a number of compounds have been shown to induce apoptosis in leukaemia, prostate cancer, lung cancer, stomach cancer, liver cancer and pancreatic cancer, suggesting that lanostane-type triterpenes may be potential chemo-preventive or anti-cancer agents.[69,70] For example, pachymic acid has been shown to induce apoptosis in lung cancer NCI-H23 and NCI-H460 cells,[71] bladder cancer EJ cells[72] and pancreatic cancer PANC-1 and MIA PaCa-2 cells.[73]

In addition, *P. cocos* polysaccharides have been investigated in cell and animal models.[74] In rats with experimentally-induced liver cancer, a polysaccharide extract reduced tumour weight and enhanced the activity of serum antioxidant enzymes.[75] Water-soluble polysaccharides inhibited growth of HL-60 leukaemia cells, and in BALB/c male mice with xenografts of sarcoma 180 cells, tumour weight was reduced, with high molecular weight polysaccharides showing greater inhibition.[76] However, the searches did not identify studies of *P. cocos* or its main constituents in CRC models.

Anti-inflammatory Effects

Extracts of *P. cocos*, and the compounds pachymic acid and dehydro-tumulosic acid have been shown to have anti-inflammatory activity in animal and cell models.[69] In LPS-stimulated RAW-264.7 cells, a 70% ethanol extract and a number of fractions were evaluated for their inhibitory effects on proinflammatory mediators (NO, iNOS, PGE2 and COX-2). Five of eight triterpenoids inhibited NO production and down-regulated iNOS expression. The most potent was a novel compound, 3-O-acetyl-16a-hydroxydehydrotrametenolic acid, which also significantly inhibited PGE2 production and reduced the protein expression of COX-2.[77] In the same model, another study found that pre-treatment with an ethanol extract reduced iNOS, COX-2, IL-1beta and TNF-alpha expression, and inactivated the NF-κB signalling pathway.[78]

Polysaccharides have also shown anti-inflammatory effects.[74] For example, a polysaccharide isolated from *P. cocos* was found to inhibit IFN-gamma-induced inflammation in human vascular endothelial cells, but showed no cytotoxicity in MCF-7 breast cancer, H-460 lung cancer, HT-29 colon cancer or CEM leukaemia cell lines.[79]

Immunoregulatory Effects

Poria cocos extracts, polysaccharides and proteins have been reported to have potentiating effects on the immune response.[69]

A novel protein, *P. cocos* immunomodulatory protein, was reported to stimulate RAW-264.7 macrophages to produce TNF-alpha and IL-1beta, as well as regulate the expression of NF-κB-related genes. In mouse peritoneal cavity macrophages, the protein showed similar activities, and was also shown to time-dependently stimulate the tyrosine phosphorylation of TLR4.[80] A chemically modified polysaccharide was reported to increase the thymus and spleen indexes and enhance macrophage phagocytosis in BALB/c mice more than the native polysaccharide, and in mice with sarcoma 180 (S-180) xenografts it showed greater reduction in tumour weight, apparently as a result of increased immune response.[75]

Antioxidant Effects

A study of four polysaccharide fractions showed concentration-dependent free-radical scavenging ability on DPPH and hydroxyl-radical scavenging activity with the PCP-M fraction (which had a lower neutral sugar content and higher uronic acid content), showing the strongest antioxidant activity.[32]

Experimental Studies on *She She Cao* 蛇舌草

The official source of *bai hua she she cao* 白花蛇舌草 (*she she cao* 蛇舌草) is the aerial parts or whole plant of *Hedyotis diffusa* Willd.[1] This plant is also called *Oldenlandia diffusa* (Willd.) Roxb. More than 170 compounds have been identified from *Hedyotis diffusa* including iridoid glycosides (such as asperuloside, asperuloside acid, geniposidic acid, alpigenoside, oldenlandoside III, scandoside and diffusosides A and B), triterpenes (such as oleanolic acid, ursolic acid, arborinone and isoarborinol), sterols (such as beta-sitosterol, stigmasterol and daucosterol), flavonoids (such as amentoflavone, quercetin, rutin and kaempferol), athraquinones (such as 2-methyl-3-methoxy anthraquinone and 2-hydroxy-1,3-dimethoxy anthraquinone), phenolic acids and their derivatives (such as p-coumaric acid, caffeic acid and ferulic acid), polysaccharides, volatile oils and other components.[81]

Effects in Cancer

In HT-29 human CRC cells, an ethanol extract of *Hedyotis diffusa* dose- and time-dependently reduced cell viability and survival via blocking cell cycle progression from the G1 to the S phase. It reduced the expression of the promoting proteins PCNA, cyclin D1 and cyclin-dependent kinase 4 (CDK4), and increased expression of the anti-proliferative protein p21.[82]

In four human CRC cell lines (HCT-8, HT-29, HCT-116 and SW-620), an ethanol extract dose- and time-dependently inhibited viability. In a xenograft of HT-29 cells in BALB/c nude mice, the extract decreased tumour volume and weight by induction of apoptosis. In tumours, Bcl-2 expression was decreased and Bax expression was increased, and the expression of the potential oncogene PIM1 was downregulated. In addition, the expression of four proteins thought to play roles in tumour angiogenesis — COX-2, iNOS, eNOS and HIF-1 alpha — were downregulated. In mouse serum, the levels of the inflammatory cytokines IL-1beta, IL-6 and TNF-alpha were significantly decreased, and the levels of IL-4 and IL-10 increased. In tumour tissues, there were significant decreases in the levels of phosphorylated AKT, ERK1/2, JNK, p38, p70S6K and STAT3, and increases in phosphorylated p53, suggesting the involvement of multiple signalling pathways.[83]

A series of extracts of *H. diffusa* were tested in four human CRC cell lines: SW-620, HT-29, HCT-116 and HCT-8. The chloroform extract had an inhibitory effect on cell viability in all cell lines with the effect being greatest in SW-620 CRC cells. Further analysis found that this extract decreased the expression of the pro-proliferative proteins PCNA, cyclin D1 and CDK4, and the anti-apoptotic Bcl-2 and survivin. In addition, it increased the expression of pro-apoptotic Bax, at both the protein and mRNA levels in SW-620 CRC cells. It also inhibited phosphorylation of AKT and ERK.[84]

An aqueous extract of *H. diffusa* showed anti-proliferative, cytotoxic, and pro-apoptotic effects in four CRC lines (HCT-116, DLD-1, HT-29 and LoVo) and in primary (patient-derived) human CRC cells. In nude mice with HCT-116 xenografts, the extract inhibited tumour growth, increased activation of AMP-activated protein kinase (AMPK), and inhibited mammalian target of rapamycin complex 1 (mTORC1), suggesting inhibition of mTOR signalling, and it activated p53 in tumour tissues.[85]

A stem-like side population (SP) of HT-29 CRC cells, HT-29 SP cells, were isolated and treated with an ethanol extract of *H. diffusa*. The extract reduced the percentage of stem-like cells in the HT-29 cell population. Within HT-29 SP cells, it inhibited cell growth and downregulated the expression of leucine-rich repeat-containing G-protein coupled receptor 5 (Lgr5), which is a marker of cancer stem cells. The extract also supressed the mRNA expression of c-Myc, b-catenin, PCNA, survivin and ATP–binding cassette, sub–family B, member 1 (ABCB1), suggesting inhibition of ABC transporter expression and the Wnt signalling pathway.[86]

To investigate the effect of an ethanol extract on the ABC family of transporters which facilitate drug resistance in CRC, expression levels of P-gp and ABCG2 were measured in the 5 fluorouracil (5 FU)-resistant CRC cell-line HCT 8/5 FU cells. When cells were treated with the extract, both the mRNA and protein expression levels were reduced in a concentration-dependent manner, suggesting that the ethanol extract was a reversing agent that targeted ABC transporters.[87] In the HCT 8/5 FU cell line, an ethanol extract time- and dose-dependently inhibited cell viability, attenuated cell adhesive ability and dose-dependently decreased migration and invasion, suggesting inhibition of metastatic potential. Downregulation of the expression of TGF-beta, mothers against decapentaplegic homolog 4 (SMAD4) and N cadherin, and upregulation of E cadherin suggest the mechanism was via the TGF-beta signalling pathway.[88] In the same cell line, another study found that an ethanol extract inhibited cell viability in a concentration- and time-dependent manner, inhibited colony formation and induced apoptosis via regulation of cyclin D1, CDK4, p21, Bcl-2 and Bax expression. It significantly increased the protein expression of phosphatase and tensin homolog (PTEN) and reduced PI3K and p-AKT, suggesting inhibition of the PI3K/AKT signalling pathway which may be a mechanism for the activation of apoptosis.[89]

An ethanol extract was found to inhibit angiogenesis in the chick embryo chorioallantoic membrane model, and to inhibit migration and tube formation in HUVECs. In HT-29 human colon carcinoma cells, it downregulated the mRNA and protein expression levels of VEGF-A.[90] In nude mice with HT-29 cell xenografts, intra-gastric administration inhibited tumour volume, compared to controls, over the 21 days of the study. Immunohistochemical staining showed the percentage of tumour cells positive for the marker CD31 was reduced in treated mice, and gel electrophoresis showed a reduction in the mRNA and protein expression of VEGF-A and its receptor VEGFR2, suggesting that tumour growth was at least partially inhibited by the Sonic hedgehog pathway.[91]

Anti-inflammatory Effects

The ethanol extract of the total flavonoids of *H. diffusa* was tested in RAW-264.7 cells. In cells treated with LPS to induce an inflammatory response, the flavonoid fraction inhibited the LPS-induced release of NO, TNF-alpha, IL6 and IL1beta, and suppressed their mRNA expression. It inhibited the excessive phosphorylation of p65 and suppressed the phosphorylation of inhibitor of kappa B (IκB)-alpha, thereby inhibiting the activation of NF-κB. In addition, it decreased the phosphorylation levels of the MAPK signalling molecules p38, JNK and ERK 1/2. These results suggest that the extract inhibited the NF-κB and MAPK signalling pathways.[92]

Immunoregulatory Effects

Extracts of *H. diffusa* and *Astragalus membranaceus* stimulated the proliferation of normal mouse spleen B cells, but not natural killer (NK) cells. The extracts stimulated mouse macrophages to produce TNF-alpha and IL-6. The immunomodulatory effects of *H. diffusa* were due mainly to the glycoprotein fraction.[93] An ethanol extract of *H. diffusa* was administered to normal BALB/c mice while the control mice received olive oil. The extract did not affect body weight or liver weight but increased spleen weight. There was no cytotoxic effect. It did not increase macrophage phagocytosis or NK cell activity. In a leukocyte population assay, it significantly increased the population of CD19 (B cells), CD11b (monocytes) and Mac-3 (macrophages) cells but did not affect the population of CD3 (T cells).[94]

Experimental Studies on *Gan Cao* 甘草

The roots of *Glycyrrhiza uralensis* Fisch., *G. inflata* Bat. and *G. glabra* L. are the official sources of *gan cao* 甘草.[1] Over 400 compounds have been isolated from *gan cao* 甘草.[95] The sweetness is mainly due to glycyrrhizic acid (also known as glycyrrhizin). Other constituents include triterpenoids (such as isoglycyrrhizin, 18Beta-glycyrrhizin, 18Alpha-glycyrrhizin and 18Beta-glycyrrhetinic acid), flavonoids and chalcones (such as liquiritin apioside, liquiritin, isoliquiritin apioside, liquiritigenin, isoliquiritigenin, licochalcones A–E, echinatin, glabridin, glycycoumarin, glyurallin B and 5-(1,1-dimethylallyl)-3,4,4'-trihydroxy-2-methoxychalcone [DTM]).[96–100]

Effects in Cancer

An ethanol extract of *G. glabra* roots time- and dose- dependently inhibited proliferation in the HT-29 colon cancer cell line and induced apoptosis. It reduced the expression of heat shock protein-90 (Hsp90), which is overexpressed in cancer cells and plays a role in metastatic processes.[101,102]

Glycyrrhizic acid

In a model of CRC development, Wistar rats were injected with DMH which induced ACF and MDF; these are considered pre-neoplastic lesions. Oral administration of glycyrrhizic acid suppressed the DMH-induced infiltration of inflammatory cells in the mucosal layer and reduced submucosal oedema, the number of MDF, the severity of submucosal oedema, crypt abscess formation and crypt ablation, suggesting that glycyrrhizic acid has chemo-preventive potential against CRC.[103]

Isoliquiritigenin and liquiritigenin

In the mouse colon cancer Colon 26 cell line and in human colon cancer COLO-320DM cells, isoliquiritigenin suppressed growth, with cytotoxic effects evident at the highest doses. At lower doses, isoliquiritigenin induced apoptosis in both cell lines and induced caspase-3 activation. In F344 rats treated with the carcinogen AOM, oral isoliquiritigenin inhibited induction of ACF in terms of the total number and number of large ACFs. It also reduced the loss of body weight induced by AOM. These results suggested isoliquiritigenin may be a chemo-preventive agent against CRC.[104]

In a model of colitis-associated tumorigenesis in BALB/c mice, which was induced by intraperitoneal injection of AOM followed by addition of DSS to drinking water, intra-gastric administration of isoliquiritigenin resulted in better maintenance of body weight, less severe colitis and decreases in the incidence, multiplicity and size of colon adenomas. A likely mechanism was M2 macrophage polarisation via the COX-2/PGE2 and IL-6 /STAT3 pathways.[105] Isoliquiritigenin also showed a demethylating effect on the death-associated protein kinase-1 (DAPK1) promoter region of DNA in HT-29 colon cancer cells, suggesting it may be a chemo-preventive agent for CRC.[106] In HCT-116 human CRC cells, liquiritigenin inhibited cell proliferation, invasion and EMT, but did not induce apoptosis. It reduced the expression of runt-related transcription factor 2 (RUNX2) and inactivated the phosphoinositide 3-kinase/protein kinase B (PI3K/AKT) pathway. These results suggest liquiritigenin may have a role in the inhibition of metastatic processes.[107]

Other compounds

Licoricidin inhibited the viability of SW-480 human colorectal adenocarcinoma cells and induced G1/S cell cycle arrest and apoptosis. In nude mice with SW-480 xenografts, treatment with licoricidin significantly reduced tumour size.[108]

In HUVECs, licochalcone A was found to inhibit proliferation, migration and tube formation, suggesting anti-angiogenic effects. It also inhibited the growth of xenografts of CT-26 colon cancer cells in BALB/c mice. Its actions involved downregulation of activated VEGFR-2.[109]

Anti-inflammatory and Antioxidant Effects

A review of the anti-inflammatory effects of *gan cao* 甘草 and its constituent compounds identified that extracts, three triterpenes and 13 flavonoids, have been shown to have anti-inflammatory properties *in vitro* (including in CRC cell lines) and/or *in vivo*. The main mechanisms identified were via decreasing TNF-alpha, inhibiting MMPs, suppressing the generation of PGE2 and scavenging free radicals.[100]

One study investigated the anti-inflammatory and antioxidant effects of six flavonoids. In RAW-264.7 mouse macrophages stimulated with LPS to induce inflammation, it found that NO secretion was reduced markedly by licochalcone B, DTM and echinatin; PGE2 secretion was reduced by licochalcone A, DTM, echinatin and glycycoumarin; and IL-6 secretion was most effectively inhibited by echinatin. Regarding antioxidant effects, licochalcone B, echinatin and glycycoumarin showed the highest radical scavenging activity in an ABTS[+] assay and were all higher than ascorbic acid. In LPS-stimulated RAW-264.7 cells, ROS production was inhibited by DTM, licochalcone B, licochalcone A and echinatin.[97]

In mouse RAW-264.7 macrophages stimulated with LPS, treatment with isoliquiritigenin at doses that did not reduce cell viability, decreased PGE2 and NO production, and dose-dependently suppressed the protein expression of COX-2 and iNOS, but not COX-1.[104]

Experimental Studies on *Ban Zhi Lian* 半枝莲

The official source of *ban zhi lian* 半枝莲 is the aerial parts or the whole plant of *Scutellaria barbata* D. Don.[1] It contains phenolic compounds including the flavones scutellarin, scutellarein, naringenin, apigenin, apigenin 5-O-β-glucopyranoside, luteolin, wogonin, 4′-hydroxy-wogonin,[110,111] carthamidin, isocarthamidin;[112] trace amounts of baicalein, p-coumaric acid,[110] hexadecanoic acid (aka palmitic acid), caryophyllene;[113] multiple diterpenoid alkaloids (such as scutebarbatines A to N)[114,115] polysaccharides; carotenoids; and chlorophylls.[116]

Scutellaria barbata is commonly used in cancer treatment, often in conjunction with *Hedyotis diffusa* (*she she cao* 蛇舌草), and is also used for inflammation and infections.[117] An investigation of National

Health Insurance data found that *ban zhi lian* 半枝莲 and *she she cao* 蛇舌草 were the most commonly used herbs by postsurgery colon cancer and breast cancer patients.[118,119] In addition, people with chronic hepatitis B who used CHMs, notably *Hedyotis diffusa*, *Scutellaria barbata* and a few other herbs, had lower risks of developing hepatocellular carcinoma over a 15-year period.[120]

Effects in Cancers

An ethanol extract of *S. barbata* was reported to inhibit growth of HT-29 human colon carcinoma cells via activation of caspase-9 and caspase-3, and increasing the ratio of the pro-apoptotic protein Bax to the anti-apoptotic protein Bcl-2 to induce apoptosis. A likely mechanism was activation of a mitochondrion-dependent pathway.[121]

In a mouse xenograft of HT-29 cells, intra-gastric administration of an ethanol extract of *S. barbata* inhibited tumour growth and reduced angiogenesis via reducing the proliferation, migration and tube formation of endothelial cells, and downregulating VEGF-A.[122] A methanol extract dose-dependently decreased the levels of phosphorylated AKT, showed cytotoxicity against LoVo cells and reduced angiogenesis in HUVECs.[123] An extract of flavanoids (including scutellarin, luteolin and apigenin) inhibited migration and tube formation in HUVECs, inhibited angiogenesis in a chick chorioallantoic membrane (CAM) assay, and suppressed the expression of VEGF in the human hepatocellular carcinoma MHCC97-H cell line, as well as in HUVECs.[124]

An investigation of the anti-metastatic effect of an ethanol extract of *S. barbata* on the migration and invasion ability of HCT-8 cells found dose-dependent reductions in cell viability, migration and invasion, and decreased expression of MMP-1, -2, -3/10, -9 and -13. In addition, there was upregulation of the tumour suppressor PTEN while the downstream proteins, phosphoinositide 3-kinase (PI3K), p-PI3K and p-AKT, were downregulated. These results suggested the PI3K/AKT and TGF-beta/SMAD signalling pathways were involved in the anti-metastatic effects of the extract.[125]

When an ethanol extract was investigated in HT-29 cells for its effects on AKT and p53, it promoted the expression of the anti-proliferative protein p21 and inhibited expression of pro-proliferative proteins PCNA, cyclin D1 and CDK4. In addition, it significantly suppressed the phosphorylation (i.e. activation) of AKT, which promotes cell survival, and increased the level of phosphorylated p53, which is a suppressor of tumour growth.[126]

The effects of an ethanol extract of *S. barbata* on the IL-6/STAT3 pathway was investigated in HT-29 cells stimulated by IL-6, to simulate the effect of IL-6 production by cells in the tumour microenvironment. The extract inhibited HT-29 cell growth and induced apoptosis, blocked G1/S progression and activated caspase-9 and caspase-3. In addition, IL-6 increased the mRNA and protein expression of Bcl-2 and decreased Bax, while adding the extract inhibited these effects. IL6 also increased the level of phosphorylated STAT3 (p-STAT3) and this increase was dose-dependently inhibited by the extract.[127]

In HT-29 tumour xenografts in nude mice, an ethanol extract of *S. barbata* suppressed tumour growth without noticeable toxicity. Analysis of the tumour cells showed induction of apoptosis by increased Bax/Bcl-2 ratio. In addition, there were increases in the levels of pSTAT3, ERK1/2 and p38, suggesting multiple cellular signalling pathways were involved.[128] In a mouse HT-29 cell xenograft model, randomised to receive an ethanol extract of *S. barbata* or saline, the extract significantly reduced tumour weight, inhibited the protein expression of the proliferation biomarker Ki-67, decreased the mRNA expression of c-Myc and survivin, decreased the protein expression of b-catenin, c-Myc and survivin, and increased adenomatous polyposis coli (APC) expression. Similar results were found in an *in vitro* study of HT-29 cells. These results suggested the extract may activate the Wnt/b-catenin pathway.[129]

When an ethanol extract of *S. barbata* (containing scutellarin, luteolin, apigenin and other compounds) was combined with low-dose 5-FU in human hepatocellular carcinoma Bel-7402 cells and human colorectal adenocarcinoma HCT-8 cells, the inhibitory effects of the combination were greater than that of either single agent. A similar result was found for tumour inhibition in a mouse model of transplanted hepatocarcinoma H-22 cells. In addition to inducing apoptosis, the extract prolonged the retention of 5-FU by modulating 5-FU metabolic enzymes.[130] In a 5-FU resistant CRC cell line (HCT-8/5-FU), an ethanol extract of *S. barbata* promoted apoptosis via downregulating cyclin D1 and Bcl-2 expression and upregulating p21 and Bax. In addition, it suppressed the aberrant activation of the PI3K/AKT pathway which has an important role in the survival of drug-resistant cells.[129]

When different solvent fractions of *S. barbata* were tested in three human colon cancer cell lines (SW-620, HT-29, HCT-8), the chloroform fraction was found to have the most potent effects on inhibiting proliferation and apoptosis.[131] In HCT-8 cells, the chloroform fraction inhibited proliferation and promoted apoptosis in a dose-dependent manner. It enhanced the mRNA expression of the gene MIR34A, and decreased its downstream target genes BCL2, NOTCH1, NOTCH2 and Jagged1 (JAG1), which are involved in promotion of cancer growth. In addition, knockdown of MIR34A by transfection of an anti-MIR34A oligonucleotide was rescued by the chloroform fraction, suggesting that MIR34A was directly targeted.[132]

In a model of tumorigenesis in rats, an extract of *S. barbata* was protective against diethylnitrosamine (DENA)-induced liver malfunction and tumour formation.[133] In a human hepatocarcinoma MHCC97H cell line, an extract of total flavonoids dose-dependently inhibited cell proliferation and invasion. A likely mechanism was decreased expression of MMP-2 and MMP-9, combined with an increase in expression of the metalloproteinases TIMP-1 and TIMP-2.[134]

In human colon cancer HCT-116 cells, the flavonoid scutellarin, dose- and time- dependently inhibited cell viability and induced apoptosis via reducing Bcl-2 and elevating Bax expression and activating caspase-3. Also, it increased phosphorylated p53 and decreased the level of its downstream protein p21. Moreover, addition of the p53 inhibitor, pifithrin-alpha, abrogated Bax increase and Bcl-2 decrease, along with the increase in caspase-3 activation associated with apoptosis. These results suggested HCT-116 cell growth was inhibited via regulation of the p53/p21 pathway.[135]

A water-soluble polysaccharide from *S. barbata* inhibited proliferation of HT-29 cells and increased the rate of apoptosis via upregulating Bax and downregulating Bcl-2. In addition, it upregulated the mRNA expression of E-cadherin and downregulated expression of N-cadherin and vimentin, suggesting it inhibited the PI3K/AKT pathway, which promotes the proliferation and survival of cancer cells.[136]

A standardised extract of *S. barbata* flavonones, including scutellarein, scutellarin, carthamidin, isocarthamidin and wogonin, showed inhibition of growth in human colon adenocarcinoma LoVo cells at the sub-G1 phase of the cell cycle.[112] Another standardised aqueous extract of *S. barbata*, called Bezielle ® (BZL101), that was developed for breast cancer, was shown to be selectively cytotoxic to cancer cells while sparing non-transformed cells. It inhibited cell proliferation and induced cell death in ER-positive BT474 and ER-negative SKBR3 cell lines.[137] A likely mechanism of action was induction of progressively higher levels of mitochondrial superoxide as well as peroxide-type ROS in the cancer cells, but not in normal cells.[138] This activity was shown by the flavonoid scutellarein, but the total extract was more potent.[139] In a phase 1 clinical trial in women with metastatic breast cancer, oral administration of the aqueous extract showed a favourable toxicity profile and evidence of clinical activity.[140] In a subsequent phase 1B dose-escalation trial in 27 women with stage IV disease, adverse events were uncommon and there was evidence of objective tumour regression in three participants and five showed disease stabilisation.[141] Although a phase 2 trial was planned, no further publications could be located.

Anti-inflammatory Effects

In BV2 microglial cells treated with LPS, pre-treatment with a methanol extract of *S. barbata* was found to significantly and dose-dependently reduce NO production and reduce the expression of iNOS, without altering cell viability.[142] In another study, RAW-264.7 macrophages were incubated with LPS, an ethanol extract (containing more flavonoids and phenolic acids), and an ethyl acetate extract (containing more chlorophylls and carotenoids) of *S. barbata,* each at varying doses. Both extracts retarded NO production dose-dependently with the ethyl acetate extract showing the greater effect. In addition, both extracts inhibited the LPS-induced increase in iNOS and NF-κB, produced decreases in PGE2, IL-1beta and IL-6 levels, reduced expression of p-ERK and p-JNK, but had little effect on levels of TNF-alpha.[116]

Antioxidant Effects

An extract of the polysaccharides of *S. barbata* showed significant superoxide radical scavenging activity using the pyrogallic acid method, free radical scavenging activity using DPPH and hydroxyl radical-scavenging activity.[143]

Experimental Studies on *Dang Shen* 党参

The herb *dang shen* 党参 is officially derived from the roots of *Codonopsis pilosula* (Franch.) Nannf., *Codonopsis pilosula* Nannf. var. *modesta* (Nannf.) L. T. Shen, and *Codonopsis tangshen* Oliv.[1] Other species used include *C. lanceolata* (*lun ye dang shen* 轮叶党参) and *C. clematidea* (*xin jiang dang shen* 新疆党参).[144,145]

Dang shen 党参 contains numerous polyacetylenes, polyenes and their glycosides (such as lobetyolinin, lobetyolin, lobetyol and cordifolioidyne B), flavonoids and their glycosides (such as neokurarinol), lignans and their glycosides (such as tangshenosides I, V, VI and VIII), alkaloids and their glycosides (such as codotubulosine A and B, codonopsinols A–C, codonopiloside A and radicamine A), terpenoids and their glycosides (such as atractylenolide II, atractylenolide III [codonolactone], codonopilates A–C and oleanolic acid), steroids and their glycosides (such as α-spinasterol, β-sitosterol and β-daucosterol), organic acids and their glycosides (such as caffeic acid, nicotinic acid and lauric acid), monosaccharides, oligosaccharides and polysaccharides.[145–148] Toxicological studies have shown no obvious toxicity or side effects.[145]

Effects in Cancer

An extract from *C. lanceolata* induced G0/G1 cell-cycle arrest and apoptosis in human colon cancer HT-29 cells.[149] A similar extract, which mainly contained lobetyolin, tangshenoside I, codonoposide I and four other compounds, inhibited tumour growth and prolonged survival time of mice bearing xenografts of hepatocarcinoma H-22 cells by inducing apoptosis and inhibiting angiogenesis via reducing serum VEGF.[150] Lobetyol induced apoptosis and cell cycle arrest time- and dose-dependently in human gastric cancer MKN45 cells. In BALB/c nude mice with MKN45 xenografts, lobetyol inhibited tumour growth. The mechanisms of action involved the MAPK signalling pathways and induction of caspase cascade.[151]

In human ovarian cancer HO-8910 cells, a water-soluble acidic polysaccharide from *C. pilosula* inhibited cell growth, cell migration and cell adhesion in a concentration-dependent manner.[152] While codonolactone (also found in *bai zhu* 白术) has shown anti-metastatic properties in MDA-MB-231 human breast cancer cells.[153] In both MDA-MB-231 and MDA-MB-468 cells, it inhibited cell invasion and migration, and it reduced tumour growth in xenografts of MDA-MB-468 cells in female mice. Notably, codonolactone inhibited the motility of metastatic breast cancer cells by inhibiting TGF-beta1-induced epithelial-mesenchymal transition.[154]

Immunoregulatory Effects

Aqueous extracts of eight herbs were tested for their effects on human lymphocytes from the blood of healthy volunteers. The extracts of *Cinnamomum cassia*, *Codonopsis pilosula*, *Oldenlandia diffusa* [*Hedyosis diffusa*] and *Rhizoma typhonii* all stimulated human lymphocytes to proliferate but did not enhance NK cell activity.[155]

The effects on cellular and humoral immune response of a water-soluble polysaccharide, that was non-toxic to mice, were investigated in ovalbumin (OVA)-immunised mice. It enhanced OVA-induced splenocyte proliferation and increased the serum levels of OVA-specific immunoglobulin IgG, IgG1, and IgG2b antibodies, suggesting it enhanced immune responses.[156] A pectic polysaccharide was found to promote lymphocyte proliferation and modulate the percentage of T cells (CD4+, CD8+, CD28+, CD152+) in a senescence-accelerated mouse model, indicating an immune-stimulating effect.[157] In BALB/c mice, with immunosuppression induced by *d*-cyclophosphamide, administration of a water-soluble polysaccharide fraction dose-dependently increased the spleen index and improved the impairment of intestinal mucosal function and the disturbance in intestinal flora.[158]

Experimental Studies on *Ban Xia* 半夏

The official source of *ban xia* 半夏 is the tubers of *Pinellia ternata* (Thunb.) Breit.[1] but *P. pedatisecta* Schott (*zhang ye ban xia* 掌叶半夏) is also used.[159] In order to reduce the toxicity and irritant effects, the raw tubers are processed to make the forms typically used in clinical practice; however, the dried unprocessed tuber also has applications in decoctions used in cancer therapy.[160] The processed forms are named according to the methods of processing as follows: *fa ban xia* 法半夏 which is processed with a solution of *Glycyrrhiza* (*gan cao* 甘草) and lime, *jiang ban xia* 姜半夏 which is boiled with ginger juice and alum, and *qing ban xia* 清半夏 which is prepared with an alum solution. It has been reported that the irritant effects of unprocessed *ban xia* 半夏 are due to raphides of calcium oxalate which form sharp crystals that damage cells. Processing with alum breaks down these crystals and also pro-inflammatory lectin proteins.[161,162] A comparison of the effects of dried unprocessed *ban xia* 半夏 and *jiang ban xia* 姜半夏 found that processing reduced, but did not attenuate, its cytotoxic effects in hepatocellular carcinoma HepG2 cells, while it enhanced its antitussive and expectorant effects in mice.[160]

Analysis of *P. ternata* (raw and processed) and *P. pedatisecta* by gas and liquid chromatography using a range of solvents found 73 peaks and identified more than 40 compounds including organic acids (succinic acid, malic acid, fumaric acid and citric acid), fatty acids (palmitic acid, linoleic acid, oleic acid, stearic acid and lin-oleic acid methyl ester), amino acids (alanine, glycine, valine, leucine, isoleucine, proline, serine, threonine, pyroglutamic acid, glutamic acid, phenylalanine, lysine and tyrosine), nucleosides (uracil, thymine, adenine and uridine), nucleic acids, phytosterols (campesterol, stigmasterol and beta-sitosterol), carbohydrate derivatives (arabinose, fructose, sorbose, mannose, glucose, sucrose and various disaccharides) and sugar alcohol derivatives (asthreitol, erythritol, xylitol, mannitol, sorbitol and myo-inositol).[163] An analysis of the volatile oil of *P. ternata* found 114 compounds of which the most abundant were beta-cubebene, atractylon, methyl eugenol and delta-cadinene.[164] In addition, *Pinellia* spp. contains lectin proteins[165] and peptides.[166]

Effects in Cancers

A lipid-soluble extract from *P. pedatisecta* was found to enhance the cytotoxicity of cis-dichlorodiammineplatinum-II (cisplatin) in human cervical cancer CaSki cells and inhibit tumour growth in a xenograft mouse model via upregulation of a series of apoptosis-associated proteins.[167] In ovarian cancer SKOV3 cells, an extract of *P. pedatisecta* induced apoptosis dose- and time-dependently.[168]

Glucocerebrosides, which are found in *P. ternata* and many other plants, are enzymatically lipolyzed in the intestines into ceramides and sphingoid bases. Of the sphingoid bases, 4,8-sphingadienine, which is well absorbed by the intestine, has shown anti-proliferative effects in a number of cancer cell lines,[169] including human colon cancer CACO-2 cells.[170] Both the ceramides and sphingoid bases induced apoptosis in HT-29 and HCT-116 cell lines.[171]

A plant lectin purified from *P. ternata* inhibited proliferation of sarcoma-180, HeLa and K-562 cells, and inhibited growth of sarcoma-180 cells in a mouse model.[172] *Pinellia ternata* agglutinin (PTA), a mannose-binding lectin from *P. ternata*, induced apoptosis in human hepatoma Bel-7404 cells.[173] A peptide with trypsin inhibitory activity isolated from *P. ternata* inhibited proliferation in human gastric adenocarcinoma BGC-823 cells and reduced tumour size in nude mice.[166] In four human cholangiocarcinoma cell lines (SNU-245, CL-6, Sk-ChA-1 and MZ-ChA-1), a purified polysaccharide from

P. ternata decreased cell viability and induced apoptosis via the intrinsic mitochondrial pathway.[174]

Experimental Studies on *E Zhu* 莪术

The herb *e zhu* 莪术 derives from the dried rhizomes of a number of *Curcuma* species. The Chinese Pharmacopoeia (2015) lists the following three species as sources: *Curcuma phaeocaulis* Val. (*peng e zhu* 蓬莪术), *Curcuma kwangsiensis* S. G. Lee et C. F. Liang (*guang xi e zhu* 广西莪术) and *Curcuma wenyujin* Y. H. Chen et C. Ling (*wen yu jin* 温郁金).[1] Instead of these three species, the *Zhong Yao Da Ci Dian* (1992) and other older sources list *Curcuma zedoaria* (Christm.) Roscoe (*peng e zhu* 蓬莪术).[159] In addition, the name *Curcuma aromatica* Salisb. is considered synonymous with *Curcuma wenyujin* Y. H. Chen et C. Ling.[175] It should be noted that there have been changes in botanical nomenclature; these curcuma species have very similar appearances; plants show regional variation; and there may be hybridisation.[176,177] The diversity of names reflects these issues rather than changes in the traditional sources of the herb. These and other *Curcuma* species have widespread uses in traditional medicine and as foods in East, Southeast and South Asia.[178–180]

There is considerable similarity between the above *Curcuma* species in terms of their constituent compounds, although there is variability in their concentrations, which can vary according to species, production location and method of processing.[181–186] Major compounds include the terpenoids (beta-elemene, delta-elemene, gamma-elemene, curdine, curcumenol, isoprocurcumenol, germacrone, furanodiene, curdione, furanodienone, curcumol, curzerenone (alsos known as zedoarone), zederone, curcuzedoalide, borneol and camphor), curcumin and other curcuminoids,[159,185,187] diarylheptanoids[188,189] and polysaccharides.[190]

Compared to *Curcuma longa* L., the source of turmeric (*jiang huang* 姜黄), the content of curcumin is relatively low in the above *Curcuma* species.[191] The effects of curcumin in cancers, including CRC, has been reviewed extensively elsewhere[192,193] so curcumin is not included in this chapter.

Effects on Tumours

In a review of *Curcuma zedoaria*, it was reported to have shown anti-mutagenic effects, and cyctotoxic and inhibitory activity in multiple cancers.[194] An essential oil from *C. zedoaria* showed anti-proliferative effects in B16BL6 (mouse melanoma) and SMMC-7721 (human hepatoma) cells. It also showed inhibition of angiogenesis in a rat aortic ring assay, in a chick embryo chorioallantoic membrane assay, in mice injected with B16BL6 cells and in a mouse model of lung metastasis. A likely mechanism was inhibition of MMP-2 and MMP-9.[195] An extract of *C. zedoaria* showed inhibition of proliferation, invasion and colony formation in human esophageal cancer TE-8 cells, and suppression of tumour formation in nude mice. Analysis of multiple proteins involved in the caspase cascade indicated induction of apoptosis, while downregulation of fibroblast growth factor receptor 1 (FGFR1) and MMP-2 suggested inhibition of angiogenesis and cell migration.[196] Extracts of *C. phaeocaulis* showed free-radical scavenging activity and anti-inflammatory activity, and significantly inhibited proliferation of SMMC-7721 (hepatocarcinoma), HepG-2 (hepatocellular carcinoma), A-549 (lung adenocarcinoma) and HeLa (endocervical adenocarcinoma) cell lines.[197]

Partially purified polysaccharide fractions from *C. zedoaria* inhibited tumour size in mice transplanted with sarcoma-180 cells without showing clastogenic effects.[198] Polysaccharides extracted from *C. kwangsiensis* were found to inhibit the proliferation of CNE-2 nasopharyngeal carcinoma cells. There were dose-dependent reductions in Bcl-2 protein expression and increases in p53 expression, indicating induction of apoptosis.[190]

Beta-elemene and delta-elemene

Of the compounds identified in *e zhu* 莪术 species, beta-elemene has received the most research attention in cancer, and this compound has been approved as an anti-cancer adjuvant drug in China.[187] In a review of beta-elemene in multiple cancers, the evidence suggests that cell cycle arrest and induction of apoptosis are likely mechanisms of action, and it has also shown anti-angiogenic activity. In addition, when combined with anti-cancer drugs, it has shown chemosensitisation of cells to cisplatin, oxaliplatin and taxanes, and has been found to sensitise multi-drug-resistant cells.[199] In hepatocellular carcinoma cells and in xenografts in nude mice, the combination of beta-elemene with oxaliplatin significantly augmented oxaliplatin-induced apoptosis by enhancing cellular uptake of oxaliplatin.[200] In cervical cancer SiHa cells, beta-elemene dose- and time-dependently inhibited proliferation and induced apoptosis via attenuation of the Wnt/b-catenin signalling pathway.[201] In two CRC cell lines (HCT-116 and HT-29), beta-elemene reduced cell viability; increased the proportions of apoptotic cells and upregulated the expression of Bax; and cleaved caspase-3 and caspase-9. Moreover, combining beta-elemene with 5-FU enhanced the sensitivity to 5-FU in both cell lines, suggesting a possible application of beta-elemene in 5-FU resistance.[202] In comparison, delta-elemene induced apoptosis in HeLa cells without inhibiting growth of normal liver WRL-68 cells.[203] It was reported to induce apoptosis in colorectal adenocarcinoma DLD-1 cells via the mitochondrial-mediated pathway.[204]

Curcumol and isocurcumenol

Curcumol induced apoptosis in human LoVo CRC cells in a dose- and time-dependent manner and inhibited tumour growth in xenograft models in nude mice.[205] Also, curcumol was reported to induce cell cycle arrest at the G0/G1 phase in human LoVo and SW-480 colon cancer cells and in human colon cancer cell xenografts in nude mice.[206]

Isocurcumenol, isolated from *C. zedoaria*, inhibited proliferation and induced apoptosis in Daltons lymphoma ascites (DLAs), lung carcinoma (A-549), nasopharyngeal carcinoma (KB) and leukaemia (K-562) cells. In mice inoculated with DLAs, treatment with isocurcumenol reduced tumour volumes and increased lifespans.[207]

Other compounds

The compounds curdione, furanodienone, curcumol and germacrone were ultrasonically extracted from *C. wenyujin*. The extract and the individual compounds were each tested for anti-proliferative activity in RKO (colon cancer) and HT-29 (colon adenocarcinoma) cells. Of the compounds, furanodienone showed the greatest inhibition of cell growth in both cell lines. However, the *C. wenyujin* extract showed greater inhibition compared to any of the compounds individually.[208] A similar result was reported for *C. phaeocaulis* using the same method.[209]

A bioassay-guided isolation of active compounds from *C. zedoaria* found that curzerenone and alismol significantly inhibited cell proliferation and induced apoptosis in three human cancer cell lines — MCF-7 (breast cancer), Ca Ski (cervical squamous cell carcinoma) and HCT-116 (CRC) — in a dose-dependent manner via activation of caspase-3.[210] In a cell migration assay of human colon cancer RKO cells, nine sesquiterpenoids derived from *C. kwangsiensis*, including newly identified compounds, were investigated for their anti-migratory activities. Of the nine compounds, compound 3 (acomadendrane-4beta,10beta-diol) showed good time-dependent activity.[211]

Anti-inflammatory Effects

In a series of animal models of inflammation, an extract of *C. wenyujin* was found to show greater anti-inflammatory and anti-nociceptive activities, compared to an extract of *Scutellaria baicalensis* Georgi (*huang qin* 黄芩), and resulted in greater reductions in the levels of TNF-alpha and IL-6.[212] Fractional extraction of an essential oil obtained from *C. wenyujin* rhizomes yielded 11 sesquiterpenes which were tested in RAW 264.7 macrophages for inhibition of LPS-induced inflammation. All compounds showed inhibition of NO production with some showing stronger activities than the positive control hydrocortisone.[213]

In LPS-activated macrophages, an extract of *C. zedoaria*, that contained curcuminoids and sesquiterpenes, inhibited TNF-alpha production.[214] In a mouse ear oedema model of inflammation, fractionated extracts of *C. zedoaria*, notably furanodiene and furanodienone, showed potent anti-inflammatory activity.[215] In an adjuvant-induced paw swelling model in mice, a methanol extract of *C. phaeocaulis* showed significant inhibitory effects on inflammation and downregulated COX-2.[191]

Immunoregulatory Effects

A pectin-type polysaccharide isolated from *C. kwangsiensis* was tested for its effects on immunosuppression induced by myeloid-derived suppressor cells (MDSCs), which can accumulate in tumour-bearing hosts. The polysaccharide was reported to promote the recovery of CD4+ and CD8+ T cells, suggesting it could reverse MDSC-mediated T cell suppression.[216]

Antioxidant Effects

In a comparison of essential oils from four *Curcuma* species (*C. phaeocaulis, C. wenyujin, C. kwangsiensis* and *C. longa*), all had DPPH free-radical scavenging ability with the highest potency being for *C. kwangsiensis*, followed by *C. wenyujin, C. phaeocaulis* and *C. longa*.[184]

Summary of Evidence from *In Vivo* and *In Vitro* Studies

This brief review included studies of the effects of each of the ten herbs in experimental models of cancer (with a focus on CRC), their effects on inflammation and the immune system, as well as reports on their antioxidant effects. The number of studies published in English in each of these areas varied considerably between herbs, with some herbs having very few papers directly relevant to CRC. For these herbs, we have briefly examined their effects in other cancers. It is important to note that this review does not include every published study and the Chinese language literature was not reviewed, so it is likely that studies on these herbs in CRC models have been missed.

The selection of herbs for this review was based on the highest frequency herbs in formulas included in the meta-analysis pool for objective tumour response (ORR) which showed that the addition of CHMs to chemotherapy improved ORR. These formulas comprised multiple herbs, and it was not possible to determine which herbs were included in the formulas in order to enhance tumour response and which herbs were included for other reasons, such as to alleviate the adverse effects of the chemotherapy, support the immune system or as components of the overall formula dynamic.

One of the most frequently used formulas in the clinical studies was *Liu jun zi tang* 六君子汤 with various modifications. Therefore, it was not surprising that its ingredients were high on the frequency list and appear in this chapter. These include *dang shen* 党参 (as a substitute for *ren shen* 人参), *bai zhu* 白术, *fu ling* 茯苓, *gan cao* 甘草 and *ban xia* 半夏. The remaining ingredient, *chen pi* 陳皮, was excluded due to its slightly lower frequency. *Huang qi* 黄芪 is a frequent addition in modified versions of this formula. A large study of prescriptions for CRC patients found modified *Liu jun zi tang* 六君子汤 to be one of the principal formulas for CRC.[118] This formula has long been used for managing a wide range of gastrointestinal disorders and for supplementing debility. The herb *ban xia* 半夏 is a frequent inclusion in formulas for nausea and vomiting, while both *dang shen* 党参 and *huang qi* 黄芪 are frequently used for debility due to *qi* deficiency. It is likely that the clinicians who designed the formulas used in the clinical trials had these functions in mind, rather than the direct effects of these herbs on cancer or inflammation. Nevertheless, the experimental studies show that a number of these herbs, notably *huang qi* 黄芪, have shown anti-cancer effects in models of CRC.

The herbs *she she cao* 蛇舌草 and *ban zhi lian* 半枝莲 are a typical herb pair in anti-cancer formulas and have long been considered to have tumour inhibitory effects in a diversity of cancers including CRC. Both have received considerable research attention in CRC and show promise for drug discovery.

Consumption of the food grain *yi yi ren* 薏苡仁 is considered cancer protective and it is a frequent addition to herbal formulas. As the adjuvant anti-cancer drug Kanglaite, *Coix* has been used in clinical trials for numerous cancers, including CRC, but injection products were excluded in Chapter 5 so the effects of Kanglaite in CRC were not evaluated. In the included experimental studies, the research focus was on *yi yi ren* 薏苡仁 for prevention of CRC development, reflecting its role as an important health food.

The various *Curcuma* species used as *e zhu* 莪术 have widespread use in both food and medicine. *E zhu* 莪术 is also a typical inclusion in herbal formulas for reducing masses and treating cancer; and one of its constituents, beta-elemene, is currently used as an anti-cancer adjuvant drug.

With regard to anti-inflammatory activity, all the herbs except *ban xia* 半夏 have shown activity, with many of the studies using similar models. With regard to immunoregulatory effects, there was a diversity of approaches to studying this complex field. Herbs used for supplementing *qi* such as *dang shen* 党参, *huang qi* 黄芪, *bai zhu* 白术 and *fu ling* 茯苓 have received considerable attention, while no studies or few studies were found for *gan cao* 甘草, *ban xia* 半夏 and the four anti-cancer herbs. It was not possible to determine whether this indicated lack of effects for these herbs or reflected research attention on other aspects of their bioactivities. Similarly, studies of antioxidant effects showed variation between herbs, but we did not search every constituent chemical for every herb, so a number of relevant studies may have been missed.

Overall, the evidence indicates the Chinese herbs listed above and their constituent compounds show activities that could directly, or indirectly, influence the progression of CRC and/or complement CRC chemotherapy. However, these results should not be over-interpreted. When used in a clinical context, the concentrations of particular constituents in the herbs are very different to those in experimental models; the degree of absorbance in humans is different; and multiple herbs are usually used in combination. Therefore, it cannot be assumed that the effects obtained in cell lines and animals with translate to the clinic.

List of Abbreviations

5-FU: 5-Fluorouracil; ABCB1: ATP-binding cassette, subfamily B, member 1; ABCG2: ATP-binding cassette, subfamily G, member 2; ABTS⁺: 2,2′-azinobis (3-ethylbenzothiazoline-6-sulfonic acid) radical cation decolourisation assay; ACF: aberrant crypt foci; AKT: protein kinase B; AMPK: AMP-activated protein kinase; AOM: azoxymethane; B7-H3 aka CD276: cluster of differentiation 276; Bax: Bcl-2-associated X protein; b-catenin: beta-catenin; Bcl-2: B-cell lymphoma 2; BCL2: gene that encodes Bcl-2; Bcl-x(L): B-cell lymphoma-extra large; bFGF: basic fibroblast growth factor; CD31: cluster of differentiation 31, aka PECAM-1: platelet endothelial cell adhesion molecule; CDK4: cyclin-dependent kinase 4; c-Myc: MYC proto-oncogene; COX-2: cyclooxygenase-2; CREB1: cAMP-responsive element-binding protein 1; DAPK1: death-associated protein kinase-1; DMH: 1,2-dimethylhydrazine; DPPH: 1,1-diphenyl-2-picrylhydrazyl; DSS: dextran sulfate sodium; E-cadherin: epithelial-cadherin; EMT: epithelial to mesenchymal transition; eNOS, endothelial nitric oxide synthase; EphB3: Ephrin type-B receptor 3; ERK: extracellular signal-regulated kinase; ETS2: ETS proto-oncogene 2; FGFR1: fibroblast growth factor receptor 1; HIF1-a: hypoxia-inducible factor 1-alpha; Hsp90: heat shock protein-90; HUVEC: human umbilical vein endothelial cell; ICAM-1: intercellular adhesion molecule 1; IFN-gamma: interferon-gamma; Ig: immunoglobulin; IL-1beta: interleukin-1 beta; iNOS: inducible nitric oxide synthase; IkB: inhibitor of kappa B; JNK: c-Jun N-terminal kinase; Lgr5: leucine-rich repeat containing G-protein coupled receptor 5; LPS: lipopolysaccharide; MAPK: mitogen-activated protein kinase; MCP-1: monocyte chemoattractant protein 1; MDF: mucin-depleted foci; miR-149: microRNA-149; MIR34A: a tumour-suppressor gene that encodes miR-34A; MMP-2: matrix metalloproteinase-2; MMP-9: matrix metalloproteinase-9; mTOR: serine/threonine-protein kinase mTOR; mTORC1: mammalian target of rapamycin complex 1; N-cadherin: neural cadherin; NF-κB: nuclear factor kappa-light-chain-enhancer of activated B cells; NK cell: natural killer cell (type of T cell); NO: nitric oxide; NOTCH3: neurogenic locus notch homolog protein 3; p38: P38 mitogen-activated protein kinases;

p53: cellular tumour antigen p53; p70S6K: 70 kDa ribosomal protein S6 kinase 1; PARP: poly-(ADP)-ribose polymerase; PCNA: proliferating cell nuclear antigen; PGE2: prostaglandin E2; P-gp: P-glycoprotein; PI3K/AKT: phosphoinositide 3-kinase/protein kinase B pathway; PIM1: proviral integration site 1 gene; PTEN: phosphatase and tensin homolog; RAS: Rat sarcoma family of oncogenes; RUNX2: runt-related transcription factor 2; SMAD4: mothers against decapentaplegic homolog 4; STAT3: signal transducer and activator of transcription 3; TGF-beta: transforming growth factor-beta; TLR4: toll-like receptor 4; TNF-alpha: tumour necrosis factor-alpha; VEGF: vascular endothelial growth factor; VEGFR-2: vascular endothelial growth factor receptor-2; VCAM-1: vascular cell adhesion molecule 1; Wnt: wingless/integrated signalling pathway.

References

1. Chinese Pharmacopoeia Commission. (2015) *Zhong Hua Ren Min Gong He Guo Yao Dian* [*Pharmacopoeia of the People's Republic of China.*] China Medical Science Press, Beijing.
2. Zhu B, Zhang QL, Hua JW, *et al.* (2018) The traditional uses, phytochemistry, and pharmacology of Atractylodes macrocephala Koidz.: A review. *J Ethnopharmacol* **226:** 143–167.
3. Lin Z, Liu YF, Qu Y, *et al.* (2015) Characterisation of oligosaccharides from bai zhu by HILIC-MS. *Nat Prod Res* **29(13):** 1194–1200.
4. Li YJ, Zhang YS, Wang ZM, *et al.* (2012) Quantitative analysis of atractylenolide I in rat plasma by LC-MS/MS method and its application to pharmacokinetic study. *J Pharm Biomed Anal* **58:** 172–176.
5. Hasada K, Yoshida T, Yamazaki T, *et al.* (2010) Quantitative determination of atractylon in Atractylodis rhizoma and Atractylodis lanceae rhizoma by H-1-NMR spectroscopy. *J Nat Med* **64(2):** 161–166.
6. Li LY, Cao FF, Su ZJ, *et al.* (2015) Assessment of the embryotoxicity of four Chinese herbal extracts using the embryonic stem cell test. *Mol Med Rep* **12(2):** 2348–2354.
7. Zhang JD, Cao G, Xia YH, *et al.* (2014) Fast analysis of principal volatile compounds in crude and processed Atractylodes macrocephala by an automated static headspace gas chromatography-mass spectrometry. *Pharmacogn Mag* **10(39):** 249–253.

8. Wang XT, Li LH, Ran XK, *et al.* (2016) What caused the changes in the usage of Atractylodis macrocephalae rhizoma from ancient to current times? *J Nat Med* **70(1):** 36–44.

9. Lin X, Xu W, Shao M, *et al.* (2015) Shenling baizhu san supresses colitis associated colorectal cancer through inhibition of epithelial-mesenchymal transition and myeloid-derived suppressor infiltration. *BMC Complement Altern Med* **15(126):** 1–15.

10. Li L, Jing L, Wang J, *et al.* (2018) Autophagic flux is essential for the downregulation of d-dopachrome tautomerase by atractylenolide I to ameliorate intestinal adenoma formation. *J Cell Commun Signal* **12(4):** 689–698.

11. Liu Y, Jia Z, Dong L, *et al.* (2008) A randomized pilot study of atractylenolide I on gastric cancer cachexia patients. *Evid Based Complement Alternat Med* **5(3):** 337–344.

12. Tian S, Yu HD. (2017) Atractylenolide II inhibits proliferation, motility and induces apoptosis in human gastric carcinoma cell lines HGC-27 and AGS. *Molecules* **22(11):** 1–10.

13. Ye Y, Wang H, Chu JH, *et al.* (2011) Atractylenolide II induces G1 cell-cycle arrest and apoptosis in B16 melanoma cells. *J Ethnopharmacol* **136(1):** 279–282.

14. Liu H, Zhu Y, Zhang T, *et al.* (2013) Anti-tumor effects of atractylenolide I isolated from Atractylodes macrocephala in human lung carcinoma cell lines. *Molecules* (Basel, Switzerland) **18(11):** 13357–13368.

15. Kang TH, Bang JY, Kim MH, *et al.* (2011) Atractylenolide III, a sesquiterpenoid, induces apoptosis in human lung carcinoma A549 cells via mitochondria-mediated death pathway. *Food Chem Toxicol* **49(2):** 514–519.

16. Wang S, Cai R, Ma J, *et al.* (2015) The natural compound codonolactone impairs tumor induced angiogenesis by downregulating BMP signaling in endothelial cells. *Phytomedicine* **22(11):** 1017–1026.

17. Liu QS, Deng R, Yan QF, *et al.* (2017) Novel beta-tubulin-immobilized nanoparticles affinity material for screening beta-tubulin inhibitors from a complex mixture. *ACS Appl Mater Interfaces* **9(7):** 5725–5732.

18. Shim AR, Dong GZ, Lee HJ, Ryu JH. (2015) Atractylochromene is a repressor of Wnt/beta-catenin signaling in colon cancer cells. *Biomol Ther (Seoul)* **23(1):** 26–30.

19. Li XJ, Liu F, Li Z, *et al.* (2014) Atractylodes macrocephala polysaccharides induces mitochondrial-mediated apoptosis in glioma C6 cells. *Int J Biol Macromol* **66:** 108–112.

20. Li CQ, He LC, Dong HY, Jin JQ. (2007) Screening for the anti-inflammatory activity of fractions and compounds from Atractylodes macrocephala Koidz. *J Ethnopharmacol* **114(2):** 212–217.
21. Li CQ, He LC, Jin JQ. (2007) Atractylenolide I and atractylenolide III inhibit lipopolysaccharide-induced TNF-alpha and NO production in macrophages. *Phytother Res* **21(4):** 347–353.
22. Wang C, Duan H, He L. (2009) Inhibitory effect of atractylenolide I on angiogenesis in chronic inflammation in vivo and in vitro. *Eur J Pharmacol* **612(1–3):** 143–152.
23. Han KH, Park JM, Jeong M, *et al.* (2017) Heme oxygenase-1 induction and anti-inflammatory actions of Atractylodes macrocephala and Taraxacum herba extracts prevented colitis and was more effective than sulfasalazine in preventing relapse. *Gut Liver* **11(5):** 655–666.
24. Ji GQ, Chen RQ, Zheng JX. (2015) Macrophage activation by polysaccharides from Atractylodes macrocephala Koidz through the Nuclear Factor-kappaB pathway. *Pharm Biol* **53(4):** 512–517.
25. Sun W, Meng K, Qi C, *et al.* (2015) Immune-enhancing activity of polysaccharides isolated from Atractylodis macrocephalae Koidz. *Carbohydr Polym* **126:** 91–96.
26. Li WY, Guo SX, Xu DN, *et al.* (2018) Polysaccharide of Atractylodes macrocephala Koidz (PAMK) relieves immunosuppression in cyclophosphamide- treated geese by maintaining a humoral and cellular immune balance. *Molecules* **23(4):** 1–15.
27. Li X, Lin J, Han W, *et al.* (2012) Antioxidant ability and mechanism of rhizoma Atractylodes macrocephala. *Molecules* **17(11):** 13457–13472.
28. Hu AJ, Zhao SN, Liang HH, *et al.* (2007) Ultrasound assisted super-critical fluid extraction of oil and coixenolide from adlay seed. *Ultrason Sonochem* **14(2):** 219–224.
29. Huang DW, Kuo YH, Lin FY, *et al.* (2009) Effect of adlay (Coix lachryma-jobi L. var. Ma-yuen Stapf) testa and its phenolic components on Cu2+-treated low-density lipoprotein (LDL) oxidation and lipopolysaccharide (LPS)-induced inflammation in Raw 264.7 macrophages. *J Agric Food Chem* **57(6):** 2259 2266.
30. Lee MY, Lin HY, Cheng FW, *et al.* (2008) Isolation and characterization of new lactam compounds that inhibit lung and colon cancer cells from adlay (Coix lachryma-jobi L. var. Ma-yuen Stapf) bran. *Food Chem Toxicol* **46(6):** 1933–1939.

31. Lin LJ, Hsiao ESL, Tseng HS, *et al.* (2009) Molecular cloning, mass spectrometric identification, and nutritional evaluation of 10 coixins in adlay (Coix lachryma-jobi L.). *J Agric Food Chem* **57(22):** 10916–10921.

32. Wang LF, Chen C, Su AX, *et al.* (2016) Structural characterization of phenolic compounds and antioxidant activity of the phenolic-rich fraction from defatted adlay (Coix lachryma-jobi L. var. Ma-yuen Stapf) seed meal. *Food Chem* **196:** 509–517.

33. Xi XJ, Zhu YG, Tong YP, *et al.* (2016) Assessment of the genetic diversity of different Job's tears (Coix lacryma-jobi L.) accessions and the active composition and anticancer effect of its seed oil. *PloS One* **11(4):** 1–22.

34. Lu Y, Li CS, Dong Q. (2008) Chinese herb related molecules of cancer-cell-apoptosis: A minireview of progress between kanglaite injection and related genes. *J Exp Clin Cancer Res* **27(31):** 1–5.

35. Shih CK, Chiang WC, Kuo ML. (2004) Effects of adlay on azoxymethane-induced colon carcinogenesis in rats. *Food Chem Toxicol* **42(8):** 1339–1347.

36. Chung CP, Hsu HY, Huang DW, *et al.* (2010) Ethyl acetate fraction of adlay bran ethanolic extract inhibits oncogene expression and suppresses dmh-induced preneoplastic lesions of the colon in F344 rats through an anti-inflammatory pathway. *J Agric Food Chem* **58(13):** 7616–7623.

37. Li SC, Chen CM, Lin SH, *et al.* (2011) Effects of adlay bran and its ethanolic extract and residue on preneoplastic lesions of the colon in rats. *J Sci Food Agric* **91(3):** 547–552.

38. Manosroi A, Sainakham M, Chankhampan C, *et al.* (2016) In vitro anticancer activities of Job's tears (Coix lachryma-jobi Linn.) extracts on human colon adenocarcinoma. *Saudi J Biol Sci* **23(2):** 248–256.

39. Manosroi A, Sainakham M, Chankhampan C, *et al.* (2016) Potent in vitro anti-proliferative, apoptotic and anti-oxidative activities of semi-purified Job's tears (Coix lachryma-jobi Linn.) extracts from different preparation methods on 5 human cancer cell lines. *J Ethnopharmacol* **187:** 281–292.

40. Son ES, Kim YO, Park CG, *et al.* (2017) Coix lacryma-jobi var. Ma-yuen stapf sprout extract has anti-metastatic activity in colon cancer cells in vitro. *BMC Complement Altern Med* **17(1):** 486.

41. Seo WG, Pae HO, Chai KY, *et al.* (2000) Inhibitory effects of methanol extract of seeds of Job's tears (Coix lachryma-jobi L. var. Ma-yuen) on nitric oxide and superoxide production in Raw 264.7 macrophages. *Immunopharmacol Immunotoxicol* **22(3):** 545–554.

42. Choi G, Han AR, Lee JH, *et al.* (2015) A comparative study on hulled adlay and unhulled adlay through evaluation of their LPS-induced anti-inflammatory effects, and isolation of pure compounds. *Chem Biodivers* **12(3):** 380–387.

43. Wang L, Chen J, Xie H, *et al.* (2013) Phytochemical profiles and antioxidant activity of adlay varieties. *J Agric Food Chem* **61(21):** 5103–5113.

44. Liu J, Hu XG, Yang Q, *et al.* (2010) Comparison of the immunoregulatory function of different constituents in Radix astragali and Radix hedysari. *J Biomed Biotechnol* **2010(479426):** 1–12.

45. Song JZ, Yiu HHW, Qiao CF, *et al.* (2008) Chemical comparison and classification of Radix astragali by determination of isoflavonoids and astragalosides. *J Pharm Biomed Anal* **47(2):** 399–406.

46. Tin MMY, Cho CH, Chan K, *et al.* (2007) Astragalus saponins induce growth inhibition and apoptosis in human colon cancer cells and tumor xenograft. *Carcinogenesis* **28(6):** 1347–1355.

47. Auyeung KKW, Mok NL, Wong CM, *et al.* (2010) Astragalus saponins modulate mTOR and ERK signaling to promote apoptosis through the extrinsic pathway in HT-29 colon cancer cells. *Int J Mol Med* **26(3):** 341–349.

48. Auyeung KK, Woo PK, Law PC, Ko JK. (2012) Astragalus saponins modulate cell invasiveness and angiogenesis in human gastric adenocarcinoma cells. *J Ethnopharmacol* **141(2):** 635–641.

49. Auyeung KKW, Law PC, Ko JKS. (2014) Combined therapeutic effects of vinblastine and astragalus saponins in human colon cancer cells and tumor xenograft via inhibition of tumor growth and proangiogenic factors. *Nutr Cancer* **66(4):** 662–674.

50. Auyeung KKW, Law PC, Ko JKS. (2012) Novel anti-angiogenic effects of formononetin in human colon cancer cells and tumor xenograft. *Oncol Rep* **28(6):** 2188–2194.

51. Wang AL, Li Y, Zhao Q, Fan LQ. (2018) Formononetin inhibits colon carcinoma cell growth and invasion by microRNA-149-mediated EPHB3 downregulation and inhibition of PI3k/AKT and STAT3 signaling pathways. *Mol Med Rep* **17(6):** 7721–7729.

52. Li L, Hou XJ, Xu RF, *et al.* (2017) Research review on the pharmacological effects of astragaloside IV. *Fundam Clin Pharmacol* **31(1):** 17–36.

53. Xie T, Li Y, Li SL, Luo HF. (2016) Astragaloside IV enhances cisplatin chemosensitivity in human colorectal cancer via regulating Notch3. *Oncol Res* **24(6):** 447–453.

54. Ye Q, Su L, Chen DG, Zheng WY, Liu Y. (2017) Astragaloside IV induced Mir-134 expression reduces EMT and increases chemotherapeutic sensitivity by suppressing Creb1 signaling in colorectal cancer cell line SW-480. *Cell Physiol Biochem* **43(4):** 1617–1626.

55. Picarda E, Ohaegbulam KC, Zang XX. (2016) Molecular pathways: Targeting B7-H3 (CD276) for human cancer immunotherapy. *Clin Cancer Res* **22(14):** 3425–3431.

56. Wang SX, Mou JG, Cui LS, *et al.* (2018) Astragaloside IV inhibits cell proliferation of colorectal cancer cell lines through down-regulation of B7-H3. *Biomed Pharmacother* **102:** 1037–1044.

57. Lai PKK, Chan JYW, Cheng L, *et al.* (2013) Isolation of anti-inflammatory fractions and compounds from the root of Astragalus membranaceus. *Phytother Res* **27(4):** 581–587.

58. Lai PKK, Chan JYW, Wu SB, *et al.* (2014) Anti-inflammatory activities of an active fraction isolated from the root of Astragalus membranaceus in RAW 264.7 macrophages. *Phytother Res* **28(3):** 395–404.

59. Zhang WJ, Frei B. (2015) Astragaloside IV inhibits NF-Kappa b activation and inflammatory gene expression in LPS-treated mice. *Mediators Inflamm* **2015(274314):** 1–11.

60. Li J, Xu L, Sang R, *et al.* (2018) Immunomodulatory and anti-inflammatory effects of total flavonoids of astragalus by regulating NF-Kappab and MAPK signalling pathways in RAW 264.7 macrophages. *Pharmazie* **73(10):** 589–593.

61. Cho WCS, Leung KN. (2007) In vitro and in vivo immunomodulating and immunorestorative effects of Astragalus membranaceus. *J Ethnopharmacol* **113(1):** 132–141.

62. Cho WCS, Leung KN. (2007) In vitro and in vivo anti-tumor effects of Astragalus membranaceus. *Cancer Lett* **252(1):** 43–54.

63. Kikuchi T, Uchiyama E, Ukiya M, *et al.* (2011) Cytotoxic and apoptosis-inducing activities of triterpene acids from Poria cocos. *J Nat Prod* **74(2):** 137–144.

64. Fu M, Wang L, Wang X, *et al.* (2018) Determination of the five main terpenoids in different tissues of Wolfiporia cocos. *Molecules* (*Basel, Switzerland*) **23(8):** 1–9.

65. Feng GF, Zheng Y, Sun Y, *et al.* (2018) A targeted strategy for analyzing untargeted mass spectral data to identify lanostane-type triterpene acids in Poria cocos by integrating a scientific information system and liquid chromatography-tandem mass spectrometry combined with ion mobility spectrometry. *Anal Chim Acta* **1033:** 87–99.

66. Wang WH, Dong HJ, Yan RY, *et al.* (2015) Comparative study of lanostane-type triterpene acids in different parts of Poria cocos (Schw.) Wolf by UHPLC-fourier transform MS and UHPLC-triple quadruple MS. *J Pharm Biomed Anal* **102:** 203–214.

67. Wang YZ, Zhang J, Zhao YL, *et al.* (2013) Mycology, cultivation, traditional uses, phytochemistry and pharmacology of Wolfiporia cocos (Schwein.) Ryvarden et Gilb.: A review. *J Ethnopharmacol* **147(2):** 265–276.

68. Ukiya M, Akihisa T, Tokuda H, *et al.* (2002) Inhibition of tumor-promoting effects by poricoic acids G and H and other lanostane-type triterpenes and cytotoxic activity of poricoic acids A and G from Poria cocos. *J Nat Prod* **65(4):** 462–465.

69. Rios JL. (2011) Chemical constituents and pharmacological properties of Poria cocos. *Planta Med* **77(7):** 681–691.

70. Rios JL, Andujar I, Recio MC, Giner RM. (2012) Lanostanoids from fungi: A group of potential anticancer compounds. *J Nat Prod* **75(11):** 2016–2044.

71. Ma J, Liu J, Lu CW, Cai DF. (2015) Pachymic acid induces apoptosis via activating ROS-dependent JNK and ER stress pathways in lung cancer cells. *Cancer Cell Int* **15(78):** 1–12.

72. Jeong JW, Lee WS, Go SI, *et al.* (2015) Pachymic acid induces apoptosis of EJ bladder cancer cells by DR5 up-regulation, ros generation, modulation of Bcl-2 and IAP family members. *Phytother Res* **29(10):** 1516–1524.

73. Cheng SJ, Swanson K, Eliaz I, *et al.* (2015) Pachymic acid inhibits growth and induces apoptosis of pancreatic cancer in vitro and in vivo by targeting ER stress. *PloS One* **10(4):** 1–20.

74. Sun YC. (2014) Biological activities and potential health benefits of polysaccharides from Poria cocos and their derivatives. *Int J Biol Macromol* **68:** 131–134.

75. Ke RD, Lin SF, Chen Y, *et al.* (2010) Analysis of chemical composition of polysaccharides from Poria cocos Wolf and its anti-tumor activity by NMR spectroscopy. *Carbohydr Polym* **80(1):** 31–34.

76. Huang QL, Jin Y, Zhang L, *et al.* (2007) Structure, molecular size and antitumor activities of polysaccharides from Poria cocos mycelia produced in fermenter. *Carbohydr Polym* **70(3):** 324–333.

77. Lee SR, Lee S, Moon E, *et al.* (2017) Bioactivity-guided isolation of anti-inflammatory triterpenoids from the sclerotia of Poria cocos using LPS-stimulated RAW264.7 cells. *Bioorganic Chem* **70:** 94–99.

78. Jeong JW, Lee HH, Han MH, *et al.* (2014) Ethanol extract of Poria cocos reduces the production of inflammatory mediators by suppressing the NF-Kappab signaling pathway in lipopolysaccharide-stimulated RAW 264.7 macrophages. *BMC Complement Altern Med* **14(101):** 1–8.

79. Lu MK, Cheng JJ, Lin CY, Chang CC. (2010) Purification, structural elucidation, and anti-inflammatory effect of a water-soluble 1,6-branched 1,3-alpha-d-galactan from cultured mycelia of Poria cocos. *Food Chem* **118(2):** 349–356.

80. Chang HH, Yeh CH, Sheu F. (2009) A novel immunomodulatory protein from Poria cocos induces Toll-like receptor 4-dependent activation within mouse peritoneal macrophages. *J Agric Food Chem* **57(14):** 6129–6139.

81. Chen R, He JY, Tong XL, *et al.* (2016) The Hedyotis diffusa Willd. (Rubiaceae): A review on phytochemistry, pharmacology, quality control and pharmacokinetics. *Molecules* **21(6):** 1–30.

82. Lin MH, Lin JM, Wei LH, *et al.* (2012) Hedyotis diffusa Willd. extract inhibits HT-29 cell proliferation via cell cycle arrest. *Exp Ther Med* **4(2):** 307–310.

83. Feng J, Jin Y, Peng J, *et al.* (2017) Hedyotis diffusa Willd. extract suppresses colorectal cancer growth through multiple cellular pathways. *Oncol Lett* **14(6):** 8197–8205.

84. Yan Z, Feng J, Peng J, *et al.* (2017) Chloroform extract of Hedyotis diffusa Willd. inhibits viability of human colorectal cancer cells via suppression of AKT and ERK signaling pathways. *Oncol Lett* **14(6):** 7923–7930.

85. Lu PH, Chen MB, Ji C, *et al.* (2016) Aqueous Oldenlandia diffusa extracts inhibits colorectal cancer cells via activating AMP-activated protein kinase signalings. *Oncotarget* **7(29):** 45889–45900.

86. Sun GD, Wei LH, Feng JY, *et al.* (2016) Inhibitory effects of Hedyotis diffusa Willd. on colorectal cancer stem cells. *Oncol Lett* **11(6):** 3875–3881.

87. Li QY, Wang XF, Shen AL, *et al.* (2015) Hedyotis diffusa Willd overcomes 5-fluorouracil resistance in human colorectal cancer HCT-8/5-fu cells by downregulating the expression of p-glycoprotein and ATP-binding casette subfamily g member 2. *Exp Ther Med* **10(5):** 1845–1850.

88. Lai ZJ, Yan ZK, Chen WJ, *et al.* (2017) Hedyotis diffusa Willld suppresses metastasis in 5-fluorouracil-resistant colorectal cancer cells by regulating the TGF-beta signaling pathway. *Mol Med Rep* **16(5):** 7752–7758.

89. Li QY, Lai ZJ, Yan ZK, *et al.* (2018) Hedyotis diffusa Willd inhibits proliferation and induces apoptosis of 5-FU resistant colorectal cancer cells by regulating the PI3k/AKT signaling pathway. *Mol Med Rep* **17(1):** 358–365.

90. Lin JM, Wei LH, Xu W, *et al.* (2011) Effect of Hedyotis diffusa Willd extract on tumor angiogenesis. *Mol Med Rep* **4(6):** 1283–1288.

91. Lin JM, Wei LH, Shen AL, *et al.* (2013) Hedyotis diffusa Willd extract suppresses sonic hedgehog signaling leading to the inhibition of colorectal cancer angiogenesis. *Int J Oncol* **42(2):** 651–656.

92. Chen YL, Lin YY, Li YC, Li CD. (2016) Total flavonoids of Hedyotis diffusa Willd inhibit inflammatory responses in LPS-activated macrophages via suppression of the NF-Kappa b and MAPK signaling pathways. *Exp Ther Med* **11(3):** 1116–1122.

93. Yoshida Y, Wang MQ, Liu JN, *et al.* (1997) Immunomodulating activity of Chinese medicinal herbs and Oldenlandia diffusa in particular. *Int J Immunopharmacol* **19(7):** 359–370.

94. Kuo YJ, Lin JP, Hsiao YT, *et al.* (2015) Ethanol extract of Hedyotis diffusa Willd affects immune responses in normal balb/c mice in vivo. *In Vivo* **29(4):** 453–460.

95. Ji S, Li ZW, Song W, *et al.* (2016) Bioactive constituents of Glycyrrhiza uralensis (licorice): Discovery of the effective components of a traditional herbal medicine. *J Nat Prod* **79(2):** 281–292.

96. Wang YC, Yang YS. (2007) Simultaneous quantification of flavonoids and triterpenoids in licorice using HPLC. *J Chromatogr B Analyt Technol Biomed Life Sci* **850(1–2):** 392–399.

97. Fu Y, Chen J, Li YJ, *et al.* (2013) Antioxidant and anti-inflammatory activities of six flavonoids separated from licorice. *Food Chem* **141(2):** 1063–1071.

98. Yin L, Guan ES, Zhang YB, *et al.* (2018) Chemical profile and anti-inflammatory activity of total flavonoids from Glycyrrhiza uralensis Fisch. *Iran J Pharm Res* **17(2):** 726–734.

99. Yang R, Li WD, Yuan BC, *et al.* (2018) The genetic and chemical diversity in three original plants of licorice, Glycyrrhiza uralensis Fisch., Glycyrrhiza inflata Bat. and Glycyrrhiza glabra L. *Pak J Pharm Sci* **31(2):** 525–535.

100. Yang R, Yuan BC, Ma YS, *et al.* (2017) The anti-inflammatory activity of licorice, a widely used Chinese herb. *Pharm Biol* **55(1):** 5–18.

101. Nourazarian SM, Nourazarian A, Majidinia M, Roshaniasl E. (2015) Effect of root extracts of medicinal herb Glycyrrhiza glabra on hsp90

gene expression and apoptosis in the HT-29 colon cancer cell line. *Asian Pac J Cancer Prev* **16(18):** 8563–8566.

102. Moser C, Lang SA, Kainz S, *et al.* (2007) Blocking heat shock protein-90 inhibits the invasive properties and hepatic growth of human colon cancer cells and improves the efficacy of oxaliplatin in p53-deficient colon cancer tumors in vivo. *Mol Cancer Ther* **6(11):** 2868–2878.

103. Khan R, Khan AQ, Lateef A, *et al.* (2013) Glycyrrhizic acid suppresses the development of precancerous lesions via regulating the hyperproliferation, inflammation, angiogenesis and apoptosis in the colon of wistar rats. *PloS One* **8(2):** 1–22.

104. Takahashi T, Takasuka N, Iigo M, *et al.* (2004) Isoliquiritigenin, a flavonoid from licorice, reduces prostaglandin E-2 and nitric oxide, causes apoptosis, and suppresses aberrant crypt foci development. *Cancer Sci* **95(5):** 448–453.

105. Zhao HX, Zhang XH, Chen XW, *et al.* (2014) Isoliquiritigenin, a flavonoid from licorice, blocks M2 macrophage polarization in colitis-associated tumorigenesis through downregulating PGE(2) and IL-6. *Toxicol Appl Pharmacol* **279(3):** 311–321.

106. Zorko BA, Perez LB, De Blanco EJC. (2010) Effects of ILTG on DAPK1 promoter methylation in colon and leukemia cancer cell lines. *Anticancer Res* **30(10):** 3945–3950.

107. Meng FC, Lin JK. (2018) Liquiritigenin inhibits colorectal cancer proliferation, invasion and epithelial to mesenchymal transition by decreasing expression of RUNT-related transcription factor 2. *Oncol Res* **27(2):** 139–146.

108. Ji S, Tang SN, Li K, *et al.* (2017) Licoricidin inhibits the growth of SW480 human colorectal adenocarcinoma cells in vitro and in vivo by inducing cycle arrest, apoptosis and autophagy. *Toxicol Appl Pharmacol* **326:** 25–33.

109. Kim YH, Shin EK, Kim DH, *et al.* (2010) Antiangiogenic effect of licochalcone A. *Biochem Pharmacol* **80(8):** 1152–1159.

110. Yao H, Li SG, Hu JA, *et al.* (2011) Chromatographic fingerprint and quantitative analysis of seven bioactive compounds of Scutellaria barbata. *Planta Med* **77(4):** 388–393.

111. Zhang ZF, He LL, Lu LY, *et al.* (2015) Characterization and quantification of the chemical compositions of Scutellaria barbatae herba and differentiation from its substitute by combining UHPLC-PDA-QTOF-MS/MS with UHPLC-MS/MS. *J Pharm Biomed Anal* **109:** 62–66.

112. Goh D, Lee YH, Ong ES. (2005) Inhibitory effects of a chemically standardized extract from Scutellaria barbata in human colon cancer cell lines, LOVO. *J Agric Food Chem* **53(21):** 8197–8204.

113. Pan R, Guo F, Lu H, *et al.* (2011) Development of the chromatographic fingerprint of Scutellaria barbata D. Don by GC-MS combined with chemometrics methods. *J Pharm Biomed Anal* **55(3):** 391–396.

114. Dai SJ, Peng WB, Shen L, *et al.* (2011) New norditerpenoid alkaloids from Scutellaria barbata with cytotoxic activities. *Nat Prod Res* **25(11):** 1019–1024.

115. Dai SJ, Wang GF, Chen M, Liu K, Shen L. (2007) Five new neo-clerodane diterpenoid alkaloids from Scutellaria barbata with cytotoxic activities. *Chem Pharm Bull* **55(8):** 1218–1221.

116. Liu HL, Kao TH, Shiau CY, Chen BH. (2018) Functional components in Scutellaria barbata D. Don with anti-inflammatory activity on RAW 264.7 cells. *J Food Drug Anal* **26(1):** 31–40.

117. Tao GY, Balunas MJ. (2016) Current therapeutic role and medicinal potential of Scutellaria barbata in traditional Chinese medicine and western research. *J Ethnopharmacol* **182:** 170–180.

118. Chao TH, Fu PK, Chang CH, *et al.* (2014) Prescription patterns of Chinese herbal products for post-surgery colon cancer patients in Taiwan. *J Ethnopharmacol* **155(1):** 702–708.

119. Yeh YC, Chen HY, Yang SH, *et al.* (2014) Hedyotis diffusa combined with Scutellaria barbata are the core treatment of Chinese herbal medicine used for breast cancer patients: A population-based study. *Evid Based Complement Alternat Med* **2014(202378):** 1–9.

120. Tsai TY, Livneh H, Hung TH, *et al.* (2017) Associations between prescribed Chinese herbal medicine and risk of hepatocellular carcinoma in patients with chronic hepatitis B: A nationwide population-based cohort study. *BMJ Open* **7(1):** 1–9.

121. Wei LH, Chen YQ, Lin JM, *et al.* (2011) Scutellaria barbata D. Don induces apoptosis of human colon carcinoma cell through activation of the mitochondrion-dependent pathway. *J Med Plant Res* **5(10):** 1962–1970.

122. Wei LH, Lin JM, Xu W, *et al.* (2012) Scutellaria barbata D. Don inhibits tumor angiogenesis via suppression of hedgehog pathway in a mouse model of colorectal cancer. *Int J Mol Sci* **13(8):** 9419–9430.

123. Zhao ZH, Holle L, Song W, *et al.* (2012) Antitumor and anti-angiogenic activities of Scutellaria barbata extracts in vitro are partially mediated by inhibition of AKT/protein kinase B. *Mol Med Rep* **5(3):** 788–792.

124. Dai ZJ, Lu WF, Gao J, *et al.* (2013) Anti-angiogenic effect of the total flavonoids in Scutellaria barbata D. Don. *BMC Complement Altern Med* **13(150):** 1–10.

125. Jin YY, Chen WJ, Yang H, *et al.* (2017) Scutellaria barbata D. Don inhibits migration and invasion of colorectal cancer cells via suppression of PI3K/AKT and TGF-beta/SMAD signaling pathways. *Exp Ther Med* **14(6):** 5527–5534.

126. Wei LH, Lin JM, Wu GW, *et al.* (2013) Scutellaria barbata D. Don induces G1/S arrest via modulation of p53 and AKT pathways in human colon carcinoma cells. *Oncol Rep* **29(4):** 1623–1628.

127. Jiang QQ, Li QY, Chen HW, *et al.* (2015) Scutellaria barbata D. Don inhibits growth and induces apoptosis by suppressing IL-6-inducible STAT3 pathway activation in human colorectal cancer cells. *Exp Ther Med* **10(4):** 1602–1608.

128. Lin JM, Chen YQ, Cai QY, *et al.* (2014) Scutellaria barbata D Don inhibits colorectal cancer growth via suppression of multiple signaling pathways. *Integr Cancer Ther* **13(3):** 240–248.

129. Wei LH, Lin JM, Chu JF, *et al.* (2017) Scutellaria barbata D. Don inhibits colorectal cancer growth via suppression of Wnt/beta-catenin signaling pathway. *Chin J Integr Med* **23(11):** 858–863.

130. Xu HL, Yu JM, Sun Y, *et al.* (2013) Scutellaria barbata D. Don extract synergizes the antitumor effects of low dose 5-fluorouracil through induction of apoptosis and metabolism. *Phytomedicine* **20(10):** 897–903.

131. Zhang L, Cai QY, Lin JM, *et al.* (2014) Chloroform fraction of Scutellaria barbata D. Don promotes apoptosis and suppresses proliferation in human colon cancer cells. *Mol Med Rep* **9(2):** 701–706.

132. Zhang L, Fang Y, Feng JY, *et al.* (2017) Chloroform fraction of Scutellaria barbata D. Don inhibits the growth of colorectal cancer cells by activating mir-34a. *Oncol Rep* **37(6):** 3695–3701.

133. Dai ZJ, Wu WY, Kang HF, *et al.* (2013) Protective effects of Scutellaria barbata against rat liver tumorigenesis. *Asian Pac J Cancer Prev* **14(1):** 261–265.

134. Dai ZJ, Wang BF, Lu WF, *et al.* (2013) Total flavonoids of Scutellaria barbata inhibit invasion of hepatocarcinoma via MMP/TIMP in vitro. *Molecules* **18(1):** 934–950.

135. Yang N, Zhao YY, Wang ZP, *et al.* (2017) Scutellarin suppresses growth and causes apoptosis of human colorectal cancer cells by regulating the p53 pathway. *Mol Med Rep* **15(2):** 929–935.

136. Sun PD, Sun D, Wang XD. (2017) Effects of Scutellaria barbata polysaccharide on the proliferation, apoptosis and emt of human colon cancer HT29 cells. *Carbohydr Polym* **167:** 90–96.
137. Klawitter J, Klawitter J, Gurshtein J, *et al.* (2011) Bezielle (BZL101)-induced oxidative stress damage followed by redistribution of metabolic fluxes in breast cancer cells: A combined proteomic and metabolomic study. *Int Cancer* **129(12):** 2945–2957.
138. Chen V, Staub RE, Fong S, *et al.* (2012) Bezielle selectively targets mitochondria of cancer cells to inhibit glycolysis and oxphos. *PloS One* **7(2):** 1–12.
139. Chen VV, Staub RE, Baggett S, *et al.* (2012) Identification and analysis of the active phytochemicals from the anti-cancer botanical extract Bezielle. *PloS One* **7(1):** 1–13.
140. Rugo H, Shtivelman E, Perez A, *et al.* (2007) Phase I trial and antitumor effects of BZL101 for patients with advanced breast cancer. *Breast Cancer Res Treat* **105(1):** 17–28.
141. Perez AT, Arun B, Tripathy D, *et al.* (2010) A phase 1b dose escalation trial of Scutellaria barbata (BZL101) for patients with metastatic breast cancer. *Breast Cancer Res Treat* **120(1):** 111–118.
142. Lee SR, Kim MS, Kim S, *et al.* (2017) Constituents from Scutellaria barbata inhibiting nitric oxide production in LPS-stimulated microglial cells. *Chem Biodivers* **14(11).**
143. Ye CL, Huang Q. (2012) Extraction of polysaccharides from herbal Scutellaria barbata D. Don (ban-zhi-lian) and their antioxidant activity. *Carbohydr Polym* **89(4):** 1131–1137.
144. He JY, Ma N, Zhu S, *et al.* (2015) The genus Codonopsis (Campanulaceae): A review of phytochemistry, bioactivity and quality control. *J Nat Med* **69(1):** 1–21.
145. Gao SM, Liu JS, Wang M, *et al.* (2018) Traditional uses, phytochemistry, pharmacology and toxicology of Codonopsis: A review. *J Ethnopharmacol* **219:** 50–70.
146. He JY, Zhu S, Goda Y, *et al.* (2014) Quality evaluation of medicinally-used Codonopsis species and Codonopsis radix based on the contents of pyrrolidine alkaloids, phenylpropanoid and polyacetylenes. *J Nat Med* **68(2):** 326–339.
147. Kim EY, Kim JA, Jeon HJ, *et al.* (2014) Chemical fingerprinting of Codonopsis pilosula and simultaneous analysis of its major components by HPLC-UV. *Arch Pharm Res* **37(9):** 1148–1158.

148. Wakana D, Kawahara N, Goda Y. (2013) Two new pyrrolidine alkaloids, codonopsinol C and codonopiloside A, isolated from Codonopsis pilosula. *Chem Pharm Bull* **61(12):** 1315–1317.

149. Wang L, Xu ML, Hu JH, *et al.* (2011) Codonopsis lanceolata extract induces G0/G1 arrest and apoptosis in human colon tumor HT-29 cells — involvement of ROS generation and polyamine depletion. *Food Chem Toxicol* **49(1):** 149–154.

150. Li W, Xu Q, He YF, *et al.* (2015) Anti-tumor effect of steamed Codonopsis lanceolata in H22 tumor-bearing mice and its possible mechanism. *Nutrients* **7(10):** 8294–8307.

151. Shen J, Lu X, Du W, *et al.* (2016) Lobetyol activate mapk pathways associated with G1/S cell cycle arrest and apoptosis in MKN45 cells in vitro and in vivo. *Biomed Pharmacother* **81:** 120–127.

152. Xin T, Zhang FB, Jiang QY, *et al.* (2012) The inhibitory effect of a polysaccharide from Codonopsis pilosula on tumor growth and metastasis in vitro. *Int J Biol Macromol* **51(5):** 788–793.

153. Wang W, Chen B, Zou RL, *et al.* (2014) Codonolactone, a sesquiterpene lactone isolated from Chloranthus henryi Hemsl, inhibits breast cancer cell invasion, migration and metastasis by downregulating the transcriptional activity of RUNX2. *Int J Oncol* **45(5):** 1891–1900.

154. Fu JJ, Ke XQ, Tan SL, *et al.* (2016) The natural compound codonolactone attenuates TGF-beta 1-mediated epithelial-to-mesenchymal transition and motility of breast cancer cells. *Oncol Rep* **35(1):** 117–126.

155. Shan BE, Yoshida Y, Sugiura T, Yamashita U. (1999) Stimulating activity of Chinese medicinal herbs on human lymphocytes in vitro. *Int J Immunopharmacol* **21(3):** 149–159.

156. Sun YX. (2009) Immunological adjuvant effect of a water-soluble polysaccharide, CPP, from the roots of Codonopsis pilosula on the immune responses to ovalbumin in mice. *Chem Biodivers* **6(6):** 890–896.

157. Zhang P, Hu LH, Bai RB, *et al.* (2017) Structural characterization of a pectic polysaccharide from Codonopsis pilosula and its immunomodulatory activities in vivo and in vitro. *Int J Biol Macromol* **104:** 1359–1369.

158. Fu YP, Feng B, Zhu ZK, *et al.* (2018) The polysaccharides from Codonopsis pilosula modulates the immunity and intestinal microbiota of cyclophosphamide-treated immunosuppressed mice. *Molecules* **23(7):** 1–13.

159. Jiangsu New Medical Academy, ed. (1986) *Zhong Yao Da Ci Dian* [*Great Compendium of Chinese Medicines.*] Shanghai Scientific and Technical Publishers, Shanghai.

160. Su T, Zhang WW, Zhang YM, *et al.* (2016) Standardization of the manufacturing procedure for Pinelliae rhizoma praeparatum cum zingibere et alumine. *J Ethnopharmacol* **193:** 663–669.

161. Yu HL, Pan YZ, Wu H, *et al.* (2015) The alum-processing mechanism attenuating toxicity of Araceae Pinellia ternata and Pinellia pedatisecta. *Arch Pharm Res* **38(10):** 1810–1821.

162. Liang ZT, Zhang J, Wong LL, *et al.* (2013) Characterization of secondary metabolites from the raphides of calcium oxalate contained in three Araceae family plants using laser microdissection and ultra-high performance liquid chromatography-quadrupole/time of flight-mass spectrometry. *Eur J Mass Spectrom* **19(3):** 195–210.

163. Lee JY, Park NH, Lee W, *et al.* (2016) Comprehensive chemical profiling of Pinellia species tuber and processed Pinellia tuber by gas chromatography-mass spectrometry and liquid chromatography-atmospheric pressure chemical ionization-tandem mass spectrometry. *J Chromatogr A* **1471:** 164–177.

164. Iwasa M, Iwasaki T, Ono T, Miyazawa M. (2014) Chemical composition and major odor-active compounds of essential oil from Pinellia tuber (dried rhizome of Pinellia ternata) as crude drug. *J Oleo Sci* **63(2):** 127–135.

165. Liu XC, Tian XP, Liu T, Liang JL. (2010) Disclosure of the tuberous lectin composed of homogeneous tetramers in Pinellia pedatisecda schott. *Appl Biochem Biotechnol* **162(4):** 1214–1223.

166. Zu G, Wang H, Wang J, *et al.* (2014) Rhizoma pinelliae trypsin inhibitor separation, purification and inhibitory activity on the proliferation of BGC-823 gastric adenocarcinoma cells. *Exp Ther Med* **8(1):** 248–254.

167. Zhang MX, Yu Y, Zhang HW, *et al.* (2017) Synergistic cytotoxic effects of a combined treatment of a Pinellia pedatisecta lipid-soluble extract and cisplatin on human cervical carcinoma in vivo. *Oncol Lett* **13(6):** 4748–4754.

168. Zhou L, Xu T, Zhang Y, *et al.* (2016) Transcriptional network in ovarian cancer cell line SKOV3 treated with Pinellia pedatisecta schott extract. *Oncol Rep* **36(1):** 462–470.

169. Rozema E, Popescu R, Sonderegger H, *et al.* (2012) Characterization of glucocerebrosides and the active metabolite 4,8-sphingadienine

from Arisaema amurense and Pinellia ternata by NMR and CD spectroscopy and ESI-MS/CID-MS. *J Agric Food Chem* **60(29):** 7204–7210.

170. Aida K, Kinoshita M, Sugawara T, *et al.* (2004) Apoptosis inducement by plant and fungus sphingoid bases in human colon cancer cells. *J Oleo Sci* **53(10):** 503–510.

171. Ahn EH, Schroeder JJ. (2002) Sphingoid bases and ceramide induce apoptosis in HT-29 and HCT-116 human colon cancer cells. *Exp Biol Med (Maywood)* **227(5):** 345–353.

172. Zuo ZY, Fan HD, Wang X, *et al.* (2012) Purification and characterization of a novel plant lectin from Pinellia ternata with antineoplastic activity. *Springerplus* **1(13):** 1–9.

173. Zhou W, Gao Y, Xu SW, *et al.* (2014) Purification of a mannose-binding lectin Pinellia ternata agglutinin and its induction of apoptosis in BEL-7404 cells. *Protein Expr Purif* **93:** 11–17.

174. Li Y, Li DJ, Chen J, Wang SG. (2016) A polysaccharide from Pinellia ternata inhibits cell proliferation and metastasis in human cholangiocarcinoma cells by targeting of CDC42 and 67 kda laminin receptor (LR). *Int J Biol Macromol* **93:** 520–525.

175. The Plant List 1.1. (2018) Available from: www.theplantlist.org/.

176. Kojima H, Yanai T, Toyota A. (1998) Essential oil constituents from Japanese and Indian Curcuma aromatica rhizomes. *Planta Med* **64(4):** 380–381.

177. Komatsu K, Sasaki Y, Tanaka K, *et al.* (2008) Morphological, genetic, and chemical polymorphism of Curcuma kwangsiensis. *J Nat Med* **62(4):** 413–422.

178. Liu YB, Roy SS, Nebie RHC, *et al.* (2013) Functional food quality of Curcuma caesia, Curcuma zedoaria and Curcuma aeruginosa endemic to northeastern India. *Plant Foods Hum Nutr* **68(1):** 72–77.

179. Xia Q, Zhao KJ, Huang ZG, *et al.* (2005) Molecular genetic and chemical assessment of Rhizoma curcumae in China. *J Agric Food Chem* **53(15):** 6019–6026.

180. Hao YF, Lu CL, Li DJ, *et al.* (2014) Protective effects of diphenylheptanes from Curcuma phaeocaulis Val. On H2O2 induced cell injury. *Food Funct* **5(7):** 1369–1373.

181. Yang FQ, Li SP, Chen Y, *et al.* (2005) Identification and quantitation of eleven sesquiterpenes in three species of Curcuma rhizomes by pressurized liquid extraction and gas chromatography-mass spectrometry. *J Pharm Biomed Anal* **39(3–4):** 552–558.

182. Deng CH, Ji J, Li N, *et al.* (2006) Fast determination of curcumol, curdione and germacrone in three species of Curcuma rhizomes by microwave-assisted extraction followed by headspace solid-phase microextraction and gas chromatography-mass spectrometry. *J Chromatogr A* **1117(2):** 115–120.

183. Zhang JS, Guan J, Yang FQ, *et al.* (2008) Qualitative and quantitative analysis of four species of Curcuma rhizomes using twice development thin layer chromatography. *J Pharm Biomed Anal* **48(3):** 1024–1028.

184. Zhang LY, Yang ZW, Chen DK, *et al.* (2017) Variation on composition and bioactivity of essential oils of four common Curcuma herbs. *Chem Biodivers* **14(11):** 1–11.

185. Wei MM, Chu C, Wang S, Yan JZ. (2018) Quantitative analysis of sesquiterpenes and comparison of three Curcuma wenyujin herbal medicines by micro matrix solid phase dispersion coupled with MEEKC. *Electrophoresis* **39(8):** 1119–1128.

186. An YW, Hu G, Yin GP, *et al.* (2014) Quantitative analysis and discrimination of steamed and non-steamed rhizomes of Curcuma wenyujin by GC-MS and HPLC. *J Chromatogr Sci* **52(9):** 961–970.

187. Lu JJ, Dang YY, Huang M, *et al.* (2012) Anti-cancer properties of terpenoids isolated from Rhizoma curcumae: A review. *J Ethnopharmacol* **143(2):** 406–411.

188. Li J, Liao CR, Wei JQ, *et al.* (2011) Diarylheptanoids from Curcuma kwangsiensis and their inhibitory activity on nitric oxide production in lipopolysaccharide-activated macrophages. *Bioorg Med Chem Lett* **21(18):** 5363–5369.

189. Chen SD, Gao JT, Liu JG, *et al.* (2015) Five new diarylheptanoids from the rhizomes of Curcuma kwangsiensis and their antiproliferative activity. *Fitoterapia* **102:** 67–73.

190. Zeng JH, Dai P, Ren LY, *et al.* (2012) Apoptosis-induced anti-tumor effect of Curcuma kwangsiensis polysaccharides against human nasopharyngeal carcinoma cells. *Carbohydr Polym* **89(4):** 1067–1072.

191. Tohda C, Nakayama N, Hatanaka F, Komatsu K. (2006) Comparison of anti-inflammatory activities of six Curcuma rhizomes: A possible curcuminoid independent pathway mediated by Curcuma phaeocaulis extract. *Evid Based Complement Alternat Med* **3(2):** 255–260.

192. Bachmeier BE, Killian PH, Melchart D. (2018) The role of curcumin in prevention and management of metastatic disease. *Int J Mol Sci* **19(6):** 1–18.

193. Jalili-Nik M, Soltani A, Moussavi S, *et al.* (2018) Current status and future prospective of curcumin as a potential therapeutic agent in the treatment of colorectal cancer. *J Cell Physiol* **233(9):** 6337–6345.

194. Lobo R, Prabhu KS, Shirwaikar A, Shirwaikar A. (2009) Curcuma zedoaria Rosc. (white turmeric): A review of its chemical, pharmacological and ethnomedicinal properties. *J Pharm Pharmacol* **61(1):** 13–21.

195. Chen WX, Lu Y, Gao M, *et al.* (2011) Anti-angiogenesis effect of essential oil from Curcuma zedoaria in vitro and in vivo. *J Ethnopharmacol* **133(1):** 220–226.

196. Hadisaputri YE, Miyazaki T, Suzuki S, *et al.* (2015) Molecular characterization of antitumor effects of the rhizome extract from Curcuma zedoaria on human esophageal carcinoma cells. *Int J Oncol* **47(6):** 2255–2263.

197. Hou Y, Lu CL, Zeng QH, Jiang JG. (2015) Anti-inflammatory, antioxidant and antitumor activities of ingredients of Curcuma phaeocaulis Val. *Excli J* **14:** 706–713.

198. Kim KI, Kim JW, Hong BS, *et al.* (2000) Antitumor, genotoxicity and anticlastogenic activities of polysaccharide from Curcuma zedoaria. *Mol Cells* **10(4):** 392–398.

199. Jiang ZY, Jacob JA, Loganathachetti DS, *et al.* (2017) Beta-elemene: Mechanistic studies on cancer cell interaction and its chemosensitization effect. *Front Pharmacol* **8:** 1–7.

200. Li XQ, Lin ZH, Zhang B, *et al.* (2016) Beta-elemene sensitizes hepatocellular carcinoma cells to oxaliplatin by preventing oxaliplatin-induced degradation of copper transporter 1. *Sci Rep* **6(21010):** 1–11.

201. Wang L, Zhao Y, Wu Q, *et al.* (2018) Therapeutic effects of beta-elemene via attenuation of the Wnt/beta-catenin signaling pathway in cervical cancer cells. *Mol Med Rep* **17(3):** 4299–4306.

202. Guo ZB, Liu ZZ, Yue HF, Wang JY. (2018) Beta-elemene increases chemosensitivity to 5-fluorouracil through down-regulating microRNA-191 expression in colorectal carcinoma cells. *J Cell Biochem* **119(8):** 7032–7039.

203. Wang XS, Yang W, Tao SJ, *et al.* (2006) The effect of delta-elemene on HeLa cell lines by apoptosis induction. *Yakugaku Zasshi* **126(10):** 979–990.

204. Xie CY, Yang W, Li M, *et al.* (2009) Cell apoptosis induced by delta-elemene in colorectal adenocarcinoma cells via a mitochondrial-mediated pathway. *Yakugaku Zasshi* **129(11):** 1403–1413.

205. Wang J, Huang FX, Bai Z, *et al.* (2015) Curcumol inhibits growth and induces apoptosis of colorectal cancer LOVO cell line via IGF-1R and p38 MAPK pathway. *Int J Mol Sci* **16(8):** 19851–19867.
206. Wang J, Li XM, Bai Z, *et al.* (2018) Curcumol induces cell cycle arrest in colon cancer cells via reactive oxygen species and AKT/GSK3 beta/cyclin D1 pathway. *J Ethnopharmacol* **210:** 1–9.
207. Lakshmi S, Padmaja G, Remani P. (2011) Antitumour effects of isocurcumenol isolated from Curcuma zedoaria rhizomes on human and murine cancer cells. *Int J Med Chem* **2011:** 253962.
208. Wang XQ, Jiang Y, Hu DD. (2016) Optimization and in vitro antiproliferation of Curcuma wenyujin's active extracts by ultrasonication and response surface methodology. *Chem Cent J* **10(32):** 1–14.
209. Wang XQ, Jiang Y, Hu DD. (2017) Antiproliferative activity of Curcuma phaeocaulis Valeton extract using ultrasonic assistance and response surface methodology. *Prep Biochem Biotechnol* **47(1):** 19–31.
210. Rahman SNSA, Wahab NA, Abd Malek SN. (2013) In vitro morphological assessment of apoptosis induced by antiproliferative constituents from the rhizomes of Curcuma zedoaria. *Evid Based Complement Alternat Med* **2013(257108):** 1–14.
211. Wang JT, Ge D, Qu HF, *et al.* (2018) Chemical constituents of Curcuma kwangsiensis and their antimigratory activities in RKO cells. *Nat Prod Res* **(Jun):** 1–7.
212. Zhou J, Qu F, Zhang HJ, *et al.* (2010) Comparison of anti-inflammatory and anti-nociceptive activities of Curcuma wenyujin YH Chen et C. Ling and Scutellaria baicalensis Georgi. *Afr J Tradit Complement Altern Med* **7(4):** 339–349.
213. Xia GY, Zhou L, Ma JH, *et al.* (2015) Sesquiterpenes from the essential oil of Curcuma wenyujin and their inhibitory effects on nitric oxide production. *Fitoterapia* **103:** 143–148.
214. Jang MK, Sohn DH, Ryu JH. (2001) A curcuminoid and sesquiterpenes as inhibitors of macrophage TNF-alpha release from Curcuma zedoaria. *Planta Med* **67(6):** 550–552.
215. Makabe H, Maru N, Kuwabara A, *et al.* (2006) Anti-inflammatory sesquiterpenes from Curcuma zedoaria. *Nat Prod Res* **20(7):** 680–685.
216. Dong CX, Zhang WS, Sun QL, *et al.* (2018) Structural characterization of a pectin-type polysaccharide from Curcuma kwangsiensis and its effects on reversing MDSC-mediated T cell suppression. *Int J Biol Macromol* **115:** 1233–1240.

7

Clinical Evidence for Acupuncture and Related Therapies

OVERVIEW

The searches identified 17 randomised controlled trials, no non-randomised controlled studies and two non-controlled studies of acupuncture and related therapies related to colorectal cancer. The therapies included manual acupuncture, electroacupuncture, warm needling, acupressure, ear acupuncture, ear acupressure and moxibustion. Most studies were for improving recovery after surgery for colorectal cancer, while three were for alleviating the adverse effects of chemotherapy. The meta-analyses focused on time to recovery of gastrointestinal function after surgery plus some data on incidence of postoperative urinary retention.

Introduction

Acupuncture is a family of techniques which stimulate acupoints to correct imbalances of energy (*qi*) and restore health to the body. Methods of stimulating acupuncture points include:

- Manual acupuncture: Insertion of an acupuncture needle into acupoints;
- Electroacupuncture: Application of electrical stimulation to acupoints;
- Warm needling: Using moxa on the end of the needle handle to warm the needles;
- Acupressure: Application of pressure to acupoints on the body;
- Ear acupuncture: Insertion of small needles into points or zones located on the ear;

- Ear acupressure: Application of pressure to points or zones located on the ear;
- Moxibustion: Burning of a herb (usually *ai ye* 艾叶 *Artemesia vulgaris* L.) close to, or on, the skin to induce a warming sensation.

Whilst many of these therapies have ancient roots, several have emerged as new techniques in the last century, including electroacupuncture and ear acupuncture.

Previous Systematic Reviews

One systematic review of acupuncture for recovery after colorectal cancer (CRC) surgery, that included seven randomised controlled trials (RCTs), concluded there was 'low' to 'moderate' quality evidence for the efficacy and safety of acupuncture for postoperative outcomes.[1] The other reviews and meta-analyses were not specific to CRC. One study concluded that acupuncture and moxibustion showed efficacy as an auxiliary treatment for cancer-related fatigue.[2] Another review concluded that no meaningful conclusion could be drawn regarding acupuncture for cancer-related fatigue[3] and a subsequent review reached a similar conclusion with regard to moxibustion.[4] One review concluded that the limited evidence suggested that moxibustion may be an effective support treatment for nausea and vomiting in cancer care[5] and another review of auricular therapy concluded it may be a promising approach for chemotherapy-induced nausea and vomiting.[6] For chemotherapy-induced leukopenia, one review found moxibustion appeared to increase white blood cell counts, but the quality of the studies was too low for firm conclusions.[7]

Identification of Clinical Studies

The searches identified 19 clinical trials of acupuncture and related therapies that met the inclusion criteria. These included 17 RCTs, no controlled clinical trials (CCTs) and two non-controlled studies (A18, A19) (Fig. 7.1).

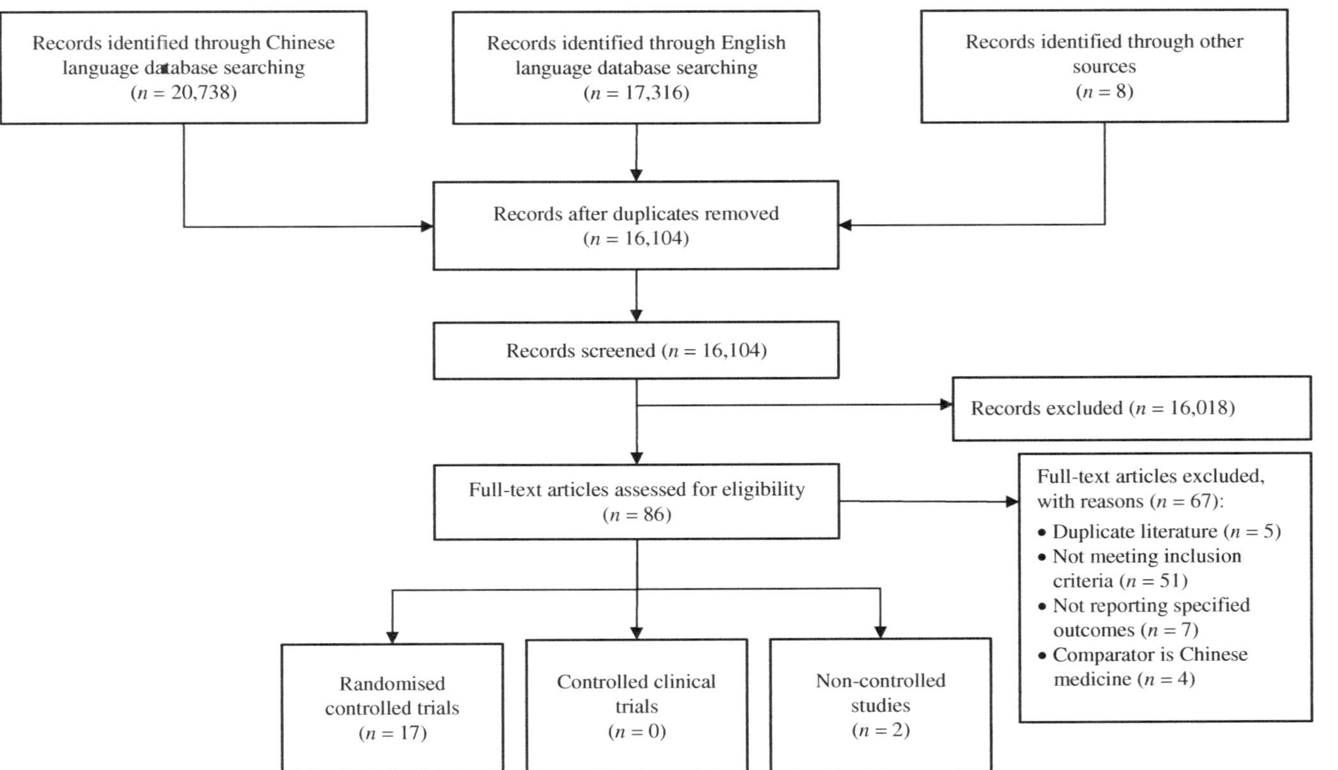

Fig. 7.1 Flowchart of Study Selection Process: acupuncture and related therapies.

The majority of studies (A1–A15, 15 studies) aimed to restore gastrointestinal functioning after surgery for CRC; one study (A16) aimed to improve recovery of urinary function after surgery for CRC; and three studies (A17–A19) were for treating adverse effects of chemotherapy. Two studies (A4, A7) involved three groups.

The test interventions included manual acupuncture (A1–A5, A16–A18), electroacupuncture (A4–A11), warm needling (A12), acupressure (A13), ear acupuncture (A5), ear acupressure (A3, A14, A15) and moxibustion (A16, A19). Three studies (A3, A5, A16) combined two or more methods. There were no studies of scalp acupuncture. Two studies (A5, A18) were conducted in the United States, 15 studies (A1–A4, A6, A8–A12, A14–A17, A19) in mainland China, one study (A7) in Hong Kong and one study (A13) in Taiwan. The studies tested the following types of acupuncture interventions:

- Manual acupuncture and/or electroacupuncture (nine RCTs, two non-controlled studies);
- Warm needling (one RCT);
- Acupuncture plus moxibustion (one RCT);
- Acupressure (one RCT);
- Ear acupressure alone (two RCTs);
- Ear acupressure plus manual acupuncture (one RCT);
- Ear acupuncture plus manual acupuncture plus electroacupuncture (one RCT);
- Moxibustion alone (one RCT).

Outline of the Data Analyses

Studies are grouped firstly by the main type of acupuncture therapy and then by the type of study (RCT, CCT or non-controlled study). Risk of bias (RoB) assessments and meta-analysis results of the 17 RCTs are presented separately in four groups for:

- Manual acupuncture, electroacupuncture, warm needling and manual acupuncture combined with moxibustion (11 RCTs);
- Acupressure (one RCT);

- Ear acupuncture and ear acupressure (with or without traditional points) (four RCTs);
- Moxibustion alone (one RCT).

Meta-analysis results of RCTs are presented for each type of acupuncture therapy for the following outcomes (if available):

- Postoperative recovery of gastrointestinal function (15 RCTs);
- Postoperative adverse reactions (four RCTs);
- Quality of life (one RCT);
- Immune function (one RCT);
- Chemotherapy-induced nausea and vomiting (one RCT).

Descriptions of any non-controlled studies and the reported results follow the RCTs in each group.

Studies of Acupuncture and Electroacupuncture

Eleven RCTs, no CCTs and two non-controlled studies used manual acupuncture, electroacupuncture, warm needling or manual acupuncture combined with moxibustion. In addition, one RCT (A3) combined ear acupressure and acupuncture on non-ear points and another RCT (A5) combined ear acupuncture, electroacupuncture and manual acupuncture. These two RCTs are included in acupuncture point calculations for RCTs in this section but the outcome results are reported separately in the section on ear acupuncture and ear acupressure.

Randomised Controlled Trials of Acupuncture and Electroacupuncture

In the 11 RCTs of manual acupuncture and/or electroacupuncture, warm needling, and acupuncture combined with moxibustion, there were 726 participants diagnosed with CRC. The age of participants ranged from 22 to 84 years, but the age range was not reported in two studies (A6, A7). Based on the reported means and standard deviations for ages, the majority of participants were aged between 50 and 80 years.

Test interventions were acupuncture using needles at traditional points in all 11 RCTs. Of these, seven RCTs (A4, A6–A11) added electroacupuncture, one (A12) used warm needling and one (A16) combined manual acupuncture with moxibustion. Two RCTs included three groups. One study (A4) compared separate manual acupuncture and electroacupuncture groups to usual postoperative care, so these groups were separated for analysis (A4.1, A4.2). Another compared electroacupuncture to sham electroacupuncture or usual postoperative care (A7). The other studies used two groups. In two RCTs (A6, A7) the control group used a sham acupuncture intervention.

All RCTs tested acupuncture for recovery after surgery. In 11 RCTs, the main outcomes related to recovery of gastrointestinal function and one RCT (A16) was for recovery of urinary function.

Syndromes

All of the 11 RCTs of acupuncture/electroacupuncture were for post-operative recovery, so there was no use of Chinese medicine syndrome differentiation.

Frequently Used Points in Randomised Controlled Trials of Acupuncture and Electroacupuncture

The points used most frequently in the 13 RCTs that used traditional acupuncture points (including the two studies that combined traditional points and ear points) were ST36 *Zusanli* 足三里, ST37 *Shangjuxu* 上巨虚, SP6 *Sanyinjiao* 三阴交, PC6 *Neiguan* 内关, LI4 *Hegu* 合谷 and SP9 *Yinlingquan* 阴陵泉 (Table 7.1).

Risk of Bias for Acupuncture and Electroacupuncture

Eleven RCTs of acupuncture/electroacupuncture are included in this RoB assessment. However, one RCT (A7) included comparisons

Table 7.1 Frequently Used Acupuncture Points in the Randomised Controlled Trials

Point Name	Frequency
ST36 *Zusanli* 足三里	13
ST37 *Shangjuxu* 上巨虚	8
SP6 *Sanyinjiao* 三阴交	5
PC6 *Neiguan* 内关	4
LI4 *Hegu* 合谷	4
SP9 *Yinlingquan* 阴陵泉	3
ST39 *Xiajuxu* 下巨虚	2
SP4 *Gongsun* 公孙	2
ST25 *Tianshu* 天枢	2
TE6 *Zhigou* 支沟	2

Analysis is based on the main points and does not include extra points added for certain symptoms.

with a sham control and a no-treatment control, so there were 12 comparisons for blinding. For sequence generation, all studies were described as 'randomised' but only eight described an appropriate method for sequence generation; one study was judged 'high' risk since patient order was used; and seven studies were judged 'low' risk (Table 7.2). The others were judged as 'unclear' risk. Two studies described the method of allocation concealment and were judged 'low' risk; the others were judged 'unclear' risk. Two studies that used a sham acupuncture intervention were judged 'low' risk for blinding the participants and outcome assessors, although the usual treatment arm in the three-armed study was 'high' risk for blinding of participants (A7). Blinding of study personnel was not described in any study, so all were judged as 'high' risk of bias since it is difficult to blind the people who perform acupuncture. There were no drop-outs or few drop-outs, so all were assessed as 'low' risk of bias for incomplete outcome data. Only one protocol could be located (A7). All outcomes were reported so it was judged 'low' risk for selective outcome reporting, whereas the other studies were judged 'unclear' risk.

Table 7.2 Risk of Bias of Randomised Controlled Trials of Acupuncture/ Electroacupuncture

Risk of Bias Domain	Low Risk *n* (%)	Unclear Risk *n* (%)	High Risk *n* (%)
Sequence generation	7 (63.6)	3 (27.3)	1 (9.1)
Allocation concealment	2 (18.2)	9 (81.8)	0 (0)
Blinding of participants*	2 (16.7)	0 (0)	10 (83.3)
Blinding of personnel[1]	0 (0)	0 (0)	11 (100)
Blinding of outcome assessors	2 (18.2)	9 (81.8)	0 (0)
Incomplete outcome data	11 (100)	0 (0)	0 (0)
Selective reporting	1 (9.1)	10 (90.9)	0 (0)

*Based on 12 groups.

[1]Blinding of personnel (acupuncturists) is challenging in manual therapies.

Electroacupuncture versus Sham Electroacupuncture

Two RCTs compared electroacupuncture to sham electroacupuncture for postoperative recovery of gastrointestinal functioning. All participants received usual postoperative care. One of the studies used laparoscopic surgery (A7) and enrolled 165 participants who were randomised equally into three groups: (1) electroacupuncture; (2) sham electroacupuncture; and (3) usual postoperative care alone. The points used were ST36 *Zusanli* 足三里, SP6 *Sanyinjiao* 三阴交, LI4 *Hegu* 合谷 and TE6 *Zhigou* 支沟 bilaterally with electrostimulation for 20 minutes, once a day from postoperative day one to day four. There were no drop-outs.

The other study used usual surgery (A6) and enrolled 40 participants to receive electroacupuncture or sham electroacupuncture bilaterally at ST36 *Zusanli* 足三里 for 30 minutes once a day on postoperative days one to four. There was one drop-out in the test group since the person did not receive surgery.

Recovery of Gastrointestinal Function

Data were available for four outcome measures and were poolable for two of these. For time to first bowel sounds, the reduction was not significant in the study of usual surgery (mean difference [MD]: –6.00 [–13.26, 1.26] hours). For time to first flatus, the reductions were not significant in either study, but the pooled result showed a significant reduction in the real electroacupuncture groups (MD: –8.00 [–14.72, –1.28] hours) without heterogeneity (I^2 = 0%). Time to first defaecation was not significantly reduced in the study of usual surgery, but there was a significant reduction in the study of laparoscopic surgery and in the pooled result (MD: –18.04 [–31.90, –4.19] hours) without heterogeneity (I^2 = 0.1%). There was no difference between groups for time to resume normal diet in the study of laparoscopic surgery (MD: –0.10 [–0.46, 0.26] days) with most participants having resumed normal diet by day four following surgery (Table 7.3).

Table 7.3 Electroacupuncture versus Sham Electroacupuncture for Recovery of Gastrointestinal Function

Outcome (Unit)	Surgery, Cancer (*N* Participants)	Effect Size (MD [95% CI]), I^2	Included Studies
Time to first bowel sounds (hours)	Usual surgery, CRC (39)	–6.00 [–13.26, 1.26]	A6
Time to first flatus (hours)	Laparoscopic surgery, CRC (110)	–7.20 [–16.22, 1.81]	A7
	Usual surgery, CRC (39)	–9.00 [–19.09, 1.09]	A6
	Pooled result (149) 2 RCTs	–8.00 [–14.72, –1.28]*, 0%	A6, A7
Time to first defaecation (hours)	Laparoscopic surgery, CRC (110)	–21.60 [–37.10, –6.11]*	A7
	Usual surgery, CRC (39)	–4.00 [–34.81, 26.81]	A6
	Pooled result (149) 2 RCTs	–18.04 [–31.90, –4.19]*, 0.1%	A6, A7
Time to resume normal diet (days)	Laparoscopic surgery, CRC (110)	–0.10 [–0.46, 0.26]	A7

*Statistically significant.

Abbreviations: CI, confidence interval; CRC, colorectal cancer; MD, mean difference; N, number; RCT, randomised controlled trial.

Acupuncture and/or Electroacupuncture versus Postoperative Care

In the nine RCTs that provided data for acupuncture/electroacupuncture plus postoperative care versus the same postoperative care, there were three comparisons for manual acupuncture, six comparisons for electroacupuncture and one comparison for manual acupuncture plus moxibustion (A16). Meta-analysis was conducted separately for acupuncture and electroacupuncture. In two studies (A1, A16) the participants all received surgery for rectal cancer. Laparoscopic surgery for CRC was used in one study of manual acupuncture plus moxibustion (A16) and one study of electroacupuncture (A7). In one study of electroacupuncture (A11), most participants received epidural anaesthesia. In two studies of manual acupuncture (A1, A2), all the participants received the Fast Track Program (FTP) of perioperative care. In the other studies, participants received usual postoperative care.

Manual Acupuncture for Recovery of Gastrointestinal Function

The pooled results showed a significant reduction in the manual acupuncture groups for time to first bowel sounds (MD: −4.83 [−8.47, −1.20] hours, I^2 = 85.5%), time to first flatus (MD: −20.51 [−39.19, −1.84] hours, I^2 = 95.3%) and time to first defaecation (MD: −16.30 [−31.35, −1.25] hours, I^2 = 95.7%), but there was considerable heterogeneity for each of these outcomes (Table 7.4). There was a significant reduction in time to first liquid intake based on a single study (MD: −0.82 [−1.43, −0.21] days).

The heterogeneity was likely due to the following differences between studies. In the two studies that used FTP, one commenced acupuncture two hours after surgery for rectal cancer (A1) while the other began acupuncture 24 hours after surgery for CRC (A2). In both studies that used FTP, most control-group participants recovered bowel sounds within 24–32 hours, so it was not surprising that commencing acupuncture at 24 hours made no difference in A2.

Table 7.4 Manual Acupuncture versus Postoperative Care for Recovery of Gastrointestinal Function

Outcome (Unit)	Surgery, Cancer (N Participants)	Effect Size (MD [95% CI]), I²	Included Studies
Time to first bowel sounds (hours)	Usual surgery, FTP, rectal cancer (84)	−7.40 [−7.97, −6.83]*	A1
	Usual surgery, FTP (30)[1]	0.00 [−4.04, 4.04]	A2
	Usual surgery, CRC (60)[1]	−5.68 [−8.47, −2.89]*	A4.1
	Pooled result (174) 3 RCTs	−4.83 [−8.47, −1.20]*, 85.5%	A1, A2, A4.1
Time to first flatus (hours)	Usual surgery, rectal cancer, FTP (84)	−28.56 [−32.45, −24.67]*	A1
	Usual surgery, FTP, CRC (30)[1]	−31.20 [−58.91, −3.49]*	A2
	Usual surgery, CRC (60)[1]	−6.49 [−11.88, −1.10]*	A4.1
	Pooled result (174) 3 RCTs	−20.51 [−39.19, −1.84]*, 95.3%	A1, A2, A4.1
Time to first defaecation (hours)	Usual surgery, FTP, rectal cancer (84)	−22.56 [−24.36, −20.76]*	A1
	Usual surgery, FTP, CRC (30)[1]	-28.80 [-62.11, 4.51]	A2
	Usual surgery, CRC (60)[1]	−5.71 [−10.25, −1.18]*	A4.1
	Pooled result (174) 3 RCTs	−16.30 [−31.35, −1.25]*, 95.7%	A1, A2, A4.1
Time to first liquid intake (days)	Usual surgery, rectal cancer, FTP (84)	−0.82 [−1.43, −0.21]*	A1

[1]Began acupuncture 24 hours after surgery.

*Statistically significant.

Abbreviations: CI, confidence interval; CRC, colorectal cancer; FTP, Fast Track Programme; MD, mean difference; N, number; RCT, randomised controlled trial.

In the study that received usual surgery for CRC (A4.1), the acupuncture commenced 24 hours after surgery, but FTP was not used and recovery times were considerably longer than in the studies that used FTP. In addition, in one study (A1) all participants received surgery for rectal surgery while the other studies specified CRC. Due to these multiple differences between studies, sensitivity analyses were not feasible.

Electroacupuncture for Recovery of Gastrointestinal Function

In the six RCTs of electroacupuncture, all participants had CRC. For electroacupuncture plus postoperative care versus postoperative care alone (Table 7.5) there were significant reductions in the acupuncture groups for

Table 7.5 Electroacupuncture versus Postoperative Care for Recovery of Gastrointestinal Function

Outcome (Unit)	Surgery, Cancer (N Participants)	Effect Size (MD [95% CI]), I^2	Included Studies
Time to first bowel sounds (hours)	Usual surgery, CRC. Pooled result (160) 3 RCTs	−9.77 [−17.35, −2.20]*, 93.6%	A9, A10, A4.2
Time to first flatus (hours)	Usual surgery, CRC (32)	−28.13 [−34.65, −21.61]*	A8
	Usual surgery, CRC (40)	−37.90 [−42.34, −33.46]*	A9
	Usual surgery, CRC (60)	−2.93 [−5.51, −0.35]*	A10
	Usual surgery, CRC (60)	−9.95 [−14.89, −5.01]*	A4.2
	Usual surgery, epidural anaesthesia, CRC (75)	3.02 [−6.44, 12.48]	A11
	Laparoscopic surgery, CRC (110)	−14.40 [−23.42, −5.39]*	A7
	Pooled result (377) 6 RCTs	−15.17 [−28.81, −1.54]*, 97.6%	A4.2, A7–A11
	Sensitivity (192) 4 RCTs	−19.65 [−37.31, −2.00]*, 98.5%	A4.2, A8–A10
Time to first defaecation (hours)	Usual surgery, CRC (60)	−5.16 [−7.98, −2.34]*	A10
	Usual surgery, CRC (60)	−12.96 [−16.67, −9.25]*	A4.2
	Usual surgery, epidural anaesthesia, CRC (76)	−0.34 [−24.71, 24.03]	A11
	Laparoscopic surgery, CRC (110)	−36.20 [−53.26, −19.14]*	A7
	Pooled result (306) 4 RCTs	−12.39 [−20.97, −3.81]*, 86%	A4.2, A7, A10, A11
	Sensitivity (120) 2 RCTs	−8.96 [−16.60, −1.32]*, 90.7%	A4.2, A10
Time to resume normal diet (days)	Laparoscopic surgery, CRC (110)	−0.80 [−1.40, −0.20]*	A7

*Statistically significant.

Abbreviations: CI, confidence interval; CRC, colorectal cancer; MD, mean difference; N, number; RCT, randomised controlled trial.

time to first bowel sounds (MD: –9.77 [–17.35, –2.20] hours, I^2 = 93.6%), time to first flatus (MD: –15.17 [–28.81, –1.54] hours, I^2 = 97.6%) and time to first defaecation (MD: –12.39 [–20.97, –3.81] hours, I^2 = 86%), with considerable heterogeneity in each pool. The time to resuming normal diet was significantly reduced in the electroacupuncture group in the study of laparoscopic surgery (MD: –0.80 [–1.40, –0.20] days).

Potential sources of between-study differences included use of epidural anaesthesia in most patients in one study (A11) and use of laparoscopic surgery in one study (A7). After these two studies were removed, time to first flatus (MD: –19.65 [–37.31, –2.00] hours, I^2 = 98.5%) and time to first defaecation (MD: –8.97 [–16.60, –1.32] hours, I^2 = 90.7%) were significantly shorter in the electroacupuncture groups, but the heterogeneity was not reduced. Another potential source of heterogeneity was variation in the recovery times in the control groups but the reasons for these differences could not be determined. In addition, variation in the acupuncture protocols is likely to have contributed to heterogeneity in the pooled results.

Postoperative Adverse Reactions

One study of manual acupuncture plus moxibustion (n = 30) reported the incidence of postoperative urinary retention. Acupuncture was used at LI4 *Hegu* 合谷, SP10 *Xuehai* 血海, ST36 *Zusanli* 足三里, SP9 *Yinlingquan* 阴陵泉, SP6 *Sanyinjiao* 三阴交 and LR3 *Taichong* 太冲, with moxibustion at RN4 *Guanyuan* 关元 and RN8 *Shenque* 神阙. There was one case in the acupuncture group (A16) and two cases in the usual care group which was not a significant difference.

Three studies reported on postoperative abdominal distension at five days after surgery and one study (A4) included two test groups. Each study used different approaches to reporting data, so pooling was not feasible (Table 7.6).

A study of manual acupuncture combined with FTP (A2) (n = 30) found two cases of medium to severe (grade II–III) abdominal distension at five days after surgery in the acupuncture group versus three cases in the usual-care group (risk ratio [RR]: 0.67 [0.13, 3.44]) which was not a significant difference. The other studies used scoring

Table 7.6 Acupuncture Therapy versus Postoperative Care for Postoperative Abdominal Distension

Surgery, Cancer (N Participants)	Acupuncture Therapy	Effect Size (MD or RR [95% CI]), I^2	Included Studies
Open surgery, FTP,[1] CRC (30)	Manual acupuncture	RR 0.67 [0.13, 3.44]	A2
Open surgery, FTP, rectal cancer (84)	Manual acupuncture	MD –0.77 [–0.80, –0.74]*	A1
Open radical surgery,[2] CRC (60)	Manual acupuncture	MD –0.27 [–0.51, –0.03]*	A4.1
Open radical surgery,[2] CRC (60)	Electroacupuncture	MD –0.53 [–0.75, –0.32]*	A4.2

[1]Acupuncture began 24 hours post-surgery.

[2]Excluding Miles surgery.

*Statistically significant.

Abbreviations: CI, confidence interval; CRC, colorectal cancer; FTP, Fast Track Programme; MD, mean difference; RR, risk ratio.

systems (A1, A4.1/4.2). These found significant reductions in abdominal distension in the manual and electroacupuncture groups, but the data were not suitable for pooling.

Quality of Life

One study of electroacupuncture ($n = 76$) for prevention of prolonged postoperative ileus reported on quality of life based on a modified Edmonton Symptom Assessment System (ESAS) which consisted of five items (pain, nausea, insomnia, abdominal distension and general sense of well-being), which were each rated using a 0–10 numeric rating scale. The authors reported no differences between groups for any outcome (A11). These data were not amenable to meta-analysis.

Warm Needling versus Postoperative Care

One RCT of 70 people with CRC (A12) employed warm needling at ST36 *Zusanli* 足三里, ST37 *Shangjuxu* 上巨虚, ST39 *Xiajuxu* 下巨虚,

SP6 *Sanyinjiao* 三阴交 and SP9 *Yinlingquan* 阴陵泉 bilaterally. Treatment commenced one day after surgery, once a day for ten days with retention for 45 minutes, during which time moxa was applied twice to the needles.

Recovery of Gastrointestinal Function

Compared to usual postoperative care for CRC, there were significant reductions in time to first bowel sounds (MD: –12.20 [–16.66, –7.74] hours), first flatus (MD: –18.55 [–23.86, –13.24] hours) and first defaecation (MD: –16.30 [–23.13, –9.48] hours) (Table 7.7).

Immune Function

The above RCT (A12) also reported data for postoperative immune function, which compared the first day versus the tenth day after surgery. The results for T cell subsets were:

- CD3+ cells – MD: 12.87 [9.24, 16.5]* %;
- CD4+ cells – MD: 4.74 [1.81, 7.67]* %;
- NK cells – MD: 2.65 [1.21, 4.09]* %;
- CD4+/CD8+ cells – MD 0.24 [–0.02, 0.5].

* Statistically significant.
Abbreviations: CD, cluster of differentiation; NK, natural killer.

Table 7.7   Warm Needling versus Postoperative Care for Recovery of Gastrointestinal Function

Outcome (Unit), Participants	Effect Size (MD [95% CI]), I^2	Included Study
Time to first bowel sounds (hours), $n = 70$	–12.20 [–16.66, –7.74]*	A12
Time to first flatus (hours), $n = 70$	–18.55 [–23.86, –13.24]*	
Time to first defaecation (hours), $n = 70$	–16.30 [–23.13, –9.48]*	

*Statistically significant.

Abbreviations: CI, confidence interval; MD, mean difference.

There was greater recovery in immune function, as measured by increases in each of the three T cell subsets. However, the increase in the ratio of CD4+ to CD8+ cells was not significant.

Frequently Reported Acupuncture Points in Meta-analyses

This section presents the acupoints frequently used in the studies included in the meta-analysis pools for recovery of gastrointestinal function in which there was a significant difference in the acupuncture groups for reduction in time to first bowel sounds, first flatus or first defaecation. The 11 included studies were divided according to whether manual acupuncture (four RCTs including one warm needling) or electroacupuncture (seven RCTs) was used. The point frequencies were calculated with each study only being included once (Table 7.8). In all studies the comparison was with usual postoperative care, and two of the studies of electroacupuncture used a sham control (A6, A7).

Table 7.8 Frequently Used Acupuncture Points in the Randomised Controlled Trials in the Meta-analysis Pools that Showed a Benefit for Recovery of Gastrointestinal Function

Type of Acupuncture (Studies)	Point Name	Frequency
Acupuncture, warm needling 4 studies[1] (A1, A2, A4.1, A12)	ST36 *Zusanli* 足三里	4
	ST39 *Xiajuxu* 下巨虚	4
	SP4 *Gongsun* 公孙	2
	PC6 *Neiguan* 内关	2
Electroacupuncture 7 studies[2] (A4.2, A6–A11)	ST36 *Zusanli* 足三里	7
	ST37 *Shangjuxu* 上巨虚	5
	SP6 *Sanyinjiao* 三阴交	2
	LI4 *Hegu* 合谷	2
	TE6 *Zhigou* 支沟	2

[1]For results of studies reporting time to first bowel sounds, first flatus or first defaecation, see Tables 7.4 and 7.6.

[2]For results of studies reporting time to first bowel sounds, first flatus or first defaecation see Tables 7.3 and 7.5.

As in the total point frequency for the RCTs (Table 7.1), ST36 *Zusanli* 足三里 was the most frequently used point overall, followed by ST37 *Shangjuxu* 上巨虚, which was mainly used in the electroacupuncture studies, and ST39 *Xiajuxu* 下巨虚 which was more frequent in the manual acupuncture studies.

GRADE for Acupuncture for Recovery of Gastrointestinal Function

Assessments using Grading of Recommendations Assessment, Development and Evaluation (GRADE) were conducted for recovery of gastrointestinal function. The following three comparisons were assessed:

- Electroacupuncture versus sham electroacupuncture;
- Manual acupuncture versus postoperative care;
- Electroacupuncture versus postoperative care.

For each comparison, outcome data were available for time to first bowel sounds, time to first flatus and time to first defaecation.

In the blinded studies that compared electroacupuncture with sham electroacupuncture, for time to first bowel sounds there was a mean reduction of six hours (MD: −6.00) in the real electroacupuncture group compared to the sham electroacupuncture control, but this was not significantly different. However, the reduction of eight hours in time to first flatus (MD: −8.00), and 18 hours in time to first defaecation (MD: −18.06) were significantly different (Table 7.9). For each outcome, the certainty of the evidence was reduced by one grade to 'moderate' due to the small sample sizes in the meta-analysis pools.

For the comparisons between groups that received manual acupuncture and groups that only received postoperative care, for time to first bowel sounds there was a mean reduction of 4.8 hours in the manual acupuncture group, compared to the control that did not receive acupuncture (MD: −4.83). There were mean reductions of 20.5 hours in time to first flatus (MD: −20.51) and 16 hours in time

Table 7.9   GRADE for Recovery of Gastrointestinal Function: Electroacupuncture versus Sham Electroacupuncture

Outcome	Absolute Effect		Relative Effect (95% CI) N Studies (N Participants)	Certainty of the Evidence GRADE
	With electro-acupuncture	Without electro-acupuncture		
Time to first bowel sounds	**7** hours	**13** hours	**MD –6.00** (–13.26 to 1.26 hours) 1 (39)	⊕⊕⊕◯ MODERATE[1]
	Average difference: 6 hours sooner (95% CI: 13.26 hours sooner to 1.26 hours later)			
Time to first flatus	**15** hours	**23** hours	**MD –8.00**[*] (–14.72 to –1.28 hours) 2 (149)	⊕⊕⊕◯ MODERATE[2]
	Average difference: 8 hours sooner (95% CI: 1.28 to 14.72 hours sooner)			
Time to first defaecation	**49.96** hours	**68** hours	**MD –18.04**[*] (–31.90 to –4.19 hours) 2 (149)	⊕⊕⊕◯ MODERATE[2]
	Average difference: 18.04 hours sooner (95% CI: 4.19 to 31.9 hours sooner)			

[*]Statistically significant result, random effect model.

[1]Single randomised controlled trial with small sample size;

[2]Two randomised controlled trials with small sample sizes.

Abbreviations: CI, confidence interval; GRADE, Grading of Recommendations Assessment, Development and Evaluation; MD, mean difference; N, number.

Study references: see Table 7.3 for included studies.

to first defaecation (MD: –16.30); all these were significantly different (Table 7.10). Since these studies were not blinded, for each outcome the certainty of the evidence was reduced by one grade. It was further reduced by one grade due to the considerable statistical heterogeneity in the meta-analyses, and by an additional grade due to the small sample size of the three included studies (i.e. fewer than 400 participants). Therefore, the resultant grade was 'very low' for certainty of the evidence.

For electroacupuncture versus postoperative care without any acupuncture, there were statistically significant differences between groups for all three outcomes in favour of the electroacupuncture groups (Table 7.11). The mean reduction of 9.8 hours in time to first

Table 7.10   GRADE for Recovery of Gastrointestinal Function: Manual Acupuncture versus Postoperative Care

Outcome	Absolute Effect		Relative Effect (95% CI) N Studies (N Participants)	Certainty of Evidence GRADE
	With acupuncture	Without acupuncture		
Time to first bowel sounds	**19.17** hours	**24** hours	**MD −4.83*** (−8.47 to −1.20 hours) 3 (174)	⊕◯◯◯ VERY LOW[1,2,3]
	Average difference: 4.83 hours sooner (95% CI: 1.2 to 8.47 hours sooner)			
Time to first flatus	**27.49** hours	**48** hours	**MD −20.51*** (−39.19 to −1.84 hours) 3 (174)	⊕◯◯◯ VERY LOW[1,2,3]
	Average difference: 20.51 hours sooner (95% CI: 1.84 to 39.19 hours sooner)			
Time to first defaecation	**62.90** hours	**79.2** hours	**MD −16.30*** (−31.35 to −1.25 hours) 3 (174)	⊕◯◯◯ VERY LOW[1,2,3]
	Average difference: 16.3 hours sooner (95% CI: 1.25 to 31.35 hours sooner)			

*Statistically significant result, random effect model.

[1]No blinding.

[2]Statistical heterogeneity was considerable.

[3]Three randomised controlled trials with small sample sizes.

Abbreviations: CI, confidence interval; GRADE, Grading of Recommendations Assessment, Development and Evaluation; MD, mean difference; N, number.

Study references: See Table 7.4 for included studies.

bowel sounds (MD: −9.77) was greater than for manual acupuncture, but the reductions of 15 hours in time to first flatus (MD: −15.17) and 13 hours in time to first defaecation (MD: −12.39) were somewhat less than for manual acupuncture. The certainty of the evidence was rated down by three grades to 'very low' for the same reasons as for manual acupuncture.

Overall, the pattern of results for each of the three GRADE assessments was similar, with each of the outcomes occurring sooner in the

Table 7.11 GRADE for Recovery of Gastrointestinal Function: Electroacupuncture versus Postoperative Care

Outcome	Absolute Effect		Relative Effect (95% CI) N Studies (N Participants)	Certainty of Evidence GRADE
	With electro-acupuncture	Without electro-acupuncture		
Time to first bowel sounds	**31.23** hours	**41** hours	**MD −9.77*** (−17.35 to −2.20 hours) 3 (160)	⊕◯◯◯ VERY LOW[1,2,3]
	Average difference: 9.77 hours sooner (95% CI: 2.2 to 17.35 hours sooner)			
Time to first flatus	**32.83** hours	**48** hours	**MD −15.17*** (−28.81 to −1.54 hours) 6 (377)	⊕◯◯◯ VERY LOW[1,2,4]
	Average difference: 15.17 hours sooner (95% CI: 1.54 to 28.81 hours sooner)			
Time to first defaecation	**73.42** hours	**85.81** hours	**MD −12.39*** (−20.97 to −3.81 hours) 4 (306)	⊕◯◯◯ VERY LOW[1,2,5]
	Average difference: 12.39 hours sooner (95% CI: 3.81 to 20.97 hours sooner)			

*Statistically significant result, random effect model.

[1] No blinding.

[2] Statistical heterogeneity was considerable.

[3] Three randomised controlled trials with small sample sizes.

[4] Six randomised controlled trials with small sample sizes.

[5] Four randomised controlled trials with small sample sizes.

Abbreviations: CI, confidence interval; GRADE, Grading of Recommendations Assessment, Development and Evaluation; MD, mean difference; N, number.

Study references: see Table 7.5 for included studies.

acupuncture therapy groups compared to the controls. However, the GRADE assessments varied considerably based on the relatively small sample sizes available, and for the second two assessments, the lack of blinding of participants and statistical heterogeneity in the meta-analysis results.

Clinical Evidence from Non-randomised Controlled Trials of Acupuncture

No non-randomised CCTs of acupuncture, electroacupuncture, ear acupuncture or acupressure were identified.

Clinical Evidence from Non-controlled Studies of Acupuncture

Two non-controlled studies of acupuncture with a total of 11 participants were identified. One retrospective study (A18) of ten cases investigated the effectiveness of acupuncture in managing oxaliplatin chemotherapy-induced peripheral neuropathy (CIPN). All patients had received chemotherapy for stage II to IV colon cancer and had developed CIPN that ranged from grade I to IV based on Common Terminology Criteria for Adverse Events version 4.0.[8] All were treated at integrative medical centres in the United States and received individualised acupuncture treatments based on syndrome differentiation and symptoms. Treatment was still ongoing in seven patients and the longest duration of treatment was two years. All but one patient had experienced reductions in CIPN grade with an average reduction of 1.5 grades. Detailed descriptions were provided for each case.

One case report from China (A17) was on abdominal acupuncture for persistent hiccups for about 15 days following chemotherapy. The acupuncture treatment involved four abdominal points: CV12 *Zhongwan* 中脘, CV10 *Xiawan* 下脘, CV4 *Guanyuan* 关元 and CV6 *Qihai* 气海, plus GV20 *Baihui* 百会, PC6 *Neiguan* 内关 and ST36 *Zusanli* 足三里. The hiccups decreased after ten minutes and stopped after 30 minutes.

Safety of Acupuncture and Electroacupuncture

Most of the RCTs did not mention adverse events (AEs) associated with acupuncture. One RCT (A11) mentioned that there were no AEs greater than CTCAE grade I.[9] Another RCT (A16) stated there were no AEs. There was no mention of AEs associated with acupuncture in the case study (A17). The case series study (A18) mentioned examples of hypersensitivity to acupuncture in the CIPN patients and described how this was managed.

Studies of Acupressure

One RCTs used acupressure on traditional points for recovery of gastrointestinal function. No CCTs or non-controlled studies of acupressure were identified. The RCT (*n* = 66) tested acupressure at ST36 *Zusanli* 足三里 which was applied bilaterally for three minutes on each point, three times per day for five days after open surgery for CRC. This was compared to a sham acupressure intervention using the same method on a non-point on each tibia (A13). There were three drop-outs in each group, three prior to the intervention, and three were excluded since they required further surgery, so data were available for 60 participants. Syndrome differentiation was not mentioned.

This study did not provide details of the randomisation method, so it was judged 'unclear' risk of bias for sequence generation and allocation concealment. Although sham acupressure was used as the control, the method of blinding was not described in detail and there was no report on assessment of unblinding, so it was judged 'unclear' risk for blinding of participants. Since it is difficult to blind personnel the judgment was 'high' risk. The use of blinded outcome assessors was stated so it was judged 'low' risk. There were drop-outs with reasons, and these were balanced between groups, so the study was judged 'low' risk for incomplete outcome data. No protocol could be located so it was judged 'unclear' risk for selective outcome reporting.

There were significant reductions in the real acupressure group for time to first flatus (MD: –0.83 [–1.36, –0.30] days) and time to first liquid intake (MD: –0.83 [–1.45, –0.22] days) but not for time to first defaecation (MD: –0.50 [–1.32, 0.32] days) or time to first solid food intake (MD: –0.57 [–1.40, 0.26] days). At 40 hours post-surgery the frequency of bowel sounds (measured by auscultation for three minutes) was higher in the real acupressure group (MD: 3.43 [0.77, 6.09] per minute) (Table 7.12). There was no mention of AEs relating to acupressure.

Table 7.12   Acupressure versus Sham Acupressure for Recovery of Gastrointestinal Function

Outcome (Unit), Participants	Effect Size (MD [95% CI])	Included Study
Time to first flatus (days), $n = 60$	–0.83 [–1.36, –0.30]*	A13
Time to first defaecation (days), $n = 60$	–0.50 [–1.32, 0.32]	
Time to first liquid intake (days), $n = 60$	–0.83 [–1.45, –0.22]*	
Time to first solid food intake (days), $n = 60$	–0.57 [–1.40, 0.26]	
Frequency of bowel sound at 40 hours,[1] $n = 60$	3.43 [0.77, 6.09]*	

[1]Frequency per minute assessed during a three-minute interval.

*Statistically significant.

Abbreviations: CI, confidence interval; MD, mean difference; n, number.

Studies of Ear Acupuncture or Ear Acupressure

Four RCTs included ear acupuncture or acupressure (with or without traditional points) as an intervention. No CCTs or non-controlled studies of ear acupuncture or ear acupressure were identified. The four RCTs enrolled 304 participants with ages ranging from 47 to 80 years but the age range was not reported in one study (A14). Based on the reported means and standard deviations for ages, the majority of participants were aged between 51 and 72 years. Following drop-outs, 295 participants completed the studies.

Two studies (A14, A15) compared ear acupressure with usual postoperative care and one RCT (A3) combined ear acupressure at the most sensitive point (*ming gan dian* 敏感点) with acupuncture at ST36 *Zusanli* 足三里. One RCT (A5) combined acupuncture on one ear point (TF4 *Shenmen* 神门) with electroacupuncture and manual acupuncture on multiple body points, so the results of this study are included separately below.

The ear points used most frequently in the four RCTs were CO7 *Dachang* 大肠, AH6a *Jiaogan* 交感, AT4 *Pizhixia* 皮质下, CO4 *Wei* 胃 and TF4 *Shenmen* 神门 (Table 7.13). None of the studies mentioned syndrome differentiation.

Table 7.13 Frequently Used Ear Points in the Randomised Controlled Trials

Point Name	Frequency[1]
CO7 *Dachang* 大肠	2
AH6a *Jiaogan* 交感	2
AT4 *Pizhixia* 皮质下	2
CO4 *Wei* 胃	2
TF4 *Shenmen* 神门	2

[1]Based on all four randomised controlled trials that used ear points, but one randomised controlled trial (A3) did not provide point names.

Risk of Bias for Studies of Ear Acupressure and Ear Acupuncture

Four RCTs were included in this assessment. Two (A5, A15) were judged 'low' risk for sequence generation, one did not provide details and was judged 'unclear' risk and one was judged 'high' risk (A14) because patients were allocated according to order of surgery. One study was 'low' risk for allocation concealment (A15), but the others did not provide information and were judged 'unclear' risk. One study (A15) was judged 'low' risk for blinding of participants and outcome assessors. All studies were judged 'high' risk for blinding of personnel. Incomplete outcome data was judged 'low' risk since the studies had either no drop-outs or few drop-outs. A protocol was available for one study (A15). There were some differences between the protocol and the published article, but all the main outcomes were included in both and the results were reported so this was judged as 'low' risk for selective reporting. The studies that had no protocols were judged 'unclear' risk (Table 7.14).

Ear Acupressure versus Postoperative Care

Three RCTs (*n* = 214) tested ear acupressure combined with postoperative care for CRC, compared to the same postoperative care

Table 7.14   Risk of Bias of Randomised Controlled Trials of Ear Acupressure and Ear Acupuncture

Risk of Bias Domain	Low Risk *n* (%)	Unclear Risk *n* (%)	High Risk *n* (%)
Sequence generation	2 (50)	1 (25)	1 (25)
Allocation concealment	1 (25)	3 (75)	0 (0)
Blinding of participants	1 (25)	0 (0)	3 (75)
Blinding of personnel[1]	0 (0)	0 (0)	4 (100)
Blinding of outcome assessors	1 (25)	3 (75)	0 (0)
Incomplete outcome data	4 (100)	0 (0)	0 (0)
Selective reporting	1 (25)	0 (0)	3 (75)

[1]Blinding of personnel (acupuncturists) is challenging in manual therapies.

without any acupressure (A3, A14, A15). One study combined ear acupressure with acupuncture at ST36 *Zusanli* 足三里 (A3).

Recovery of Gastrointestinal Function

In the three RCTs there were significant reductions in the ear acupressure groups in the pooled results for time to first bowel sounds (MD: –7.92 [–9.82, –6.03] hours, I^2 = 54.7%), time to first flatus (MD: –15.67 [–20.77, –10.57] hours, I^2 = 94.1%) and time to first liquid intake (MD: –19.72 [–20.22, –19.22], hours I^2 = 0%). The time to first defaecation was only reported by one RCT (A15), which found a significantly shorter time in the ear acupressure group (MD: –9.28 [–16.74, –1.83] hours) (Table 7.15).

Due to the moderate to considerable heterogeneity in the outcomes for times to first bowel sounds and flatus, sensitivity analyses were conducted based on removal of the single study of colon cancer (A15). This produced the following pooled results for time to first bowel sounds (MD: –8.66 [–9.86, –7.46] hours, I^2 = 0%) and first flatus (MD: –19.80 [–20.29, –19.31] hours, I^2 = 0%). These results indicate significant reductions in the ear acupressure groups, compared to controls with no heterogeneity.

Table 7.15 Ear Acupressure versus Postoperative Care for Recovery of Gastrointestinal Function

Outcome (Unit)	Surgery, cancer (*N* Participant)	Effect Size (MD [95% CI]), I^2	Included Studies
Time to first bowel sounds (hours)	Usual surgery, CRC (78)	–8.51 [–9.95, –7.08]*	A14
	Usual surgery, colon cancer (60)	–4.83 [–8.25, –1.41]*	A15
	Usual surgery, CRC[1] (76)	–9.00 [–11.18, –6.83]*	A3
	Pooled result (214) 3 RCTs	–7.92 [–9.82, –6.03]*, 54.7%	A3, A14, A15
	Sensitivity (154)	–8.66 [–9.86, –7.46]*, 0%	A3, A14
Time to first flatus (hours)	Usual surgery, CRC (78)	–19.85 [20.35, –19.35]*	A14
	Usual surgery, colon cancer (60)	–6.73 [–11.16, –2.30]*	A15
	Usual surgery, CRC[1] (76)	–18.70 [–21.01, –16.39]*	A3
	Pooled result (214) 3 RCTs	–15.67 [–20.77, –10.57]*, 94.1%	A3, A14, A15
	Sensitivity (154) 2 RCTs	–19.80 [–20.29, –19.31]*, 0%	A3, A14
Time to first defaecation (hours)	Usual surgery, colon cancer (60)	–9.28 [–16.74, –1.83]*	A15
Time to first liquid intake (hours)	Usual surgery, CRC (78)	–19.76 [–20.27, –19.25]*	A14
	Usual surgery, CRC[1] (76)	–18.90 [–21.20, –16.60]*	A3
	Pooled result (154) 2 RCTs	–19.72 [–20.22, –19.22]*, 0%	A3, A14

*Statistically significant.

[1]Ear acupressure at sensitive point plus acupuncture at ST36.

Abbreviations: CI, confidence interval; CRC, colorectal cancer; MD, mean difference; RCT, randomised controlled trial.

Ear Acupuncture plus Acupuncture and Electroacupuncture versus Sham Interventions

One RCT (A5) enrolled 90 people due to undergo colorectal surgery to receive a combination of ear acupuncture plus acupuncture and electroacupuncture versus sham interventions for postoperative recovery. Both groups received usual postoperative care. Seven pairs of bilateral points were used: TF4 ear *Shenmen* 神门, ST36 *Zusanli* 足三里, PC6 *Neiguan* 内关, LI4 *Hegu* 合谷, SP6 *Sanyinjiao* 三阴交, SP9 *Yinlingquan* 阴陵泉 and ST25 *Tianshu* 天枢, with insertion for 30 minutes and electrical stimulation (2 Hertz, 0.5 millisecond square wave pulses) on ST36 *Zusanli* 足三里 (negative) and PC6 *Neiguan* 内关 (positive). Treatment began on postoperative day one and was applied twice a day for three days. In the sham group, needles were taped on same points with no insertion twice a day and the electrostimulator had the current disabled. There were seven dropouts in the real group (*n* = 39) and two drop-outs in the control group (*n* = 42), all prior to the intervention.

Assessments of recovery of gastrointestinal function were based on the following two composite measures: GI3 (the later of the following two events — time that the patient first tolerated solid food, *and* time that the patient first passed flatus *or* a bowel movement); and GI2 (the later of the following two events — time patient first tolerated solid food *and* time patient first passed a bowel movement). There were no significant differences between groups for GI3 (MD: 3.00 [–26.12, 32.12] hours, *n* = 81) or GI2 (MD: –3.00 [–31.74, 25.74] hours, *n* = 81). The authors noted that the standard deviations were unexpectedly wide for both measures. There was no difference between groups for emetic episodes before GI recovery (GI-3).

GRADE for Ear Acupressure for Recovery of Gastrointestinal Function

Assessments of ear acupressure versus postoperative care for recovery of gastrointestinal function using GRADE were conducted for the following four outcomes:

- Time to first bowel sounds;
- Time to first flatus;
- Time to first defaecation;
- Time to first liquid intake.

For each outcome there were significant reductions in the groups that received ear acupressure compared to the groups that received postoperative care without any acupressure (Table 7.16). In the ear acupressure group, first bowel sounds appeared 7.9 hours earlier on average (MD: –7.92) compared to the control groups, but the certainty of this evidence was reduced by two grades to 'low' since the three included studies were not blinded and the overall sample size was small. For time to first flatus, the difference between groups was more than 15 hours (MD: –15.67) but this was based on the same three unblinded studies with small sample sizes plus the meta-analysis result showed considerable heterogeneity, so the evidence was reduced by three grades to 'very low.' For time to first defaecation, data were only available from one unblinded study with a small sample size, so the average reduction of more than nine hours (MD: –9.28) in the ear acupressure group was graded as 'low' certainty. Similarly, for the two studies that reported on time to first liquid intake, the mean reduction of over 19 hours (MD: –19.72) was graded as 'low' certainty due to the lack of blinding and small sample size, although there was no heterogeneity in the meta-analysis.

Safety of Ear Acupuncture and Ear Acupressure

Adverse events associated with ear acupuncture were not mentioned in the study of ear acupuncture plus acupuncture and electroacupuncture (A5). Also, none of the three studies of ear acupressure mentioned AEs.

Studies of Moxibustion

One RCT, no CCTs and no non-controlled studies of moxibustion were identified. The RCT (*n* = 60) investigated the effects of moxibustion alone in conjunction with chemotherapy. Moxibustion was at ST36 *Zusanli* 足三里 and PC6 *Neiguan* 内关 bilaterally and CV12 *Zhongwan* 中脘 (in this order) using a moxa stick for five minutes on each point, followed by one minute of massage (*an mo* 按摩) on the point. Treatment was once a day from one day before, until three

Table 7.16 GRADE for Recovery of Gastrointestinal Function: Ear Acupressure versus Postoperative Care

Outcome	Absolute Effect		Relative Effect (95% CI) N Studies (N Participants)	Certainty of the Evidence GRADE
	With CHM	Without CHM		
Time to first bowel sounds	**11.78** hours	**19.70** hours	**MD –7.92*** (–9.82 to –6.03 hours) 3 (214)	⊕⊕○○ LOW[1,2]
	Average difference: 7.92 hours sooner (95% CI: 6.03 to 9.82 hours sooner)			
Time to first flatus	**26.03** hours	**41.70** hours	**MD –15.67*** (–20.77 to –10.57 hours) 3 (214)	⊕○○○ VERY LOW[1,2,3]
	Average difference: 15.67 hours sooner (95% CI: 10.57 to 20.77 hours sooner)			
Time to first defaecation	**43.29** hours	**52.57** hours	**MD –9.28*** (–16.74 to –1.83 hours) 1 (60)	⊕⊕○○ LOW[1,4]
	Average difference: 9.28 hours sooner (95% CI: 1.83 to 16.74 hours sooner)			
Time to first liquid intake	**23.88** hours	**43.60** hours	**MD –19.72*** (–20.22 to –19.22 hours) 2 (154)	⊕⊕○○ LOW[1,5]
	Average difference: 19.72 hours sooner (95% CI: 19.22 to 20.22 hours sooner)			

*Statistically significant result, random effect model.

[1]No blinding.

[2]Three randomised controlled trials with small sample sizes.

[3]Statistical heterogeneity was considerable.

[4]One randomised controlled trial with small sample size.

[5]Two randomised controlled trials with small sample sizes.

Abbreviations: CI, confidence interval; GRADE, Grading of Recommendations Assessment, Development and Evaluation; MD, mean difference; N, number.

Study references: see Table 7.15 for included studies.

days after, chemotherapy. There was no syndrome differentiation. The total duration of therapy was 12 weeks (six cycles). All participants received adjuvant chemotherapy with FOLFOX4 plus the anti-nausea drug ondansetron (A19). The control group received FOLFOX4 plus ondansetron without moxibustion.

This study did not report sufficient details on methodological aspects, so it was judged 'unclear' risk for sequence generation and allocation concealment. The study was not blinded so it was 'high' risk for blinding of participants and personnel and 'unclear' risk for outcome assessors. There were no drop-outs and all outcomes in the method were reported so it was judged 'low' risk for incomplete outcome data. No protocol could be located so it was judged 'unclear' risk for selective outcome reporting.

The outcome was based on the World Health Organisation (WHO) criteria for grading of nausea and vomiting.[10] At the end of the treatment period there were no cases of grade III/IV in the moxibustion group and three cases in the control group. For all grades, there were seven cases in the moxibustion group and 15 in the control which was a significant difference (RR: 0.47 [0.22, 0.98]). There was no report of any AEs.

Clinical Evidence for Commonly Used Acupuncture Interventions

The points recommended in one of the guidelines for intestinal obstruction after CRC surgery include PC6 *Neiguan* 内关 on the arm, ST36 *Zusanli* 足三里 on the leg, and ST25 *Tianshu* 天枢, CV13 *Shangwan* 上脘, CV12 *Zhongwan* 中脘 and CV10 *Xiawan* 下脘 on the abdomen (see Chapter 2). In the RCTs, the main points on the leg were ST36 *Zusanli* 足三里 and ST37 *Shangjuxu* 上巨虚; and on the arm the two main points were PC6 *Neiguan* 内关 and LI4 *Hegu* 合谷. Points on the abdomen were uncommon in the RCTs with ST25 *Tianshu* 天枢 being used in only two studies.

In the RCTs, the use of electroacupuncture in a number of studies would have required the use of at least two points since two electrodes are required. Since ST36 *Zusanli* 足三里 is a key point, it is likely that ST37 *Shangjuxu* 上巨虚 was selected as the second point since it has a similar function and this pair is convenient for electroacupuncture since these points are close together. The relatively few abdominal points used in the RCTs may reflect the inconvenience of these points immediately postsurgery in a hospital setting.

As Table 7.8 indicates, both ST36 *Zusanli* 足三里 and ST37 *Shangjuxu* 上巨虚 were frequently used points in studies that showed significant improvements in postoperative gastrointestinal function based on meta-analysis of RCT data. PC6 *Neiguan* 内关 and LI4 *Hegu* 合谷 were less frequently used in these studies.

In the case of ear acupuncture, the guidelines did not provide any recommendations for recovery of gastrointestinal function. For nausea and vomiting, the guidelines recommended acupuncture at PC6 *Neiguan* 内关, ST36 *Zusanli* 足三里, SP4 *Gongsun* 公孙, LR3 *Taichong* 太冲, BL21 *Weishu* 胃俞, CV14 *Juque* 巨阙 and BL17 *Geshu* 膈俞 (Chapter 2). Of the RCTs of acupuncture, none reported data for this outcome, but the single RCT of moxibustion (A19) used both ST36 *Zusanli* 足三里 and PC6 *Neiguan* 内关 and found a significant reduction in all grades.

For urinary retention, the guidelines recommended acupuncture at SP6 *Sanyinjiao* 三阴交, BL28 *Pangguangshu* 膀胱俞, KI3 *Taixi* 太溪 and SP9 *Yinlingquan* 阴陵泉 (Chapter 2). In the case of the single RCT for urinary retention after CRC surgery (A16), acupuncture was used at two of these points, SP9 *Yinlingquan* 阴陵泉 and SP6 *Sanyinjiao* 三阴交, as well as at other points. However, there were too few cases in either group for any conclusions with regard to effectiveness.

Overall, the guidelines and the RCTs used similar points, suggesting that the RCTs generally reflected the clinical practice of acupuncture for these conditions.

Summary of Clinical Evidence for Acupuncture and Related Therapies

The majority of the studies focused on the effects of manual and/or electroacupuncture on measures of gastrointestinal function recovery. Of the RCTs, the pooled results for two sham controlled studies of electroacupuncture showed significant reductions in time to first flatus and first defaecation (Table 7.3), with no heterogeneity in the results. However, the relatively small sample size ($n = 140$) somewhat limited our confidence in the result.

In the nine studies that did not use a sham acupuncture method to blind participants, there were significant improvements in time to first bowel sounds, flatus and defaecation for both the manual acupuncture (Table 7.4) and electroacupuncture (Table 7.5) groups; however, these two meta-analysis pools showed considerable heterogeneity with regard to the magnitude, but not the direction, of the effect. This appears likely due to differences between studies in the surgical and conventional postoperative care used, and differences in the acupuncture methods. The size of the meta-analysis pool for manual acupuncture was relatively small ($n = 174$) but the sample was over 300 for two of the outcomes for electroacupuncture. Similar results were found for the single of study of warm needling (Table 7.7) and the single RCT of acupressure reported a significant reduction in time to first flatus, but not in time to first defaecation (Table 7.12). Overall, most of the RCTs of acupuncture and related interventions using traditional points indicated reductions in at least some of the measures of gastrointestinal functional recovery after CRC surgery.

Notably, all these studies had the point ST36 *Zusanli* 足三里 in common. In textbooks and guidelines (see Chapter 2), acupuncture and related therapies are recommended for CRC, mainly for managing symptoms. ST36 *Zusanli* 足三里 was the most frequently used point for most symptoms, including postoperative ileus, abdominal distension and abdominal pain. There is considerable overlap in the points recommended in the guidelines and those used in these studies.

In the three RCTs of ear acupressure, which did not use any traditional points, significant improvements were found for all measures of recovery of gastrointestinal function (Table 7.15). Heterogeneity was evident in some outcomes, but this was due to the different effect sizes in the single study of colon cancer.

Of the other postoperative outcomes, only abdominal distension at five days after surgery was tested in multiple RCTs. Two of the three studies showed reductions in the manual acupuncture groups compared to usual postoperative care alone, but the data were not suitable for meta-analysis. In addition, a single RCT of incidence of postoperative urinary retention (A16) found too few cases in either group for a meaningful result regarding the effectiveness of manual acupuncture plus moxibustion. For quality of life postsurgery, a single study (A11) reported no significant effect of electroacupuncture on the modified ESAS. The single study of warm needling (A12) found increases in T cell subsets suggestive of improved immune function.

Only one RCT of moxibustion reported on the AEs of chemotherapy (A19). It found a benefit for combining moxibustion with the anti-nausea drug ondansetron for nausea and vomiting associated with FOLFOX4. In addition, single non-controlled studies reported benefits for acupuncture in managing oxaliplatin chemotherapy-induced peripheral neuropathy (A18) and persistent hiccups following chemotherapy (A17).

Overall, the results of the meta-analyses of multiple RCTs suggested that manual acupuncture and electroacupuncture interventions were effective in reducing the time to recovery of gastrointestinal function recovery following surgery for CRC. The evidence was strongest for electroacupuncture, since this was based on sham-controlled studies with little heterogeneity plus a larger number of non-blinded RCTs, which although there was considerable heterogeneity in the pooled results, showed a consistent direction in effect. This is not to say that manual acupuncture was less effective. It is likely that some trial designers favored electroacupuncture over manual acupuncture since it was more feasible to implement a sham intervention using a disabled electrostimulator than attempt blinding of manual acupuncture. Hence, there was a lack of blinded studies of manual acupuncture. It should be noted that blinding of the personnel who deliver the acupuncture is difficult.

Ear acupressure shows evidence based on multiple studies, but these were small and not blinded. Evidence for other acupuncture therapies was relatively sparse and none were blinded, so our conclusions regarding warm needling and moxibustion were tentative while we wait for further studies.

There were inadequacies in the methodological reporting quality in most the studies. Some studies did not describe the method of randomisation and it is possible that lack of blinding in the majority of studies could have influenced assessments in favour of the acupuncture interventions. These issues should be considered when interpreting results and making clinical decisions.

References

1. Kim KH, Kim DH, Kim HY, Son GM. (2016) Acupuncture for recovery after surgery in patients undergoing colorectal cancer resection: A systematic review and meta-analysis. *Acupunct Med* **34(4):** 248–256.
2. He XR, Wang Q, Li PP. (2013) Acupuncture and moxibustion for cancer-related fatigue: A systematic review and meta-analysis. *Asian Pac J Cancer Prev* **14(5):** 3067–3074.
3. Posadzki P, Moon TW, Choi TY, *et al.* (2013) Acupuncture for cancer-related fatigue: A systematic review of randomized clinical trials. *Support Care Cancer* **21(7):** 2067–2073.
4. Lee S, Jerng UM, Liu Y, *et al.* (2014) The effectiveness and safety of moxibustion for treating cancer-related fatigue: A systematic review and meta-analyses. *Support Care Cancer* **22(5):** 1429–1440.
5. Lee MS, Choi TY, Park JE, *et al.* (2010) Moxibustion for cancer care: A systematic review and meta-analysis. *BMC Cancer* **10(130):** 1–8.
6. Tan JY, Molassiotis A, Wang T, Suen LK. (2014) Current evidence on auricular therapy for chemotherapy-induced nausea and vomiting in cancer patients: A systematic review of randomized controlled trials. *Evid Based Complement Alternat Med* **2014(430796):** 1–14.
7. Choi TY, Lee MS, Ernst E. (2015) Moxibustion for the treatment of chemotherapy-induced leukopenia: A systematic review of randomized clinical trials. *Support Care Cancer* **23(6):** 1819–1826.
8. National Institutes of Health and National Cancer Institute. (2008) Common terminology criteria for adverse events (CTCAE), version 4. National Institutes of Health, Bethesda, MD.

9. Trotti A, Colevas AD, Setser A, *et al.* (2003) CTCAE v3.0: Development of a comprehensive grading system for the adverse effects of cancer treatment. *Semin Radiat Oncol* **13(3):** 176–181.

10. Miller AB, Hoogstraten B, Staquet M, Winkler A. (1981) Reporting results of cancer treatment. *Cancer* **47(1):** 207–214.

List of Clinical Studies Included in Chapter 7

Study Number	Reference
A1	佟宛云, 阿依古丽, 徐乐. (2014) 穴位针刺对直肠癌术后胃肠蠕动功能的影响. 中医药导报 **20(12):** 39–41.
A2	王慧敏. (2011) 针刺对结直肠癌快速康复术后胃肠功能恢复的影响. 学位论文. 南京中医药大学, pp. 10–28.
A3	谭双, 郑婵美. (2015) 耳穴贴压结合针刺足三里对大肠癌术后胃肠功能恢复的临床研究. 北方药学 **12(12):** 112–113.
A4	肖超. (2014) 电针促进结直肠癌术后胃肠功能恢复的临床研究. 学位论文. 湖南中医药大学, pp. 1–14.
A5	Deng G, Wong WD, Guillem J, *et al.* (2013) A phase II, randomized, controlled trial of acupuncture for reduction of postcolectomy ileus. *Ann Surg Oncol* **20:** 1164–1169.
A6	Zhang ZD, Wang QY, Li MY, *et al.* (2014) Electroacupuncture at ST36 accelerates the recovery of gastrointestinal motility after colorectal surgery: A randomised controlled trial. *Acupunct Med* **32(3):** 223–226.
A7.1	Ng SSM, Leung WW, Hon SSF, *et al.* (2013) Electro-acupuncture for ileus after laparoscopic colorectal surgery: A randomised sham-controlled study. *Hong Kong Med J* **19(6):** 33–35.
A7.2	Ng SSM, Leung WW, Mak TWC, *et al.* (2013) Electroacupuncture reduces duration of postoperative ileus after laparoscopic surgery for colorectal cancer. *Gastroenterology* **144(2):** 307–313.
A8	牛春风, 李东朝, 高永红. (2008) 电针穴位治疗对大肠癌根治术后肠蠕动的影响. 长春中医药大学学报 **24(1):** 83.
A9	司纪广, 丁悦森. (2015) 电针恢复大肠癌根治术后胃肠功能临床研究. 实用中医药杂志 **31(8):** 754–755.
A10	杨俊杰. (2011) 电针刺下合穴对结直肠癌术后患者胃肠道功能影响的研究. 学位论文. 广州中医药大学, pp. 10–20.

(Continued)

(*Continued*)

Study Number	Reference
A11	Meng ZQ, Garcia MK, Chiang JS, *et al.* (2010) Electro-acupuncture to prevent prolonged postoperative ileus: A randomized clinical trial. *World J Gastroenterol* **16(1):** 104–111.
A12	张双燕, 杜业勤. (2011) 温针灸对肠癌术后患者胃肠功能及免疫功能的影响. 中国针灸 **31(6):** 513–517.
A13	Chao HL, Miao SJ, Liu PF, *et al.* (2013) The beneficial effect of ST-36 (zusanli) acupressure on postoperative gastrointestinal function in patients with colorectal cancer. *Oncol Nurs Forum* **40(2):** 61–68.
A14	陆金英, 金惠明. (2011) 耳穴贴压对大肠癌术后胃肠功能恢复的效果观察. 中国中医急症 **20(12):** 2061–2062.
A15	王鄂明. (2012) 耳穴贴压对结肠癌术后胃肠功能恢复的影响. 学位论文. 广州中医药大学, pp. 15–23.
A16	严银波. (2011) 针灸促进腹腔镜下直肠癌腹会阴联合切除术后排尿功能恢复的临床研究. 学位论文. 南京中医药大学, pp. 11–31.
A17	柏巧玲, 黄顺贵. (2004) 腹针治疗化疗后呃逆 1 例. 中国临床医生**32(9):** 51.
A18	Valentine-Davis B, Altshuler LH. (2015) Acupuncture for oxaliplatin chemotherapy-induced peripheral neuropathy in colon cancer: A retrospective case series. *Med Acupunct* **27(3):** 216–223.
A19	向培. (2011) 艾灸减轻结肠癌术后辅助化疗所致恶心呕吐效果观察. 中国中医急症 **20(8):** 1327–1328.

8

Clinical Evidence for Other Chinese Medicine Therapies

OVERVIEW

The searches identified two randomised controlled trials, no non-randomised controlled studies and no non-controlled studies of other Chinese medicine therapies. In both studies the therapy was the *an mo* 按摩 style of Chinese remedial massage, and one study also included a hot water foot bath. Both were for improving recovery after surgery for colorectal cancer. The meta-analyses focused on time to recovery of gastrointestinal function and incidence of abdominal distension following surgery.

Introduction

In addition to Chinese herbal medicine and acupuncture therapies, Chinese medicine (CM) includes a range of other therapies to treat disease and maintain health. These include:

- Chinese remedial massage (*tui na* 推拿 and *an mo* 按摩): This involves pressing, rubbing and other manual techniques on meridians, acupoints, muscles and skin areas using different parts of the palms and fingers and varying degrees of force;
- Chinese exercise therapies: Including various styles of *tai chi* 太極 (*tai ji quan* 太极拳), various forms of *dao yin yang sheng gong* 导引养生功 and various types of *qi gong* 气功. These therapies tend to be holistic systems that coordinate body posture and movement, breathing and meditation that are used for maintaining or recovering health, developing spirituality and/or martial arts training.

Previous Systematic Reviews

One systematic review, that included a range of CM therapies including Chinese remedial massage (*tui na* 推拿), *qi gong* 气功 and *tai chi* 太极 for all types of cancers, concluded that *tui na* 推拿 relieved gastrointestinal discomfort. Based on four studies, Chinese remedial massage reduced time to first flatulence and intestinal peristaltic sounds following surgery, but there were no separate meta-analysis results provided for Chinese remedial massage in colorectal cancer (CRC).[1,2]

Identification of Clinical Studies

The searches identified two randomised controlled trials (RCTs), no controlled clinical trials (CCTs) and no non-controlled studies that met the inclusion criteria (Fig. 8.1).

Both the RCTs tested the effectiveness of an *an mo* 按摩 form of Chinese remedial massage for the management of postoperative abdominal distension and recovery of gastrointestinal function. One study tested the combination of *an mo* 按摩 plus usual postoperative care versus usual care (O1). The other study used *an mo* 按摩 plus foot baths using hot water, in addition to usual care versus usual care (O2). Both studies were conducted in China. In total, 120 people participated in the two studies. Neither study mentioned syndrome differentiation. No studies of *tai chi* 太极, *qi gong* 气功 or Chinese food therapy were included.

An mo Remedial Massage

Two studies of Chinese *an mo* 按摩 remedial massage for CRC were included (O1, O2). Both were RCTs. The mostly frequently used locations for *an mo* 按摩 were ST36 *Zusanli* 足三里 and LI4 *Hegu* 合谷, which were used in both studies.

Randomised Controlled Trials

One RCT (O1) (*n* = 40) tested *an mo* 按摩 remedial massage in people aged 33 to 72 years, who had just received laparoscopic surgery

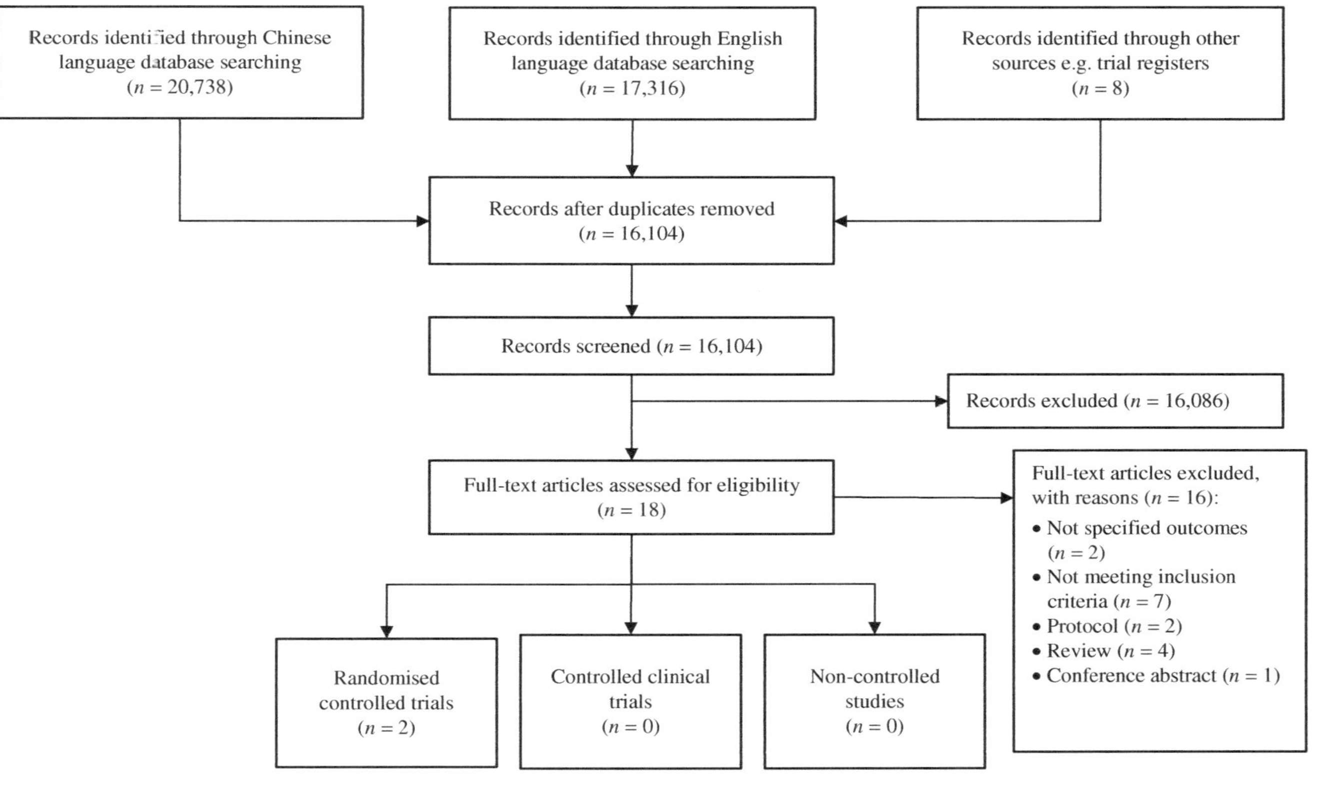

Fig. 8.1 Flowchart of Study Selection Process: other Chinese medicine therapies.

for CRC to determine whether this treatment improved postoperative abdominal distension, as well as measures of recovery of gastrointestinal function. The *an mo* 按摩 therapy involved massage at ST36 *Zusanli* 足三里 and LI4 *Hegu* 合谷 for 10–15 minutes per session, commencing six hours after surgery and repeated every four to six hours thereafter.

The other RCT (O2) tested a similar *an mo* 按摩 intervention in 80 people (mean age of 60.40 years in the *an mo* 按摩 group and 59.83 years in the control group) with the addition of a foot bath. The *an mo* 按摩 commenced eight hours after surgery at ST36 *Zusanli* 足三里, LI4 *Hegu* 合谷, and ST37 *Shangjuxu* 上巨虚 twice a day (morning and evening) with *an mo* 按摩 on each point for three to four minutes. The foot bath involved soaking both feet in hot water (40–45°C) for 20 minutes prior to sleep. Treatment continued until first passage of flatus. In both RCTs the control groups received usual postoperative care without *an mo* 按摩 treatment or foot bath.

Risk of Bias

Both studies were described as randomised but one study (O1) made no mention of the method for sequence generation, while the other study (O2) alternately allocated patients to groups according to when the surgery was performed (Table 8.1). The first

Table 8.1   Risk of Bias of Randomised Controlled Trials: *An Mo Remedial Massage*

Risk of Bias Domain	Low Risk *n* (%)	Unclear Risk *n* (%)	High Risk *n* (%)
Sequence generation	0 (0)	1 (50)	1 (50)
Allocation concealment	0 (0)	2 (100)	0 (0)
Blinding of participants	0 (0)	0 (0)	2 (100)
Blinding of personnel*	0 (0)	0 (0)	2 (100)
Blinding of outcome assessor	0 (0)	2 (100)	0 (0)
Incomplete outcome data	2 (100)	0 (0)	0 (0)
Selective reporting	0 (0)	2 (100)	0 (0)

*Blinding of personnel is challenging in manual therapies.

study (O1) was judged as 'unclear' risk and the second study (O2) was judged as 'high' risk. Neither study mentioned allocation concealment or blinding. Both studies were assessed as 'unclear' risk for allocation concealment and 'high' risk of bias for blinding of participants and personnel and unclear for outcome assessors. Both studies were assessed as 'low' risk for incomplete outcome data as there were no drop-outs and all data on the outcomes specified in the methods were available. For selective outcome reporting, both studies were assessed as 'unclear' risk as no protocols were identified.

Results

Outcome data suitable for meta-analysis were available for three measures of time to recovery of gastrointestinal function and incidence of postoperative abdominal distension.

Time to First Bowel Sounds

A significant reduction in time to first bowel sounds, based on assessments using a stethoscope, was found in the pooled result for the two studies (mean difference [MD]: –8.00 [–10.08, –5.92] hours, I^2 = 34.5%) with a mean reduction to the commencement of bowel sounds of eight hours (Table 8.2).

Time to First Passage of Flatus

Time to first passage of flatus was based on reports by patients in both studies. There were no significant differences between groups (MD: –5.12 [–16.06, 5.82] hours) in the first study (O1), but there was a significant reduction in time in the group that received *an mo* 按摩 plus foot bath compared to the group that received usual care alone (MD: –21.60 [–22.33, –20.87] hours) in the second study (O2) (Table 8.2). The pooled time to first passage of flatus was not significantly different between groups (MD: –14.30 [–30.35, 1.74] hours), but the heterogeneity was substantial (I^2 = 88.5%).

Table 8.2 *An Mo* Remedial Massage: Recovery of Gastrointestinal Function

Included Studies	*N* Participants	Effect Size (MD [95% CI)]), I^2
Time to first bowel sounds (hours)		
O1	40	−6.02 [−9.91, −2.14]*
O2	80	−8.57 [−9.70, −7.44]*
Pooled result (2 studies)	120	−8.00 [−10.08, −5.92]*, 34.5%
Time to first passage of flatus (hours)		
O1	40	−5.12 [−16.06, 5.82]
O2	80	−21.60 [−22.33, −20.87]*
Pooled result (2 studies)	120	−14.30[−30.35, 1.74], 88.5%
Time to first defaecation (hours)		
O2	80	−36.07 [−37.19, −34.95]*

*Statistically significant.

Abbreviations: CI, confidence interval; MD, mean difference; N, number.

Time to First Defaecation

Only one study (O2) reported time to first defaecation based on patient records. There was a significant reduction in the *an mo* 按摩 plus foot bath group, compared to usual care alone (MD: −36.07 [−37.19, −34.95] hours) (Table 8.2).

Postoperative Abdominal Distention

Both studies reported incidence of abdominal distension based on reports by patients. One study (O1) reported no significant difference between groups (relative risk [RR]: 0.67 [0.29, 1.54]), while the other study (O2) reported a significant reduction in the *an mo* 按摩 plus foot bath group, compared to usual care alone (RR: 0.17 [0.08, 0.36]) (Table 8.3). The pooled result for the two studies showed no significant difference between groups (RR: 0.33 [0.09, 1.31]) but there was substantial heterogeneity (I^2 = 83.2%).

Safety of *An Mo* Remedial Massage

Neither study mentioned adverse events associated with the *an mo* 按摩 or foot bath.

Table 8.3 *An Mo* **Remedial Massage: Postoperative Abdominal Distention**

Included Studies	*N* Participants	Effect Size (RR [95% CI]) I^2
O1	40	0.67 [0.29, 1.54]
O2	80	0.17 [0.08, 0.36]*
Pooled result (2 studies)	120	0.33 [0.09, 1.31] 83.2%

*Statistically significant.

Abbreviations: CI, confidence interval, N, number; RR, risk ratio.

Summary of Clinical Evidence for Other Chinese Medicine Therapies

Only two studies of other CM therapies for CRC met all inclusion and exclusion criteria. These both tested *an mo* 按摩 remedial massage for postoperative abdominal distension and recovery of gastrointestinal function. Both studies used similar *an mo* 按摩 interventions and a number of the same outcome measures, so data pooling was feasible. The smaller of the two studies (O1) (*n* = 40) showed a significant reduction in time to first bowel sounds in the *an mo* 按摩 group compared to the control group, but no significant difference in time to first passage of flatus. In the larger study (O2) (*n* = 80) there were significant reductions in time for each of the three measures of recovery of gastrointestinal function and in incidence of abdominal distension. There was considerable heterogeneity in the pooled results. It is notable that the time to recovery of gastrointestinal function was much shorter in the first study (O1) and the incidence of abdominal distension was much lower in the control group, than in the control group in the second study (O2). The first study employed laparoscopic surgery. Although the type of surgery was not specified in the second study, it is likely that usual surgical methods were employed. In cases where laparoscopic surgery is applicable, the incidence of postsurgical complications has been reported to be lower and hospital stays shorter, compared to open surgery.[3] So it appears likely that the difference in surgical methods used in the two studies was an important contributor to the statistical heterogeneity of the pooled outcomes.

Whether the addition of *an mo* 按摩 on ST37 *Shangjuxu* 上巨虚 and the foot bath improved the outcomes in the second study (O2) is difficult to assess since the type of surgery was different and the overall time to recovery was much shorter in the laparoscopic surgery study, so the two studies were not directly comparable. It is notable that a recent RCT of foot massage concluded that reflexology foot massage in CRC patients reduced incidence of distension and urinary frequency, and improved quality of life.[4]

Overall, the results suggest that *an mo* 按摩 on ST36 *Zusanli* 足三里 and LI4 *Hegu* 合谷 assists in reducing recovery of bowel sounds following both laparoscopic and usual surgery for CRC.

In textbooks and guidelines (see Chapter 2), *tui na* 推拿 techniques, which are very similar to those described as *an mo* 按摩 in the preceding two studies, are recommended for recovery of intestinal function in CRC. In addition, there is considerable overlap in the acupoints recommended in the guidelines and those used in these studies.

References

1. Tao W, Luo X, Cui B, *et al.* (2015) Practice of traditional Chinese medicine for psycho-behavioral intervention improves quality of life in cancer patients: A systematic review and meta-analysis. *Oncotarget* **6(37):** 39725–39739.
2. Tao WW, Jiang H, Tao XM, *et al.* (2016) Effects of acupuncture, tui na, tai chi, qigong, and traditional Chinese medicine five-element music therapy on symptom management and quality of life for cancer patients: A meta-analysis. *J Pain Symptom Manage* **51(4):** 728–747.
3. Degiuli M, Mineccia M, Bertone A, *et al.* (2004) Outcome of laparoscopic colorectal resection. *Surg Endosc* **18(3):** 427–432.
4. Uysal N, Kutlutürkan S, Uğur I. (2017) Effects of foot massage applied in two different methods on symptom control in colorectal cancer patients: Randomized control trial. *Int J Nurs Pract* **23(3):** 1–11.

List of Clinical Studies Included in Chapter 8

Study Number	References
O1	陈运丽. (2008) 穴位按摩对腹腔镜下结直肠癌根治术后腹胀的作用. 中国误诊学杂志 **8(31):** 7627–7628.
O2	陆金英. (2010) 穴位按摩联合足浴对肠癌术后患者肠蠕动恢复的影响. 护理学报 **17(4B):** 61–62.

9

Clinical Evidence for Combination Therapies

OVERVIEW

The searches identified eight randomised controlled trials, zero non-randomised controlled studies and four non-controlled studies that used combinations of Chinese medicine therapies. All studies used Chinese herbal medicine, administered orally or topically. The main combination was with acupuncture while three studies used moxibustion. Other therapies including *an mo* 按摩, *qi gong* 气功, *tai chi* 太极 and dietary therapy were used in single studies. Most studies were for improving recovery after surgery for colorectal cancer. Meta-analyses were conducted for measures of time to recovery of gastrointestinal function after surgery.

Introduction

Combination therapies are defined as two or more Chinese medicine (CM) interventions administered together, for example Chinese herbal medicine (CHM) plus acupuncture. No previous systematic review of CHM combined with acupuncture, or other CM therapies for colorectal cancer (CRC) could be located.

Identification of Clinical Studies

The searches identified eight randomised controlled studies (RCTs), no non-randomised controlled clinical trial (CCT), and four non-controlled studies (Fig. 9.1). Two non-controlled studies (C1, C2) tested the

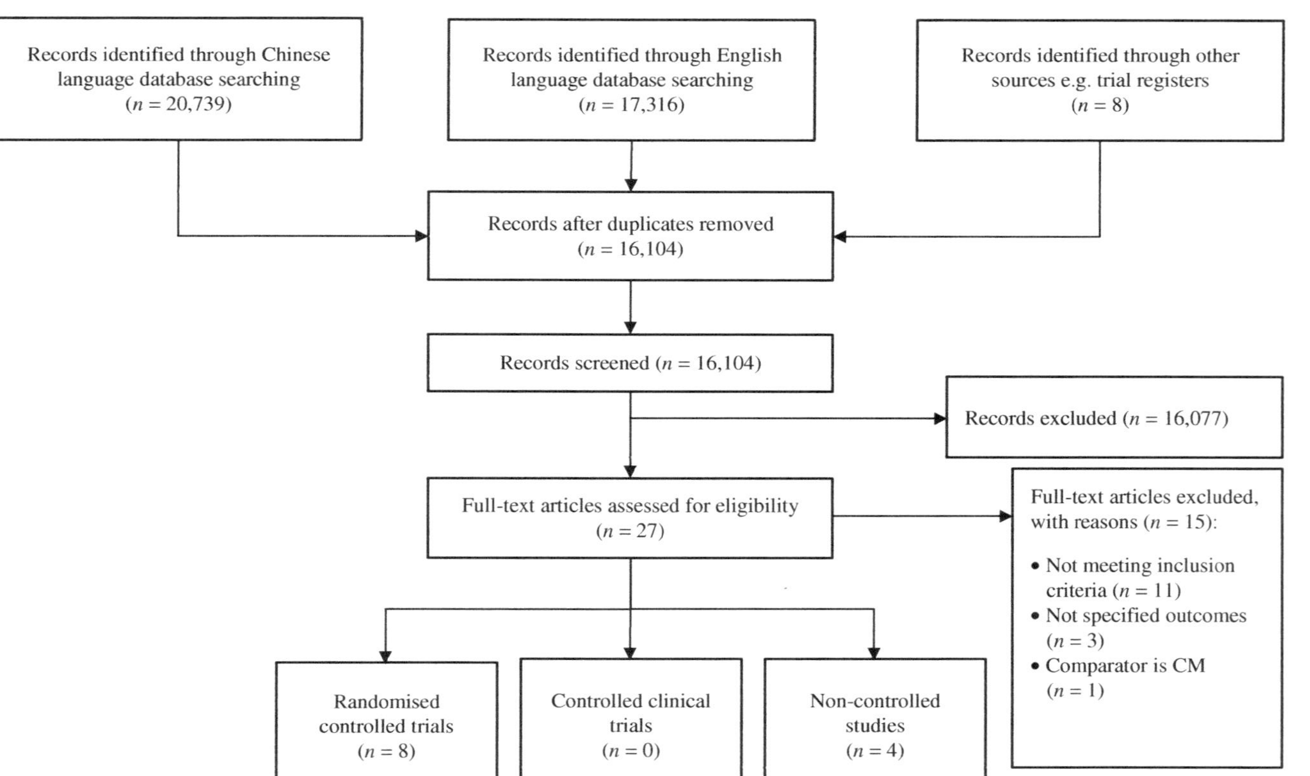

Fig. 9.1   Flowchart of Study Selection Process: Combination Therapies

Table 9.1 Summary of Combination Therapy Interventions

Combination Therapy Interventions	No. of Studies	Included Studies
Oral CHM + acupuncture	2	C1, C2
Oral CHM + topical CHM[1] + acupuncture	2	C3, C4
Oral CHM + acupuncture + qi gong 气功 + tai chi 太极 + diet	1	C5
Oral CHM + moxibustion	1	C6
CHM enema + acupuncture	2	C7, C8
Topical CHM[2] + moxibustion	2	C9, C10
Topical CHM[3] + moxibustion + an mo 按摩	1	C11
Topical CHM[1] + electroacupuncture	1	C12

[1]Fomentation.

[2]Fomentation (C9), cataplasm (C10).

[3]Cataplasm.

Abbreviations: CHM, Chinese herbal medicine.

combination of oral CHM and acupuncture. Two studies (C3, C4), including one RCT (C3), used both oral and topical CHM combined with acupuncture. One cohort study (C5) tested a combination of CM therapies including oral CHM, acupuncture, *qi gong* 气功, *tai chi* (*tai ji* 太极), diet and other therapies based on patient needs. One RCT (C6) combined oral CHM and moxibustion, two RCTs (C7, C8) combined CHM enema with acupuncture, two RCTs (C9, C10) combined topical CHM with moxibustion, one (C11) combined topical CHM with moxibustion plus *an mo* 按摩 massage, and one RCT (C12) combined topical CHM with electroacupuncture (Table 9.1).

Outline of the Data Analyses

Studies are grouped by the type of study (RCT or non-controlled study) and by the type of CHM and acupuncture therapy. Meta-analysis results of RCTs are presented for each type of combination therapy for the following outcomes (if available):

- Recovery of gastrointestinal function;
- Postoperative complications;

- Postoperative immune function;
- Postoperative diarrhoea;
- Karnofsky Performance Status;
- Quality of life.

The results of the single cohort study (C5) and descriptions of the case series and case studies follow the RCTs.

Randomised Controlled Trials of Combination Therapies

The searches located eight parallel group RCTs of CM combination therapy (Fig. 9.1). The RCTs tested various combinations of oral and/ or topical CHM and acupuncture or moxibustion. In seven RCTs the outcomes were for postoperative recovery of gastrointestinal function and other postoperative conditions. One RCT (C10) was for supporting people who were not suitable for surgery, chemotherapy or other CRC-specific therapy. All the RCTs were conducted in mainland China. The included studies enrolled 610 participants. The age of participants ranged from 28 to 84 years.

For the purpose of meta-analysis, the studies were broadly grouped according to whether oral CHM was used (C3, C6), whether the CHM was via enema *guan chang* 灌肠 (C7, C8), or whether the CHM was only applied to the skin as a fomentation *yun tang* 熨烫 (C3, C9, C12) or a cataplasm *yao gao* 药膏 (C10, C11). One study used both oral and topical CHM (C3).

Groups were further subdivided according to whether acupuncture (C3, C7, C8) or moxibustion (C6, C9, C10, C11) was used. All studies used usual care as the comparator. One study (C12) used four groups, but the other comparison was included in Chapter 5. One of these studies (C3) specified the use of a Fast Track Programme (FTP) of perioperative care.

Syndromes

Only one study (C10) reported on CM syndromes. The mentioned syndrome was *qi* and Blood dual deficiency *qi xue kui xu* 气血亏虚, which was an inclusion criterion.

Formula, Herb and Acupuncture Point Frequencies

Each RCT used a different CHM formula but these included a number of herbs as common ingredients. The most frequently used herbs in the oral formulas were *dang shen* 党参, *sheng ma* 升麻, *dang gui* 当归, *chai hu* 柴胡, *bai zhu* 白术, *chen pi* 陈皮 and *huang qi* 黄芪 (Table 9.2).

The most frequently used herbs in the topical formulas (not including enemas) were *wu zhu yu* 吴茱萸, followed by *dan shen* 丹参, *bing pian* 冰片, *bai jie zi* 白芥子 and *xi xin* 细辛 (Table 9.3).

Table 9.2   Oral Herbs Frequently Used in the Combined Interventions

Herb Name	Scientific Name	No. of Studies
Dang shen 党参	*Codonopsis pilosula* (Franch.) Nannf.	3
Sheng ma 升麻	*Cimicifuga foetida* L.	3
Dang gui 当归	*Angelica sinensis* (Oliv.) Diels	3
Chai hu 柴胡	*Bupleurum chinense* DC.	3
Bai zhu 白术	*Atractylodes macrocephala* Koidz.	3
Chen pi 陈皮	*Citrus reticulata* Blanco	3
Huang qi 黄芪	*Astragalus membranaceus* (Fisch.) Bge.	3
Shan yao 山药	*Dioscorea opposita* Thunb.	2
Gou qi zi 枸杞子	*Lycium barbarum* L.	2
Gan cao 甘草[1]	*Glycyrrhiza uralensis* Fisch.	2
Shan zha 山楂	*Crataegus pinnatifida* Bge.	2
Bai shao 白芍	*Paeonia lactiflora* Pall.	2
Sha ren 砂仁	*Amomum villosum* Lour.	2
Shen qu 神曲	*Massa medicata fermentata*	2
Fu ling 茯苓	*Poria cocos (Schw.)* Wolf	2
Yi yi ren 薏苡仁	*Coix lacryma-jobi* L. var. *mayuen* (Roman.) Stapf	2
Ji xue teng 鸡血藤	*Spatholobus suberectus* Dunn	2
Mai ya 麦芽	*Hordeum vulgare* L.	2

[1]One used *zhi gan cao* 炙甘草.

The use of some herbs may be restricted in some countries. Readers are advised to comply with relevant regulations.

Table 9.3 Topical Herbs Frequently Used in the Combined Interventions

Herb Name	Scientific Name	No. of Studies
Wu zhu yu 吴茱萸	*Euodia rutaecarpa* (Juss.) Benth.	4
Dan shen 丹参	*Salvia miltiorrhiza* Bge.	2
Bing pian 冰片	Borneol	2
Bai jie zi 白芥子	*Sinapis alba* L.	2
Xi xin 细辛	*Asarum sieboldii* Miq.	2

The use of some herbs may be restricted in some countries. Readers are advised to comply with relevant regulations.

Table 9.4 Points for Acupuncture or Electroacupuncture and Moxibustion Frequently Used in the Combined Interventions

Points for Acupuncture/Electroacupuncture		Points for Moxibustion	
Point Name	No. of Studies	Point Name	No. of Studies
ST36 *Zusanli* 足三里	4	ST36 *Zusanli* 足三里	4
ST37 *Shangjuxu* 上巨虚	3	CV8 *Shenque* 神阙	3
ST39 *Xiajuxu* 下巨虚	2	ST25 *Tianshu* 天枢	2
CV12 *Zhongwan* 中脘	2	CV6 *Qihai* 气海	2
ST25 Tianshu 天枢	2		

In the two RCTs that used enemas (C7, C8), the herbs used in both the enema formulas were *da huang* 大黄, *mang xiao* 芒硝, *hou pu* 厚朴, *lai fu zi* 莱菔子, *dang shen* 党参, *mu xiang* 木香 and *huang qi* 黄芪.

The most frequently used points for acupuncture or electroacupuncture were ST36 *Zusanli* 足三里 and ST37 *Shangjuxu* 上巨虚, and the most frequently used points for moxibustion were ST36 *Zusanli* 足三里 and CV8 *Shenque* 神阙 (Table 9.4).

Risk of Bias

All eight studies were described as randomised but only four described an appropriate method for sequence generation so these were judged 'low' risk for this item (Table 9.5). The others were judged as 'unclear' risk. No study mentioned allocation concealment,

Table 9.5   Risk of Bias of Randomised Controlled Trials: Combination Therapies

Risk of Bias Domain	Low Risk *n* (%)	Unclear Risk *n* (%)	High Risk *n* (%)
Sequence generation	4 (50)	4 (50)	0 (0)
Allocation concealment	0 (0)	8 (100)	0 (0)
Blinding of participants	0 (0)	2 (25)	6 (75)
Blinding of personnel*	0 (0)	0 (0)	8 (100)
Blinding of outcome assessor	0 (0)	8 (100)	0 (0)
Incomplete outcome data	7 (87.5)	0 (0)	1 (12.5)
Selective reporting	0 (0)	8 (100)	0 (0)

*Blinding of personnel is challenging in manual therapies.

so all studies were assessed as 'unclear' risk. No study mentioned blinding, but both enema studies used a control enema of normal saline which we assume was intended to blind participants. Since it is not clear whether blinding was achieved, these were judged 'unclear' risk. The other studies were judged 'high' risk of bias for blinding of participants. All studies were judged 'high' risk for blinding of personnel and 'unclear' risk for blinding of outcome assessors. Seven studies were assessed as 'low' risk for incomplete outcome data as there were no drop-outs and all data on the outcomes mentioned in the method sections of the articles were available. One study had eight drop-outs but did not report the reasons and it was not clear which groups the drop-outs were in, so it was judged 'high' risk. No protocols were identified for any included studies, so all studies were assessed as 'unclear' risk of bias for selective reporting. Overall the methodological reporting was inadequate, so results should be interpreted with caution as none of the studies were free from potential bias.

Clinical Evidence for Oral Chinese Herbal Medicine plus Acupuncture/Moxibustion with or without Chinese Herbal Medicine Fomentation Therapy

Two RCTs (C3, C6) investigated orally administered CHM plus acupuncture or moxibustion at traditional points. One of these studies (C3) also added a fomentation. Each of these studies employed different comparisons and/or outcome measures so it was not possible to pool data.

Recovery of Gastrointestinal Function

One RCT (C3, 80 participants) used an oral decoction for three days prior to surgery. The ingredients were *huang qi* 黄芪, *ji xue teng* 鸡血藤, *yi yi ren* 薏苡仁, *shan ci gu* 山慈菇, *dang shen* 党参, *teng li gen* 藤梨根, *bai zhu* 白术, *sheng ma* 升麻, *chai hu* 柴胡, *dang gui* 当归, *fu ling* 茯苓, *bai shao* 白芍, *shan yao* 山药, *gou qi zi* 枸杞子, *chen pi* 陈皮, *shen qu* 神曲, *mai ya* 麦芽, *shan zha* 山楂, *sha ren* 砂仁 and *zhi gan cao* 炙甘草. After surgery the oral decoction was modified by removing *shan ci gu* 山慈菇 and *teng li gen* 藤梨根, and adding *hou pu* 厚朴, *mang xiao* 芒硝 and *zhi shi* 枳实. Following first defaecation, *mang xiao* 芒硝 was removed. The decoction was used for seven days postsurgery.

Acupuncture was commenced 12 hours after surgery at ST36 *Zusanli* 足三里, ST37 *Shangjuxu* 上巨虚 and ST39 *Xiajuxu* 下巨虚, one to two times per day (30 mins retention time).

In addition, a fomentation was made by powdering *wu zhu yu* 吴茱萸, *rou gui* 肉桂 and *ding xiang* 丁香, placing the herbs in a cloth bag, heating the bag and placing it on the abdomen for 20 to 30 minutes once or twice per day. The acupuncture and topical CHM were continued until gastrointestinal function recovered. Both groups received perioperative care according to the FTP but the control group received no CM therapies. There were significant reductions in time to first flatus (mean difference [MD]: −13.25 [−19.92, −6.59] hours) and time to first defaecation (MD: −13.61 [−19.30, −7.92] hours) in the CM combination therapy group (Table 9.6).

Postoperative Complications

The above RCT (C3) reported on postoperative complications. In the CM combination therapy group, there were significant reductions in the incidence of three of the five postoperative complications

Table 9.6   Oral Chinese Herbal Medicine plus Acupuncture plus Chinese Herbal Medicine Fomentation for Recovery of Gastrointestinal Function

Intervention (*N* Participants)	Outcome	Effect Size (MD [95% CI]) (hours)	Included Studies
Oral CHM + acupuncture + CHM fomentation (80)	Time to first flatus	−13.25 [−19.92, −6.59]*	C3
	Time to first defaecation	−13.61 [−19.30, −7.92]*	

*Statistically significant.

Abbreviations: CHM, Chinese herbal medicine; CI, confidence interval; MD, mean difference.

measured: urinary retention (relative risk [RR]: 0.67 [0.12, 3.78], *n* = 80), incision infection (RR: 0.50 [0.16, 1.53], *n* = 80) and anastomotic fistula (RR; 0.88 [0.35, 2.18], *n* = 80). The other two measures were not assessable, since there were no cases of bowel obstruction or gastric retention in either group. These complications all resolved following treatment.

Postoperative Immune Function

The above RCT (C3) also reported data for postoperative immune function. At seven days after surgery there was greater recovery in immune function in the CM combination therapy group, as measured by increases in levels of immunoglobulin (Ig)A (MD: 0.46 [0.22, 0.70] g/L, *n* = 80), IgG (MD: 0.50 [0.16, 1.53] g/L, *n* = 80), and IgM (MD: 0.88 [0.35, 2.18] g/L, *n* = 80).

Postoperative Diarrhoea

Another RCT (C6) (*n* = 46) combined modified *Bu zhong yi qi tang* 补中益气汤 (*huang qi* 黄芪, *dang shen* 党参, *bai zhu* 白术, *chai hu* 柴胡, *dang gui* 当归, *sheng ma* 升麻, *gan cao* 甘草 and *chen pi* 陈皮) once a day with moxibustion on CV8 *Shenque* 神阙 and ST36 *Zusanli* 足三里 once a day for 30 minutes on each point. Treatment continued for two weeks with the aim of reducing postoperative diarrhoea. The control group received usual treatment for diarrhoea with oral loperamide hydrochloride and a probiotic containing a combination of live *Bifidobacterium, Lactobacillus* and *Enterococcus* in capsules for two weeks, but these were not administered in the combined CM group. More people showed complete recovery from diarrhoea within three to seven days in the combined CM group compared to controls (RR: 2.00 [0.70, 5.73], *n* = 46).

Karnofsky Performance Status

The above RCT (C6) reported data for Karnofsky Performance Status (KPS). After seven days postsurgery, more people in the combined CM group showed improvements of 10 points or more (RR: 1.60 [0.93, 2.74], *n* = 46) and fewer people showed declines of 10 points or more (RR: 0.10 [0.01, 0.72], *n* = 46).

Chinese Herbal Medicine Enema plus Acupuncture

Two RCTs (C7, C8) investigated CHM enema plus acupuncture for postoperative recovery of gastrointestinal function in rectal cancer patients. Therefore, the results of these studies could be pooled (Table 9.7). Both of the studies used a CHM enema compared with normal saline enema in the control groups.

One study specifically recruited 120 people with postoperative intestinal paralysis (C7) and treated them with an enema decoction (*da huang* 大黄, *mang xiao* 芒硝, *hou pu* 厚朴, *lai fu zi* 莱菔子, *zhi ke* 枳壳, *niu xi* 牛膝, *dang shen* 党参, *mu xiang* 木香, *huang qi* 黄芪 and *dang gui* 当归) once or twice a day. In addition, they received acupuncture at ST36 *Zusanli* 足三里, ST25 *Tianshu* 天枢, CV12 *Zhongwan* 中脘, CV6 *Qihai* 气海, CV4 *Guanyuan* 关元, ST37 *Shangjuxu* 上巨虚 and ST39 *Xiajuxu* 下巨虚 once per day (30 min. retention time). All treatments commenced 12 hours after surgery and until gastrointestinal function recovered. Both groups received usual postoperative care, but the control group did not receive any CM therapies.

The other RCT (C8) (*n* = 50) combined an enema using *Jia wei da cheng qi tang* 加味大承气汤 (*da huang* 大黄, *hou pu* 厚朴, *mang*

Table 9.7   Chinese Herbal Medicine Enema plus Acupuncture for Recovery of Gastrointestinal Function

Outcome (Unit)	Participant Type (No.)	Effect Size (MD [95% CI]), I²	Included Studies
Time to first bowel sounds (hours)	With postoperative intestinal paralysis (120)	−17.37 [−18.91, −15.83]*	C7
	General postoperative patients (50)	−8.66 [−11.40, −5.92]*	C8
	Pooled result (170)	−13.09 [−21.63, −4.56]*, 96.6%	C7, C8
Time to first flatus (hours)	With postoperative intestinal paralysis (120)	−12.23 [−14.11, −10.35]*	C7
	General postoperative patients (50)	−15.91 [−20.40, −11.43]*	C8
	Pooled result (170)	−13.48 [−16.90, −10.01]* 54.5%	C7, C8
Time to first defaecation (hours)	With postoperative intestinal paralysis (120)	−12.79 −18.50, −7.08]*	C7
	General postoperative patients (50)	−11.09 [−15.51, −6.67]*	C8
	Pooled result (170)	−11.73 [−15.22, −8.23]*, 0%	C7, C8
Time to normal bowel sounds (hours)	General postoperative patients (50)	−16.59 [−20.20, −12.98]*	C8

*Statistically significant.

Abbreviations: CI, confidence interval; MD, mean difference.

xiao 芒硝, *zhi shi* 枳实, *mu xiang* 木香, *lai fu zi* 莱菔子, *huang qi* 黄芪, *dan shen* 丹参 and *dang shen* 党参) twice a day with acupuncture at ST36 *Zusanli* 足三里, ST37 *Shangjuxu* 上巨虚, ST25 *Tianshu* 天枢 and CV12 *Zhongwan* 中脘 once a day for 30 minutes. All treatments commenced 12 hours after surgery and continued for seven days. Both groups received usual perioperative care.

Recovery of Gastrointestinal Function

The pooled results showed that time to first bowel sounds was significantly shorter in the combined CM therapy groups, compared to the control groups (MD: −13.09 [−21.63, −4.56] hours), but there was considerable heterogeneity (I^2 = 96.6%). This was likely due to the differences in the participant groups. In study C7 all participants had postoperative intestinal paralysis which was identified after surgery, so these patients could be expected to take longer to recover than the participants in study C8 who were general postoperative patients. This difference was evident in the mean recovery times in the control groups of 34.6 hours versus 24 hours, respectively. Also, the patients in C8 received therapy within 12 hours after surgery but therapy in C7 commenced after they had been identified with postoperative intestinal paralysis.

The pooled result for time to first flatus was significantly reduced (MD: −13.48[−16.90, −10.01] hours) in the CHM enema plus acupuncture groups with moderate heterogeneity (I^2 = 54.5%), which appears to be due to differences in patient groups. For time to first defaecation, there was a significant reduction in the pooled result of the CHM enema plus acupuncture groups (MD: −11.73 [−15.22, −8.23] hours) with no heterogeneity.

Time to normal bowel sounds was only reported by the seven-day study (C8). There were significant improvements in the combined CHM enema plus acupuncture group (MD: −16.59 [−20.20, −12.98] hours).

Topical Chinese Herbal Medicine plus Moxibustion, with or without *An Mo*

One RCT (C9) combined a CHM fomentation with moxibustion on a slice of ginger, one (C10) combined a CHM cataplasm with moxibustion on ginger, and one (C11) combined a CHM cataplasm with moxibustion plus *an mo* 按摩 remedial massage.

Recovery of Gastrointestinal Function

Two of the RCTs (C9, C10) combined topical CHMs with moxibustion on ginger for postoperative recovery of gastrointestinal function, so the results of these studies were pooled where possible (Table 9.8).

Table 9.8 Topical Chinese Herbal Medicine plus Moxibustion for Recovery of Gastrointestinal Function

Outcome (Unit)	Cancer (*N* Participants)	Effect Size (MD [95% CI]), I^2	Included Studies
Time to first bowel sounds (hours)	Rectal cancer (60)	–15.72 [–18.50, –12.94]*	C9
	General CRC (150)	–8.77 [–10.79, –6.75]*	C10
	Pooled result (210)	–12.18 [–18.99, –5.37]*, 93.6%	C9, C10
Time to first flatus (hours)	Rectal cancer (60)	–20.64 [–23.17, –18.11]*	C9
	General CRC (150)	–8.90 [–11.78, –6.02]*	C10
	Pooled result (210)	–14.79 [–26.30, –3.29]*, 97.2%	C9, C10
Time to first defaecation (hours)	General CRC (150)	–11.30 [–15.60, –7.00]*	C10

*Statistically significant.

Abbreviations: CI, confidence interval; CRC, colorectal cancer; MD, mean difference.

One RCT (*n* = 60) used a fomentation called *Cu dong san* 促动散 that was made by the author. The ingredients were *wu zhu yu* 吴茱萸, *hui xiang* 茴香, *hou pu* 厚朴, *wu yao* 乌药, *mu xiang* 木香 and *chuan xiong* 川芎. These were powdered and mixed and the dry powder was placed in a cloth bag. The bag was heated and placed on the abdomen for 20 minutes. In addition, participants received moxibustion on slices of ginger at CV8 *Shenque* 神阙 (3–5 cones) and ST36 *Zusanli* 足三里 (5–10 cones). Both treatments commenced six hours after sphincter-preserving surgery for rectal cancer. Treatments were administered twice a day and continued for three days (C9).

In the other RCT (C10) (*n* = 150), cataplasms were made using powdered *wu zhu yu* 吴茱萸, *dan shen* 丹参, *xi xin* 细辛, *bai jie zi* 白芥子 and *bing pian* 冰片, mixed with scallion juice (*cong zhi* 葱汁) to make a paste which was applied to gauze. Moxibustion on ginger was applied to CV8 *Shenque* 神阙, CV4 *Guanyuan* 关元, CV 6 *Qihai* 气海, ST25 *Tianshu* 天枢 and ST36 *Zusanli* 足三里 once a day, five cones per point. Following the moxibustion, a cataplasm was placed on each point with infrared being applied for 15 minutes to warm each point. The cataplasms were retained for four to five hours. Treatment commenced six hours after surgery for CRC and continued for 20 days. In both studies all groups received usual care but the control groups did not receive CM therapies.

The pooled results for time to first bowel sounds (MD: −12.18 [−18.99, −5.37], I^2 = 93.6%) and time to first flatus (MD: −14.79 [−26.30, −3.29], I^2 = 97.2%) were significantly shorter in the topical CHM plus moxibustion groups, than in the control groups, but the heterogeneity was considerable for both outcomes. The heterogeneity was likely influenced by differences in the patient groups. For example, there was considerably longer bowel sound recovery time in the control groups in C9 (47.09 hours), who received sphincter-preserving surgery for rectal cancer, compared to C11 (37.11 hours), who received usual surgery for CRC.

Time to first defaecation was reported by the 20-day study only (C11). This was significantly shorter than in the control group (MD: −11.30 [−15.60, −7.00] hours).

Karnofsky Performance Status and Quality of Life

Another RCT (C11) (n = 60) was for improving quality of life in advanced CRC. This study used a similar method to study C10. Cataplasms were made using powdered *huang qi* 黄芪, *xi xin* 细辛, *bai jie zi* 白芥子, *bing pian* 冰片, *dan shen* 丹参, *wu ling zhi* 五灵脂 and other ingredients, mixed with yellow wine (*huang jiu* 黄酒) to make a paste which was applied to gauze.

Moxibustion was applied to CV6 *Qihai* 气海, ST25 *Tianshu* 天枢 and ST36 *Zusanli* 足三里 for 10 to 15 minutes followed by *an mo* 按摩 massage on the same points. After this, a cataplasm was applied to each point and retained for four to five hours. All treatments continued for 14 days. Both groups received best supportive care. At the end of treatment there was an improvement in KPS scores in the CM group (MD: 9.00 [5.32, 12.68], n = 60) but there was no significant difference between groups for total scores on The European Organization for Research and Treatment of Cancer Quality of Life Questionnaire (EORTC QLQ-C30)[1] (MD: 8.20 [−2.37, 18.77], n = 60).

Table 9.9 Topical Chinese Herbal Medicine plus Electroacupuncture for Recovery of Gastrointestinal Function

Outcome (Unit)	Effect Size (MD [95% CI])	Included Studies
Time to first bowel sounds (hours)	5.71 [–15.63, 27.05]	C12
Time to first flatus (hours)	3.59 [–6.96, 14.14]	
Time to first defaecation (hours)	11.64 [–17.60, 40.88]	

Abbreviations: CI, confidence interval; MD, mean difference.

Topical Chinese Herbal Medicine plus Electroacupuncture

One RCT (C12) (*n* = 36) used *wu zhu yu* 吴茱萸 in a heated cloth bag placed on the abdomen for 30 minutes plus electroacupuncture at ST36 *Zusanli* 足三里 for 30 minutes for postoperative recovery of gastrointestinal function. Both treatments commenced one day after surgery, were administered twice a day (9 am and 4 pm) and continued for six days. Both groups received usual postoperative care but the control group did not receive CM therapies (Table 9.9).

There were no significant differences in time to first bowel sounds (MD: 5.71 [–15.63, 27.05] hours), time to first flatus (MD: 3.59 [–6.96, 14.14] hours) and time to first defaecation (MD: 11.64 [–17.60, 40.88] hours) in the CM combination therapy group compared to controls.

Clinical Evidence from Non-controlled Studies of Combination Therapy

The four non-controlled studies of combination therapy included one cohort study (C5), two case series studies (C2, C4) and one case study (C1). All of the studies used different herbs and groups of points, with ST36 *Zusanli* 足三里 being used in two studies. Each study is described separately.

The longitudinal cohort study (C5) compared a cohort of 193 people in California, the United States, who had received CM combination treatment as an adjunctive treatment to chemotherapy and/ or radiotherapy, following surgical resection to control cohorts from the Kaiser Permanente Northern California and California Cancer Registries. The treatment cohort were all patients who received CM during 1987–1992, following a regimen designed to supplement their conventional therapy. Treatments included acupuncture, CHM, *qi gong* 气功, vitamins, imagery, exercise, *tai chi* 太极, yoga, diet and other practices, based on the stage of therapy and the needs of the particular person.

Ten-year survival time was the main outcome and a comparison was conducted between people who followed the programme for a short time and those who adhered to the programme for a long time. Covariates included cancer stage (I–IV), age and sex. Kaplan-Meier plots showed longer survival in the CM cohort for all cancer stages compared to the control cohorts from the cancer registries. Cox proportional hazards regression did not find a significant difference between short-term and long-term adherents to the programme, but the CM combination cohort showed significantly longer survival for stages I, II and IV, with a similar trend for stage III.

One case series (C2) reported on the combination of oral CHM (infusion of *hui xiang* 茴香 and *hu po* 琥珀) plus acupuncture at EX-CA-c *Liniaoxue* 利尿穴 (an extra point also called *Zhixie* 止泻) and BL28 *Pangguangshu* 膀胱俞, plus other points according to the condition, in 21 people with postoperative urinary retention. The authors reported recovery after one to 12 treatments.

The other case series (C4) reported on five people with postoperative ileus who received the usual treatment plus the oral CHM modified *Wen pi tang* 温脾汤 (*fu zi* 附子, *gan jiang* 干姜, *bai zhu* 白术, *fu ling* 茯苓, *dang shen* 党参, *da huang* 大黄, *mang xiao* 芒硝, *lai fu zi* 莱菔子, *zhi ke* 枳壳, *hou pu* 厚朴, *dang gui* 当归, *chi shao* 赤芍, *bai shao* 白芍 and *gan cao* 甘草) combined with acupuncture at ST36 *Zusanli* 足三里, PC6 *Neiguan* 内关 and ST44 *Neiting* 内庭 for 30 to 45 minutes per day, continued for three to five days. In addition, the herbal residues were placed in a cloth bag, which was heated and placed on the abdomen once per day. The author reported all the people recovered after three to five days of treatment.

The case report (C1) was on one patient who suffered from delayed diarrhoea after adjuvant chemotherapy. The combined therapy was a modified decoction called *Tong xie yao fang* 痛泻要方 (*fang feng* 防风, *fu zi* 附子, *bai zhu* 白术, *bai shao* 白芍, *chen pi* 陈皮, *cao dou kou* 草豆蔻, *rou dou kou* 肉豆蔻, *sha ren* 砂仁, *gan jiang* 干姜, *long gu* 龙骨, *mu li* 牡蛎, *zhi gan cao* 炙甘草 and *huo xiang* 藿香) one packet per day in three doses, plus acupuncture at BL23 *Shenshu* 肾俞, BL20 *Pishu* 脾俞, BL25 *Dachangshu* 大肠俞, BL26 *Guanyuanshu* 关元俞, ST36 *Zusanli* 足三里, ST37 *Shangjuxu* 上巨虚 and LR3 *Taichong* 太冲 for 20 minutes per day. After ten days of treatment, the patient was reported to have recovered.

Safety of Combination Therapies

Three RCTs (C3, C10, C12) specified there were no obvious adverse events. The other RCTs, and the non-controlled studies, did not mention adverse events.

Summary of Clinical Evidence for Combination Therapies

Most of the evidence was from the RCTs that combined CHM with an acupuncture therapy and used the parameter of postoperative recovery as the main outcome measure. Only one study used syndrome differentiation and all studies used different CHM interventions. Four out of eight RCTs were judged 'low' risk of bias for sequence generation and none were adequately blinded, so there was potential for bias in the reported outcomes.

For measures of postoperative recovery of gastrointestinal function, there were significant improvements in the groups that received:

- Oral CHM plus acupuncture plus CHM fomentation (one RCT);
- CHM enema plus acupuncture (two RCTs);
- Topical CHM plus moxibustion (two RCTs);
- But not for one RCT of topical CHM plus electroacupuncture.

There were fewer postoperative complications in one RCT of CHM plus acupuncture plus CHM fomentation. In addition, postoperative diarrhoea improved in one RCT of oral CHM plus moxibustion.

For KPS there were improvements in the groups that received:

- Oral CHM plus moxibustion (one RCT);
- Moxibustion plus *an mo* 按摩 massage plus CHM cataplasm (one RCT).

For the Cancer Quality of Life Questionnaire (EORTC QLQ-C30) there was no significant difference between groups for moxibustion plus *an mo* 按摩 massage plus CHM cataplasm (one RCT). There were improvements in postoperative immune function after treatment with oral CHM plus acupuncture plus CHM fomentation (one RCT). The single cohort study was well designed and showed a correlation between the use of combined CM therapies and improved ten-year survival rate.

Two of the non-controlled studies were for postoperative recovery, with one reporting that oral CHM plus acupuncture was effective for postoperative urinary retention, while the other found that people with postoperative ileus improved with oral CHM plus acupuncture plus CHM fomentation. The remaining study was a single case of an oral CHM plus acupuncture resolving diarrhoea following chemotherapy. For safety outcomes, there was insufficient data for any assessments.

Comparison with Other Chapters

When compared to the therapeutic recommendations in Chapter 2, the only oral CHM that appeared in the guidelines was *Bu zhong yi qi tang* 补中益气汤, which was used for postoperative diarrhoea which is a similar condition to that in the guideline. This formula was also used in multiple studies in Chapter 5.

However, few formulas had formal names in Chapter 5 or Chapter 9, so the frequently included herbal ingredients provide a better indication of similarity. The herbs frequently used in the oral formulas in Chapter 9 are distinctly similar to those in Chapter 5 for postoperative recovery (see Table 5.1), suggesting that despite the diversity in formula names, the oral CHMs in the combination studies were similar to those in the RCTs in Chapter 5. Regarding topical herbs for postoperative recovery, *wu zhu yu* 吴茱萸 was commonly used in both Chapter 5 and Chapter 9, but there were too few studies in these groups for other meaningful comparisons.

The frequently mentioned acupuncture points were all recommended for various symptoms associated with CRC. When compared to the points frequently used in the RCTs in Chapter 7, all but the point CV12 *Zhongwan* 中脘 appear in both Table 7.1 and Table 9.4 for acupuncture. Therefore, the acupuncture points used in these studies tend to reflect those in the RCTs in Chapter 7 and the points recommended in the textbooks.

Overall, the results of the studies included in this chapter for combinations of CHM (oral and/or topical) plus acupuncture and/or moxibustion tended to reflect those for postoperative recovery in Chapter 5 (CHM) and Chapter 7 (acupuncture). However, the meta-analysis pools were small and none of the studies were properly blinded, so our confidence in the accuracy of the effect sizes is low. No RCTs were located for combinations of other CM therapies such as as diet therapy or exercise therapies.

Reference

1. Aaronson NK, Ahmedzai S, Bergman B, *et al.* (1993) The European Organization for Research and Treatment of Cancer QLQ-C30: A quality-of-life instrument for use in international clinical trials in oncology. *J Natl Cancer Inst* **85(5):** 365–376.

List of Clinical Studies Included in Chapter 9

Study Number	References
C1	刘俊涛, 韩红, 周文波. (2013) 痛泻要方联合针灸临床治愈结肠癌术后化疗后迟发性腹泻 1 例报告. 实用中医内科杂志 **27(1):** 111–112.

(Continued)

(*Continued*)

Study Number	References
C2	杨楣英. (1991) 针灸治愈直肠癌根治性手术后尿潴留. 四川中医 **(11):** 51.
C3	刘铁龙, 路越. (2015) 中医药干预在结直肠癌围手术期 FTP 模式中的应用. 山东中医杂志 **34(9):** 686–689.
C4	曹志遥, 尹伯约. (2009) 温脾汤加减及针刺配合西医治疗直肠癌术后肠梗阻 5 例分析. 中国肛肠病杂志 **29(7):** 58.
C5	McCullock M, Broffman M, van der Laan M, *et al.* (2011) Colon cancer survival with herbal medicine and vitamins combined with standard therapy in a whole-systems approach: Ten-year follow-up data analyzed with marginal structural models and propensity score methods. *Integr Cancer Ther* **10(3):** 240–259.
C6	余胜珠, 杨光华, 付尚志. (2011) 补中益气汤加减配合艾灸治疗大肠癌术后腹泻的临床观察. 现代中西医结合杂志 **20(27):** 3427–3428.
C7	李志强. (2013) 中西医结合治疗直肠癌术后肠麻痹的 60 例临床观察分析. 中医临床研究 **5(2):** 24–25.
C8	粟艳琴. (2015) 中药保留灌肠配合针灸促进直肠癌术后胃肠功能恢复的疗效观察. 中医药导报 **21(17):** 26–28.
C9	高恒清, 印丽华, 应征. (2014) 隔姜灸联合腹部熨烫促进直肠癌保肛术后胃肠道功能恢复的临床研究. 中国烧伤创疡杂志 **26(5):** 371–374.
C10	邹波峰, 宋海英. (2016) 穴位隔姜灸联合中药贴敷促进大肠癌术后胃肠功能恢复及周围血象影响临床研究. 辽宁中医药大学学报 **18(1):** 123–126.
C11	蒋益兰, 苏乙花, 赵晔, 李剑英. (2014) 艾灸联合穴位敷贴法改善晚期大肠癌患者生活质量的临床观察. 湖南中医杂志 **30(5):** 11–14.
C12	郑军营. (2011) 以吴茱萸热熨为主的中医外治法对结直肠癌术后胃肠功能恢复的影响. 学位论文. 广州中医药大学, pp. 12–21.

10

Summary and Conclusions

OVERVIEW

This chapter summarises the main findings of the previous chapters and provides cross-references between chapters for syndrome differentiation, herbal formulas, acupuncture and related therapies, acupuncture points, and other Chinese medicine therapies. The main results of the meta-analyses of the clinical trials are discussed, as well as the quality of the evidence and its limitations. The implications of the findings of the previous chapters are discussed with regard to the clinical management of colorectal cancer using Chinese medicine. Future directions are proposed for further clinical and experimental research.

Introduction

The conventional management of colorectal cancer (CRC) can involve a number of stages including surgical resection and postoperative recovery, chemotherapy and the management of any associated adverse events, radiotherapy or chemo-radiotherapy, and/or supportive or palliative care. At each of these stages in the CRC journey, various Chinese medicine (CM) therapies may be used as adjuncts to conventional management.

The 'whole-evidence' approach used in this series has identified the main contemporary clinical recommendations for the use of CM in CRC (Chapter 2) and how CRC was managed in the classical medical literature (Chapter 3). The evidence from clinical trials is assessed in Chapters 5, 7, 8 and 9 and experimental evidence on the main herbs used in the studies included in Chapter 5 is reviewed in Chapter 6.

Contemporary clinical guidelines and textbooks include the selection of Chinese herbal medicine (CHM) formulas based on CM syndrome differentiation. There is a focus on orally administered CHMs with modifications based on the person's current condition, and manufactured medicines (*zhong cheng yao* 中成药) with specific actions. In addition, herbal enemas, suppositories, sitz baths, hand and foot baths, and topical cataplasms, fomentations and powders are suggested for specific symptoms. Manual acupuncture, electroacupuncture, moxibustion and ear acupressure can be used to alleviate certain symptoms. In addition, exercise therapies (such as *tai chi* 太极) and various types of *qi gong* 气功, manual therapies (such as *tui na* 推拿), and dietary therapies can be used to maintain physical and psychological health and manage certain symptoms. These approaches are typically used in conjunction with conventional treatment and monitoring in the integrative management of CRC. In the following sections, the recommendation in the contemporary CM guidelines and textbooks (Chapter 2) are cross-referenced to the findings of Chapters 5, 7, 8 and 9 to identify points of similarity and difference.

Chinese Medicine Syndrome Differentiation

The *Guideline of Diagnosis and Treatment of Tumours in TCM* (2008)[1] identified six main syndromes and the associated guiding CHM formulas (Table 2.1) with additional syndromes and formulas from the textbooks (Table 2.2). Since a number of syndrome names contain multiple concepts and overlap, the principal components of the syndromes were identified and these were used for the purpose of comparison (Table 10.1). The acupuncture studies in Chapter 7 were mainly for recovery after surgery and none mentioned syndromes, so the majority of the data were from studies of CHM in Chapter 5 plus two from Chapter 9.

Of the syndromes included in Chapter 2, Spleen deficiency (*pi xu* 脾虚) was by far the most common syndrome in the clinical studies

Table 10.1   Summary of Chinese Syndromes Included in Chapter 2, Chapter 5 and Chapter 9

Syndrome Names[1]	Chapter 2	Chapter 5 (No. of Studies)			Chapter 9[2] (No. of Studies)
		RCT	CCT	Non-controlled	RCT
Spleen deficiency: *Pi xu* 脾虚	Yes	28	3	1	0
Blood stasis: *Yu xue* 瘀血; stasis: *Yu* 瘀	Yes	16	1	1	0
Dampness: *Shi* 湿	Yes	14	0	1	0
Kidney deficiency: *Shen xu* 肾虚	Yes	8	0	0	0
Qi deficiency: *Qi xu* 气虚	Yes	7	1	0	1
Blood deficiency: *Xue xu* 血虚	Yes	5	0	0	1
Heat: *Re* 热	Yes	5	0	1	0
Qi stagnation: *Qi zhi* 气滞	Yes	5	0	0	0
Cancer toxin: *Ai du* 癌毒; toxin: *Du* 毒	Yes	2	1	0	0
Healthy qi deficiency: *Zheng qi xu* 正气虚	No	2	0	0	0
Phlegm: *Tan* 痰	No	2	0	0	0
Yin deficiency: *Yin xu* 阴虚; Liver and Kidney *yin* deficiency: *Gan shen yin xu* 肝肾阴虚	Yes	2	0	0	0
Yang deficiency: *Yang xu* 阳虚	Yes	0	0	0	0
Spleen and Stomach deficiency: *Pi wei xu ruo* 脾胃虚弱	No	0	2	0	0
Spleen deficiency and sunken qi: *Pi xu xia xian* 脾虚下陷; sunken middle *qi*: *Zhong qi xia xian* 中气下陷	No	1	0	1	0

[1]Some studies included more than one syndrome.

[2]The non-controlled studies in Chapter 9 did not mention any specific syndromes and there was no mention of syndrome differentiation in the acupuncture studies in Chapter 7.

Abbreviations: CCT, non-randomised controlled clinical trial; RCT, randomised controlled trial.

(n = 32). Of the other deficiency syndromes, *qi* deficiency (*qi xu* 气虚) was fairly frequent (n = 9), followed by Kidney deficiency (*shen xu* 肾虚) (n = 8) and Blood deficiency (*xue xu* 血虚) (n = 6), with *yin* deficiency (*yin xu* 阴虚) being infrequent (n = 2) and *yang* deficiency (*yang xu* 阳虚) not being mentioned. Of the pathogens, the most common were Blood stasis (*yu* 瘀血) (n = 18) and dampness (*shi* 湿) (n = 15), followed by heat (*re* 热) (n = 6) and *qi* stagnation (*qi zhi* 气滞) (n = 5), with cancer toxin (*ai du* 癌毒) being relatively infrequent (n = 3). There were no syndromes that appeared frequently in the clinical studies but not in Chapter 2, so the syndromes mentioned in the clinical studies tended to reflect those in the guidelines and textbooks.

Chinese Herbal Medicine

In contemporary CM, the use of CHM in conjunction with conventional medicine is common practice in China. This integrative approach ensures accurate diagnosis of CRC and can enable early detection. In contrast, diagnosis in pre-modern times was based on the clinical presentation so it is not possible to be certain which of the conditions described in the classical literature (Chapter 3) would now be diagnosed as CRC. Nevertheless, it seems reasonable to conclude that at least some of the conditions called *zang du* 脏毒 were of gastrointestinal tract bleeding due to CRC and the masses affecting the intestines in the conditions described as *ji ju* 积聚 or *zheng jia* 症/癥瘕 were sometimes cases of CRC. In terms of CHM treatments, there are some similarities, but there are also considerable differences between the classical and contemporary approaches. These differences reflect advances in the understanding of CRC and the shift to an integrative approach to management that involves combinations of surgery, chemotherapy, radiotherapy and CHM. In the past, CHM was the primary treatment for restraining bleeding and reducing masses, but now CHM mainly plays a supportive role, so the frequently used herbs and formulas in Chapter 3 are different to those used in the clinical trials in Chapter 5.

In Chapter 5, the meta-analysis results of RCTs for postoperative recovery indicated that orally administered CHMs improved measures of gastrointestinal recovery when combined with usual care (Table 5.3), the Fast Track Programme (FTP) (Table 5.4) and enteral nutrition (Table 5.5). The Grading of Recommendations Assessment, Development and Evaluation (GRADE) assessments were 'very low' to 'low' (Table 5.9), mainly due to lack of blinding and relatively small sample sizes. Significant improvements were also evident for postoperative abdominal distension, nausea and vomiting, and Karnofsky Performance Status (KPS) (Table 5.6), but not for other measures. A few randomised controlled trials (RCTs) that tested topically applied CHMs also reported improvements in time to recovery of gastrointestinal function.

When orally administered CHMs were combined with various chemotherapy regimens for CRC, there were small, but significant, increases in objective response rate (ORR) based on the World Health Organisation (WHO) criteria and Response Evaluation Criteria in Solid Tumours (RECIST). The meta-analysis results had large sample sizes without heterogeneity (GRADE: 'moderate', Table 5.70). This indicates that the combination of chemotherapy plus CHM improved the response of tumours to treatment. However, it was not possible to determine if this was due to improved response to the chemotherapy, additional anti-tumour effects of the CHMs, immune-enhancing effects of the CHMs, or whether it was a consequence of the alleviation of chemotherapy–related adverse events (AEs) thereby enabling better compliance with chemotherapy. Whether this translated into improved survival was difficult to assess since there were few studies with longer-term data. The available data suggest some improvement in survival rates (Table 5.26), median survival time (MST, Table 5.27), median progression-free survival (mPFS, Table 5.28) and other measures; however, statistical tests were not feasible, so we could not determine if the apparent differences between groups were meaningful.

It is notable that when the experimental studies on the herbs used most frequently in the studies that reported on ORR were reviewed in Chapter 6, there was considerable evidence that herbs such as *huang qi* 黄芪, *she she cao* 蛇舌草 and *ban zhi lian* 半枝莲 show anti-proliferative, anti-angiogenic, and other cancer-inhibitory properties in cell and animal models of CRC.

Measures of quality of life improved in the combination therapy groups (Table 5.30), as did KPS (Tables 5.31 and 5.32). Immune status, in terms of T cell subsets, showed significant improvements (Tables 5.33–5.37), but the results were mixed, leading to considerable heterogeneity in the pooled results.

For the alleviation of AEs associated with chemotherapy, there were significant reductions in severe (grade III + IV) chemotherapy-induced nausea and vomiting (CINV) (Tables 5.39, 5.41) and in all grades of CINV based on large samples. Heterogeneity was absent for grade III + IV events but evident for all grades (WHO criteria). Since GRADE assessments were for all grades of CINV, the certainty of evidence was 'low' (Table 5.71).

There were improvements in a number of measures of chemotherapy-related myelosuppression. These included significant reductions in grade III + IV and all grades of leukopenia (Table 5.46, 5.47), based on large sample sizes, and reductions in grade III + IV and all grades of neutropenia, based on smaller but still substantial sample sizes (Tables 5.48 and 5.49). There were improvements in the incidences of reduced haemoglobin (Tables 5.51 and 5.52) and thrombocytopenia (Tables 5.53 and 5.54). For each of these outcomes, the GRADE assessment was 'moderate' (Table 5.72). For the data on a range of other outcomes see Chapter 5.

Chemotherapy-induced peripheral neurotoxicity (CIPN) was significantly reduced in the combination therapy groups for severe events and all grades of events based on the WHO criteria (Tables 5.57 and 5.58) and Levi's criteria (Table 5.59), but not on the National Cancer Institute-Common Terminology Criteria for Adverse Events (NCI-CTCAE) (Table 5.60), which had the smallest data set. The GRADE assessments were WHO criteria — 'moderate'; Levi's criteria — 'low'; and NCI-CTCAE criteria — 'low' (Table 5.73). There was evidence for a significant reduction in hand and foot syndrome (WHO criteria, all grades) in the sensitivity analysis, but the results for the NCI-CTCAE criteria showed no differences between groups.

In a few studies, CHMs were applied topically in conjunction with chemotherapy. For all levels of CIPN, CHM hand and foot baths showed significant reductions in the incidence of events (Table 5.82), but the certainty of these results was 'low' due to relatively small sample sizes and heterogeneity.

For CHM combined with radiotherapy there were only three RCTs and there were only two RCTs of CHM combined with chemo-radiotherapy. A number of benefits were reported in these studies, but meta-analysis was only feasible for post-radiotherapy immune function, which found increases in some T cell subsets (Table 5.95).

In the supportive and/or palliative care of people with advanced CRC, only three RCTs were available and meta-analysis was only feasible for KPS, which showed a significant improvement in the CHM groups compared to usual care alone. There were also seven case-series studies. Survival outcomes were reported in two of the RCTs and four of the case-series studies (Table 5.99). This tended to be improved in the CHM groups in both the RCTs and the non-controlled studies, but meta-analysis was not feasible.

Data on the safety of the CHMs were lacking in many studies. There were few opportunities for meta-analysis of the safety of CHM for postoperative recovery, CHM combined with radiotherapy or chemo-radiotherapy, and CHM in supportive or palliative care. For CHM combined with chemotherapy, the meta-analysis results indicate that there were no reductions in the response of the tumour to chemotherapy in the groups that combined CHM with chemotherapy and there were no significant increases in hepatotoxicity (Tables 5.63–5.66), nephrotoxicity (Tables 5.67 and 5.68), or skin rash.

Chinese Herbal Medicine Formulas in Key Clinical Guidelines and Textbooks, Classical Literature and Clinical Studies

In this overview of which CHM formulas appeared in multiple chapters, Table 10.2 lists all the CHM formulas from Chapter 2 and all formulas that appeared in two or more clinical studies. Modified versions of formulas are grouped together. These formulas were

Table 10.2   Summary of Oral Chinese Herbal Medicine Formulas Included in Chapter 2, Chapter 3, Chapter 5 and Chapter 9

Formula Names	Chapter 2	Chapter 3 (No. of Citations)	Chapter 5 (No. of Studies)			Chapter 9[1] (No. of Studies)
			RCT	CCT	Non-controlled	RCT
Liu jun zi tang 六君子汤*	Yes	4	5	0	1	0
Huai jiao wan 槐角丸, *Huai hua san* 槐花散, *Huai jiao di yu tang* 槐角地榆汤*	Yes (all 3)	26	0	0	0	0
Ge xia zu yu tang 膈下逐瘀汤*	Yes	0	1	0	0	0
Zhi bai di huang wan 知柏地黄丸, *Liu wei di huang wan* 六味地黄汤*	Yes	0	2	0	0	0
Bu zhong yi qi tang 补中益气汤	Yes	1	2	0	1	1
Bai tou weng tang 白头翁汤*	Yes	0	2	0	1	0
Li zhong wan 理中丸*	Yes	0	0	0	0	0
Si wu tang 四物汤, *Tao hong si wu tang* 桃红四物汤*	Yes	4	4	0	0	0
Shen ling bai zhu san 参苓白术散*	Yes	0	2	0	0	0
Si shen wan 四神丸	Yes	0	0	0	0	0
Ba zhen tang 八珍汤, *Shi quan da bu tang* 十全大补汤*	Yes[2]	0	2	0	0	0
Si jun zi tang 四君子汤*	Yes	1	4	2	0	0
Si mo tang 四磨汤	No	0	2	0	0	0

Formula Names	Chapter 2	Chapter 3 (No. of Citations)	Chapter 5 (No. of Studies)			Chapter 9[1] (No. of Studies)
			RCT	CCT	Non-controlled	RCT
Da cheng qi tang 大承气汤, *Jia wei hou pu san wu tang* 加味厚朴三物汤*	No	0	3[a]	0	1	1[b]
Da jian zhong tang 大建中汤	No	0	0	2	0	0
Da chai hu tang 大柴胡汤	No	0	2	0	0	0
Ling gui zhu gan tang 苓桂术甘汤	No	0	2	0	0	0
You gui wan 右归丸	No	0	2	0	0	0
Fu fang ban mao jiao nang 复方斑蝥胶囊	Yes	0	2	0	0	0
Hua chan su pian/jiao nang 华蟾素片/胶囊	Yes	0	1	0	0	0

*Modified formula; (a) Included one that used topical CHM (H23) and one study of the related formula *Jia wei hou pu san wu tang* 加味厚朴三物汤 (H14); (b) Used CHM enema.

[1]The non-controlled studies in Chapter 9 did not mention any of these formulas.

[2]*Shi quan da bu tang* 十全大补汤, which includes all the ingredients of *Ba zhen tang* 八珍汤, was in Chapter 2 whereas variants of *Ba zhen tang* 八珍汤 were mentioned in the clinical studies in Chapter 5.

Abbreviations: CCT, non-randomised controlled clinical trial; CHM, Chinese herbal medicine; RCT, randomised controlled trial.

cross-referenced to the formulas used in the clinical trials in Chapter 5 and Chapter 9.

Of the CHM formulas included in the guideline and textbooks (Chapter 2), 11 (including modified versions) were test interventions in at least one clinical study. Of these, the most frequently used were *Liu jun zi tang* 六君子汤 (including modifications) and the related formula *Si jun zi tang* 四君子汤 (including modifications) which each appeared in six studies. This is consistent with Spleen deficiency and *qi* deficiency being the dominant syndromes. Modified versions of *Si wu tang* 四物汤 or *Tao hong si wu tang* 桃红四物汤 appeared in four RCTs, reflecting the importance of Blood stasis as an aspect of CRC syndromes. *Bu zhong yi qi tang* 补中益气汤 appeared in four studies of postoperative diarrhoea, including one that mentioned the syndrome sunken middle *qi*. Modified versions of *Bai tou weng tang* 白头翁汤 were used in three studies, whereas the other formulas from Chapter 2 were used in two or fewer studies.

Of the formulas not included in Chapter 2, *Da cheng qi tang* 大承气汤 was used in four studies, while the formulas *Si mo tang* 四磨汤, *Da jian zhong tang* 大建中汤, *Da chai hu tang* 大柴胡汤, *Ling gui zhu gan tang* 苓桂术甘汤 and *You gui wan* 右归丸 were each used in two studies.

A number of the formulas in Chapter 2 were also included in the classical literature (Chapter 3). The related formulas *Huai jiao wan* 槐角丸, *Huai hua san* 槐花散 and *Huai jiao di yu tang* 槐角地榆汤, which are used to restrain bleeding, appeared as variants or in combination with other formulas in 26 classical citations, but not in any of the clinical studies. Other formulas that appeared in the classical literature, as well as in the clinical studies, were *Liu jun zi tang* 六君子汤 (*n* = 4) and *Si jun zi tang* 四君子汤 (*n* = 1), multiple variations of *Si wu tang* 四物汤 (*n* = 6), and *Bu zhong yi qi tang* 补中益气汤 with additions (*n* = 1).

There were a few opportunities for meta-analysis of specific formulas. Modified *Liu jun zi tang* 六君子汤 showed significant reductions in measures of postoperative recovery of gastrointestinal function based on two RCTs (GRADE: 'very low', Table 5.14). One of these two RCTs showed significant increases in immunoglobulin levels but the other did not, so there were no significant differences in the pooled results (Table 5.11). The pooled results from two RCTs of *Si mo tang* 四磨汤

did not show a significant improvement (GRADE: 'very low' to 'low', Table 5.13). For postoperative diarrhoea, *Bu zhong yi qi wan/tang* 补中益气丸/汤 plus anti-diarrhoea medicines versus anti-diarrhoea medicines alone did not show a significant improvement (Table 5.12). When combined with chemotherapy, the pooled result for two RCTs of *Liu jun zi tang* 六君子汤 (including modified versions) showed no significant improvement in KPS (Table 5.113). In all of these meta-analyses the sample sizes were small and the studies were not blinded, so it is difficult to draw any conclusions regarding the certainty of the effects.

Acupuncture and Related Therapies

A range of acupuncture interventions (manual acupuncture, electroacupuncture, ear acupressure and moxibustion) are included in the guideline and textbooks (Chapter 2) for the management of a diversity of symptoms associated with CRC. The traditional methods, manual acupuncture and moxibustion, were both mentioned frequently in the classical literature (Chapter 3) and appeared in RCTs in Chapters 7 and 9 (Table 10.3). Overall, moxibustion was used less

Table 10.3 Summary of Acupuncture-related Therapies Included in Chapter 2, Chapter 3, Chapter 7 and Chapter 9

Acupuncture Therapy[1]	Chapter 2	Chapter 3 (No. of Citations)	Chapter 7 (No. of Studies)[2]		Chapter 9 (No. of Studies)[2]	
			RCT	Non-controlled	RCT	Non-controlled
Acupuncture/ electroacupuncture	Yes	54	12	2	8	3
Moxibustion	Yes	29	3[a]	0	5	0
Ear acupuncture/ear acupressure	Yes	0	4	0	0	0

Including one study of warm needling (A12).

[1]Some studies used more than one intervention e.g. acupuncture plus moxibustion. These are counted separately in this table.

[2]There were no non-randomised controlled clinical trials (CCT) of acupuncture in Chapters 7 or 9. Abbreviations: RCT, randomised controlled trial.

frequently and was often combined with acupuncture. The modern acupuncture methods of electroacupuncture and ear acupuncture/ ear acupressure were included in multiple RCTs; however, ear acupuncture/ear acupressure was infrequent with only two RCTs of ear acupressure alone and the other two RCTs being of ear acupuncture/ ear acupressure combined with acupuncture on traditional points.

In the classical literature, acupuncture/moxibustion was used for abdominal masses (*ji ju* 积聚 and/or *zheng jia* 症/癥瘕). It was unclear whether the authors intended that acupuncture be used to reduce the mass, but there were clear mentions of acupuncture for the relief of pain and symptoms such as abdominal distension. For *zang du* 脏毒, the acupuncture was mainly used to restrain bleeding and relieve pain.

In the clinical studies in Chapter 7, manual acupuncture, electroacupuncture, acupressure, warm needling, and ear acupuncture/ ear acupressure were all used for recovery after surgery for CRC. The meta-analysis results showed significant improvements in at least some measures of gastrointestinal function in the sham controlled studies of electroacupuncture (two RCTs, GRADE: 'moderate', Table 7.9), the unblinded studies of manual acupuncture (three RCTs, GRADE: 'very low', Table 7.10), the unblinded studies of electroacupuncture (three to six RCTs, GRADE: 'very low', Table 7.11), the single study of warm needling, the single sham controlled study of acupressure, and the studies of ear acupressure (three RCTs, GRADE: 'very low' to 'low', Table 7.16).

In Chapter 9, acupuncture therapies were combined with CHMs for recovery of gastrointestinal function in a number of studies. There were significant improvements in at least some measures in studies of oral CHM plus acupuncture plus CHM fomentation (one RCT, Table 9.6); CHM enema plus acupuncture (two RCTs, Table 9.7); and topical CHM plus moxibustion (two RCTs, Table 9.8); but not for topical CHM plus electroacupuncture (one RCT, Table 9.9).

Overall, the evidence was broadly consistent across the types of acupuncture therapy and suggests that these therapies shortened the time to recovery of gastrointestinal function following surgery. The certainty of the evidence was highest for electroacupuncture since there were multiple sham-controlled studies available for meta-analysis. However, there was considerable variation between studies in the magnitude of the effects, so it was not possible to determine which type of acupuncture therapy was more effective than another. In addition, there was limited evidence in Chapter 7 that acupuncture reduced postoperative abdominal distension (two RCTs) and moxibustion reduced the incidence of all grades nausea and vomiting associated with FOLFOX4 chemotherapy (one RCT). In Chapter 9, CHM plus moxibustion improved postoperative diarrhoea and KPS (one RCT).

Acupuncture Points Used in Key Clinical Guidelines and Textbooks, Classical Literature and Clinical Studies

This section summarises the use of specific acupuncture points in Chapters 2, 3, 7 and 9. Due to the large number of different acupuncture points, only those from Chapter 2 that were also mentioned in at least one of the other chapters are included in the summary in Table 10.4, along with points that appeared in two or more citations in Chapter 3.

Table 10.4 Summary of Acupuncture Points Included in Chapter 2, Chapter 3, Chapter 7 and Chapter 9

Points[1]	Chapter 2	Chapter 3 (No. of Citations)	Chapter 7 (No. of Studies)[2]		Chapter 9 (No. of Studies)[2]	
			RCT	Non-controlled	RCT	Non-controlled
Acupuncture/electroacupuncture/moxibustion						
ST36 *Zusanli* 足三里	Yes	0	14	1	7	2
ST37 *Shangjuxu* 上巨虚	Yes	0	8	0	3	1
SP6 *Sanyinjiao* 三阴交	Yes	0	5	0	0	0
PC6 *Neiguan* 内关	Yes	0	4	1	0	1
LI4 *Hegu* 合谷	Yes	0	4	0	0	0
SP9 *Yinlingquan* 阴陵泉	Yes	0	3	0	0	0
ST39 *Xiajuxu* 下巨虚	Yes	0	2	0	2	0

(Continued)

Table 10.4 (***Continued***)

Points[1]	Chapter 2	Chapter 3 (No. of Citations)	Chapter 7 (No. of Studies)[2]		Chapter 9 (No. of Studies)[2]	
			RCT	Non-controlled	RCT	Non-controlled
SP4 *Gongsun* 公孙	Yes	0	2	0	0	0
ST25 *Tianshu* 天枢	Yes	0	2	0	4	0
CV10 *Xiawan* 下脘	Yes	1	0	1	0	0
CV12 *Zhongwan* 中脘	Yes	0	1	1	2	0
CV13 *Shangwan* 上脘	Yes	1	0	0	0	0
BL20 *Pishu* 脾俞	Yes	3	0	0	0	1
CV6 *Qihai* 气海	Yes	0	0	1	3	0
GV20 *Baihui* 百会	Yes	1	0	1	0	0
BL17 *Geshu* 膈俞	Yes	3	0	0	0	0
CV4 *Guanyuan* 关元	Yes	0	0	1	2	0
TE6 *Zhigou* 支沟	No	1	2	0	0	0
KI17 *Shangqu* 商曲	No	19	0	0	0	0
SP12 *Chongmen* 冲门	No	8	0	0	0	0
BL22 *Sanjiaoshu* 三焦俞	No	5	0	0	0	0
CV8 *Shenque* 神阙	Yes	0	0	0	3	0
BL57 *Chengshan* 承山	No	7	0	0	0	0
GV1 *Changqiang* 长强	No	5	0	0	0	0
BL18 *Ganshu* 肝俞	No	4	0	0	0	0
BL52 *Zhishi* 志室	No	2	0	0	0	0
PC8 *Laogong* 劳宫	No	2	0	0	0	0
Ear acupuncture/ear acupressure						
CO7 *Dachang* 大肠	No	0	2	0	0	0
AH6a *Jiaogan* 交感	Yes	0	2	0	0	0
AT4 *Pizhixia* 皮质下	No	0	2	0	0	0
CO4 *Wei* 胃	Yes	0	2	0	0	0
TF4 Ear *shenmen* 神门	No	0	2	0	0	0

[1]Some studies used more than one intervention e.g. acupuncture plus ear acupuncture. These are counted separately in this table.

[2]There were no non-randomised controlled clinical trials (CCT) of acupuncture in Chapters 7 or 9.

Abbreviations: RCT, randomised controlled trial.

This comparison shows that only five of the points from Chapter 2 also appeared in Chapter 3. Most were located on the midline of the abdomen (CV10 *Xiawan* 下脘 and CV13 *Shangwan* 上脘) or adjacent to the thoracic spine on the back (BL20 *Pishu* 脾俞 and BL17 *Geshu* 膈俞) and were used for distension and/or pain in Chapter 3. In comparison, Chapter 2 suggested CV10 *Xiawan* 下脘 and CV13 *Shangwan* 上脘 as two of a number of points for intestinal obstruction after CRC surgery, together with CV12 *Zhongwan* 中脘 which is located between the other two points and has a similar function. In Chapter 2, BL20 *Pishu* 脾俞 was suggested as one of the points for abdominal distension and pain and for diarrhoea, while BL17 *Geshu* 膈俞 was for nausea and vomiting, and both of these points were suggested for types of myelosuppression.

The other point in both Chapters 2 and 3 was GV20 *Baihui* 百会 at the vertex of the head. Although its specific use was not given in the citation in Chapter 3, as it was one of four points, it is likely it was intended to restrain gastrointestinal bleeding by lifting the weak middle *qi* (*zhong qi* 中气). In Chapter 2, it was still one of the points for blood in the stool and was also used for diarrhoea.

In the clinical studies, three of these five points were used but they were relatively infrequent and only one of the other points from Chapter 3, TE6 *Zhigou* 支沟, was used in the clinical trials. By far the most frequently used points were ST36 *Zusanli* 足三里 and other Stomach channel points on the lower leg, ST37 *Shangjuxu* 上巨虚 and ST39 *Xiajuxu* 下巨虚. This was hardly surprising since the main focus of the acupuncture trials was on recovery of gastrointestinal function and the interventions were applied following CRC surgery so abdominal points would not be suitable. Other points on the leg used in these studies included SP6 *Sanyinjiao* 三阴交 and SP9 *Yinlingquan* 阴陵泉. PC6 *Neiguan* 内关 and LI4 *Hegu* 合谷 were used as arm points for postoperative recovery. It is important to note that these acupuncture points have a range of applications, for example PC6 *Neiguan* 内关 was also for relieving nausea and vomiting and LI4 *Hegu* 合谷, SP6 *Sanyinjiao* 三阴交 and SP9 *Yinlingquan* 阴陵泉 were all used in the study of urinary retention; however, there were few studies of these other outcomes. Each of these points were included in Chapter 2, even though there was no specific recommendation for the management of postoperative ileus or recovery of gastrointestinal function.

It was not possible to make assessments of the relative effectiveness of specific acupoints, since most studies of postoperative recovery used multiple, but overlapping, sets of points. The majority of the studies included ST36 *Zusanli* 足三里 but the high frequency of this point should not be misinterpreted as an indication of its superior efficacy.

In the case of ear points, both AH6a *Jiaogan* 交感 and CO4 *Wei* 胃 were in Chapter 2 and in Chapter 7 where they were used, along with other points, for recovery of gastrointestinal function. The RCTs appeared to show improvements in a number of outcomes but it was not possible to determine which ear points were more or less effective.

Other Chinese Medicine Therapies

This section summarises the evidence from Chapters 2, 3, 8 and 9 for the use of other CM therapies.

In Chapter 2, a number of textbooks mentioned the application of *qi gong* 气功, *tai chi* 太极 and related therapies for improving physical and mental well-being in cancer patients. These were not described in detail since there are a large number of *qi gong* 气功 methods in use and these tend not to be specific for CRC. The classical literature (Chapter 3) also mentioned a number of exercise methods which were specifically aimed at reducing abdominal masses, some of which resemble modern forms of *qi gong* 气功 (Table 10.5).

In the clinical studies, none were located that investigated specific Chinese exercise therapies for CRC. The cohort study in Chapter 9 (C5) that examined survival in people who received CM for CRC included *qi gong* 气功 and *tai chi* 太极, along with CHM and acupuncture in the mix of therapies the cohort received; however, it was not possible to determine which CM therapies led to the reported improvements in survival.

Table 10.5   Summary of other Chinese Medicine Therapies Included in Chapter 2, Chapter 3, Chapter 8 and Chapter 9

Other Therapy[1]	Chapter 2	Chapter 3 (No. of Citations)	Chapter 8 (No. of Studies)[2]	Chapter 9 (No. of Studies)[3]	
			RCT	RCT	Non-controlled
Exercises including *tai chi* 太极, *dao yin* 导引 and *qi gong* 气功	Yes	3	0	0	1
Therapeutic massage including *tui na* 推拿 and *an mo* 按摩	Yes	0	2	1	0
Dietary interventions	Yes	1	0	0	1

[1]Some studies or citations used more than one intervention. These are counted separately in this table.

[2]There were no CCTs or non-controlled studies in Chapter 8.

[3]There were no CCTs in Chapter 9.

Abbreviations: CCT, non-randomised controlled clinical trial; RCT, randomised controlled trial.

One book in Chapter 2 provided a *tui na* 推拿 intervention that aimed to assist in the recovery of stomach and intestine function and improve health. No therapeutic massage interventions were located in the classical literature. In Chapter 8, the pooled results from two RCTs (O1, O2) that investigated *an mo* 按摩 therapies found improved measures of postoperative recovery, but no significant change in the rate of postoperative abdominal distension. In Chapter 9, one RCT in advanced CRC (C11) that combined *an mo* 按摩 with moxibustion and a CHM cataplasm, found an improvement in KPS but no significant difference between groups on a measure of quality of life.

In Chapter 2, multiple books provided 13 recipes for special foods that could be used to relieve certain symptoms associated with CRC and/or supplement weaknesses. In the classical literature, only one dietary/fasting method was found for reducing abdominal masses, but this was not similar to modern methods. No RCTs of specific dietary interventions were located but there was a general mention of the use of diet in the cohort study (C5) in Chapter 9.

Overall, the only meta-analysis results from clinical studies of other therapies were from two small RCTs of *an mo* 按摩 therapeutic massage for postoperative recovery. These employed massage methods on acupoints similar to those used in the acupuncture studies (Chapter 7) and the combination therapy studies (Chapter 9) and reported results consistent with the studies in these chapters.

Limitations of the Evidence

Each chapter aimed to provide a detailed overview of the current state of the evidence at the time of writing; however, there are a number of limitations to the scope and depth of the coverage.

New guidelines and new clinical and experimental studies of relevance to CRC are being published frequently. New research can result in changes to practice, and when additional studies are added to a meta-analysis, these will inevitably change the effect sizes. In addition, new experiments will shed further light on the mechanisms of action of herbs and their constituent compounds. Consequently we recommend that readers supplement the information in these chapters with searches of the recent literature.

Considering the complexity of the conventional management of CRC, Chapter 1 should be viewed as a brief general introduction to the field, the main guidelines and the main therapies. For further information, readers could consult the most recent versions of the guidelines and review articles on particular topics. Similarly, Chapter 2 relies on a limited range of the available literature and should be considered illustrative of contemporary CM approaches to the integrative management of CRC. For more detailed information, the reader could consider recent books on the management of CRC and authoritative review articles.

Chapter 3 was based on searches of the *Zhong Hua Yi Dian* 中华医典, which was at the time the largest digital collection of CM books. However, this collection does not include every CM book published in the pre-modern era, nor does it include fragmentary texts, or texts recently recovered in archaeological excavations. In the case of the term *zang du* 脏毒, the data were based on a complete search of this term alone. However, due to the prohibitively large number of citations of the terms *ji ju* 积聚 and *zheng jia* 症/癥瘕 (aggregations and accumulations), the search results were focused by combining these terms with *chang* 肠 (intestine). This approach inevitably led to some omissions of citations relevant to CRC, so the data for these terms should be considered as a sample. Consequently, there may have been other citations in the classical literature that were consistent with CRC but were not found in these searches. Another limitation is the low diagnostic precision possible in the classical literature. At best, the identified citations may have been CRC due to the absence of a more likely explanation. Since none of the citations could be identified as CRC with certainly, the reader should exercise appropriate caution when interpreting the results of this chapter.

In Chapters 5, 7, 8 and 9, the participants in the RCTs were all diagnosed with CRC. Studies of mixed cancers and studies with unclear diagnostic criteria were excluded. Moreover, studies were required to provide data on well-established clinical outcomes. Consequently, a large number of studies did not meet all the inclusion criteria. This was especially the case for non-RCTs, leading to a relatively small number of such studies. With regard to the meta-analysis results, data were available for a large number of comparisons and outcomes in Chapter 5, but the volume of data was highly variable across outcomes and chapters. When there were many studies available, we subgrouped the data according to the type of CRC and/ or conventional therapy in order to provide more fine-grained analyses, in addition to the overall meta-analysis results. Nevertheless, readers should note that every study had its own individual characteristics which cannot all be captured in consolidated data. Since all studies are identifiable via the study numbers and the lists at the end of each chapter, we encourage readers to follow up on their areas of interest by referring to the original studies.

Differences between studies led to elevated statistical heterogeneity in some meta-analysis pools. The use of random effects models in all meta-analyses at least partially mitigated the effects of heterogeneity. Sensitivity analyses were used where possible to identify likely sources of heterogeneity, but this was not always successful. When heterogeneity was 50% or higher, our confidence in the effect size estimate was diminished.

Risk of bias was an issue in the majority of studies. About half of the studies included in the main comparisons for CHM (Chapter 5) and acupuncture therapies (Chapter 7) provided adequate data on the method of sequence generation but the only adequately blinded studies were a few sham-controlled RCTs of acupuncture therapies. This lack of blinding is likely to have elevated effect size estimates, more so when more subjective outcomes were involved such as quality of life, but less so when the outcome was based on laboratory reports such as ORR. Nevertheless, lack of blinding limits our confidence in the estimates of effect sizes and we urge caution when interpreting the meta-analysis results. Another issue was the lack of protocols in the majority of studies which made it difficult to determine the extent of selective reporting of outcome measures.

The safety of the interventions used in the studies was not well reported. In the case of CHMs combined with chemotherapies, data were reported for a large number of AEs known to be associated with chemotherapies. The pooled results showed either reductions in the integrative therapy groups or no differences between groups; however, such consolidated data could not determine the proportion of AEs attributable to the CHMs. Also, the range of AEs reported in the RCTs was highly variable, suggesting that publications may only be reporting on a few of the available outcomes. Therefore, it was not possible to make accurate assessments of the numbers and types of AEs associated with the groups that received CM interventions, usually in conjunction with conventional interventions, compared to the AEs in the control groups.

The CHM interventions used in the clinical studies were variable in terms of their ingredients and form (pill, capsule, granule, decoction, etc.). It was not feasible to include full details of all the CHM interventions. Some are described where space permits; otherwise, the main ingredients are summarised in the tables. Few studies provided adequate data on the quality standards of the CHM interventions. Most simply provided ingredient lists in Chinese, and/or manufacturer names. In the herb frequency tables, the Chinese names have been converted to scientific names but some herbs can be derived from multiple species, so there may be regularisation errors in the tables in favour of the dominant species.

Implications for Practice

The clinical guideline and expert recommendations summarised in Chapter 2 form a basis for syndrome differentiation and the prescription of appropriate CHM formulas. In addition, CHM interventions are typically modified according to the presentation of the particular person and the circumstances of their CRC treatment, including the concomitant use of conventional therapies. It is notable that the majority of the clinical studies were of the integrative management of CRC and even when CHM was used as a stand-alone therapy, it was in the context of overall integrative management and oversight. Similarly, acupuncture was used as an adjunctive therapy, mainly to hasten recovery after surgery. Hence, we caution against interpreting the results of the meta-analyses as indicating the effectiveness of CHM or acupuncture for CRC. Rather, these results indicate that CHM and acupuncture therapies can have beneficial roles in the overall integrative management of CRC.

Notably, both CHM and acupuncture therapies appear to enhance recovery after surgery for CRC and the data for acupuncture is partly based on blinded studies, lending greater credence to the reported effects. Considering the relative simplicity of the acupuncture therapies, hospitals could consider incorporating these interventions into their programmes for postoperative recovery.

In the alleviation of chemotherapy-related AEs, addition of CHMs to the chemotherapies showed a number of benefits. For alleviation of nausea and vomiting the results showed significant reductions in WHO grade III+IV events without heterogeneity. Similarly, there was evidence for relief of WHO grade III+IV diarrhoea, both based on samples of over 1,000 participants. These results suggest that CHM could be considered an option for people who have insufficient relief from conventional anti-emetics or anti-diarrhoea medications. In the case of measures of myelosuppression, the meta-analysis result indicated improvements in grade III + IV leukopenia and thrombocytopenia based on substantial sample sizes, as well as improvements in other measures. Severe myelosuppression may lead to the cessation of chemotherapy,[2] so clinicians could consider the use of CHM in people who develop myelosuppression in order to enable completion of the chemotherapy.

The results for ORR showed that when CHMs were combined with chemotherapies, there was no reduction in the effectiveness of the chemotherapy with regard to reduction of the tumour. Conversely, the CHMs may confer a small benefit. This suggests that when CHMs are used to alleviate chemotherapy-related AEs, they do not counter the benefits of the chemotherapy. This result should not be misinterpreted as an indication that the CHMs on their own were responsible for the increase in ORR. Although the experimental studies suggest that a number of CHMs contain specific compounds that control proliferation in cell and animal models, the clinical evidence does not focus on single herbs or single compounds. It is important to note that frequency lists of ingredients in clinical studies do not imply that the higher frequency herbs are more effective. These are summary data to inform clinicians and researchers. In the clinical setting it remains unclear which CHMs can reduce tumour growth, under what circumstances there is response, and what degree of tumour response can be achieved. Therefore, we strongly caution against the exclusive use of CHM or other CM therapy in the management of CRC and suggest that integrative approaches should be considered.

Implications for Research

The majority of the studies were not blinded so it was likely that this led to overestimations of effect sizes. Although blinding is difficult when CHM decoctions are used, it is feasible for CHMs that have been manufactured into pills or capsules.[3] For acupuncture therapies, a number of 'sham' methods and devices have been developed,[4,5] some of which were used in the clinical studies in Chapter 7. However, there remain questions regarding whether these methods are truly inert and whether they can achieve effective blinding[6] so future studies may consider the addition of a control arm (unblinded) which employs conventional management alone. It is also important that the effectiveness of blinding should be assessed and the results reported.

Future clinical studies should conform to all aspects of clinical trial methodology, with regard to trial registration and the provision of a protocol and the monitoring of safety by an independent committee. In addition, RCTs should employ rigorous methods for the generation of the randomisation sequence and the concealment of allocation, and use proper statistical methods for dealing with dropouts and other types of missing data.[7] Each of these aspects is important in reducing the risk of bias in the results in order to obtain meaningful estimates of the clinical effects of the interventions.

In the case of studies of CHMs, complete and sufficiently detailed information on the nomenclature, amounts and quality of the herbal ingredients and the processes involved in manufacture and or preparation should be provided.[8,9]

In general, the clinical trial reports were brief and did not provide all the information required by the Consolidated Standards of Reporting Trials (CONSORT)[10] or the extensions for herbal medicine,[11] or acupuncture.[12,13] Inadequate reporting was at least partially due to most Chinese journals not endorsing CONSORT or an equivalent guideline for trial reporting standards.[14] Researchers should work to improve reporting standards since this is likely to lead to broader dissemination of study results internationally.

Although there have been a considerable number of RCTs of CHMs for CRC, these tested a diversity of formulas and only a few studies employed the same formulas. Also, while there have been studies that employed formula selection based on syndrome differentiation, these did not provide data for the individual formulas so it was not possible to assess the effectiveness of particular formulas for a particular outcome. Further research is needed to determine the relative effects of different formulas, and different approaches to formula selection, on a range of outcomes in the integrative management of CRC. Such research would facilitate the development of evidence-based guidelines that relate to the stage of CRC and the type of conventional management the person is receiving.

Another clinical area requiring further research is the longer-term outcomes of CM use. A few RCTs provided data on survival outcomes and some longer-term cohort studies have indicated that CHM use improves outcomes[15,16] but these studies were mostly for advanced CRC. Additional long-term studies are needed to determine which people benefit from the addition of CM therapies to their conventional treatment and which therapies are the most effective.

With regard to experimental research, the studies discussed in Chapter 6 indicate that a number of herbs and/or their constituent compounds have pro-apoptotic effects and effects on cell migration and adhesion, inhibit angiogenesis, reduce pro-inflammatory mediators, scavenge free radicals, and/or have various effects on immune response. Also, some herbs appear to enhance the effects of chemotherapeutic agents or counter the effects of drug resistance. However, much of this research is motivated by the search for new compounds that could be developed into drugs, so fractions or single compounds are frequently used and the concentrations of the compounds used in the experiments are high. Consequently, it is difficult to determine the extent to which these experiments reflect the actions of the herbs when ingested by humans. While drug discovery is clearly an important goal of experimental research, it is also important to investigate the likely mechanisms of action of herbs in humans, and the effects of combinations of herbs, in order to gain further insight into their clinical actions.

References

1. 中华中医药学会. (2008) 肿瘤中医诊疗指南 [Guideline of Diagnosis and Treatment of Tumours in TCM.] 北京: 中国中医药出版社.
2. Crawford J, Dale DC, Lyman GH. (2004) Chemotherapy-induced neutropenia: Risks, consequences, and new directions for its management. *Cancer* **100(2):** 228–237.

3. Bian ZX, Moher D, Dagenais S, *et al.* (2006) Improving the quality of randomized controlled trials in Chinese herbal medicine, part II: Control group design. *Zhong Xi Yi Jie He Xue Bao* **4(2):** 130–136.

4. Zhang CS, Yang AW, Zhang AL, *et al.* (2014) Sham control methods used in ear-acupuncture/ear-acupressure randomized controlled trials: A systematic review. *J Altern Complement Med* **20(3):** 147–161.

5. Zhang CS, Tan HY, Zhang GS, *et al.* (2015) Placebo devices as effective control methods in acupuncture clinical trials: A systematic review. *PLoS One* **10(11):** e0140825.

6. Zhang GS, Zhang CS, Tan HY, *et al.* (2018) Systematic review of acupuncture placebo devices with a focus on the credibility of blinding of healthy participants and/or acupuncturists. *Acupunct Med* **36(4):** 204–214.

7. Ellenberg SS. (2012) Protecting clinical trial participants and protecting data integrity: Are we meeting the challenges? *PloS Med* **9(6):** e1001234.

8. Wolsko PM, Solondz DK, Phillips RS, *et al.* (2005) Lack of herbal supplement characterization in published randomized controlled trials. *Am J Med* **118(10):** 1087–1093.

9. Leung KS, Bian ZX, Moher D, *et al.* (2006) Improving the quality of randomized controlled trials in Chinese herbal medicine, part III: Quality control of Chinese herbal medicine used in randomized controlled trials. *Zhong Xi Yi Jie He Xue Bao* **4(3):** 225–232.

10. Schulz KF, Altman DG, Moher D. (2010) Consort 2010 statement: Updated guidelines for reporting parallel group randomised trials. *J Pharmacol Pharmacother* **1(2):** 100–107.

11. Gagnier JJ, Boon H, Rochon P, *et al.* (2006) Reporting randomized, controlled trials of herbal interventions: An elaborated consort statement. *Ann Intern Med* **144(5):** 364–367.

12. MacPherson H, White A, Cummings M, *et al.* (2002) Standards for reporting interventions in controlled trials of acupuncture: The STRICTA recommendations. *J Altern Complement Med* **8(1):** 85–89.

13. MacPherson H, Altman DG, Hammerschlag R, *et al.* (2010) Revised standards for reporting interventions in clinical trials of acupuncture (STRICTA): Extending the Consort statement. *J Evid Based Med* **3(3):** 140–155.

14. Chen M, Cui J, Zhang AL, *et al.* (2017) Adherence to consort items in randomized controlled trials of integrative medicine for colorectal

cancer published in Chinese journals. *J Altern Complement Med* **24(2):** 115–124.

15. Yang YF, Ge JZ, Wu Y, *et al.* (2008) Cohort study on the effect of a combined treatment of traditional Chinese medicine and western medicine on the relapse and metastasis of 222 patients with stage II and III colorectal cancer after radical operation. *Chin J Integr Med* **14(4):** 251–256.

16. Xu Y, Mao JJ, Sun L, *et al.* (2017) Association between use of traditional Chinese medicine herbal therapy and survival outcomes in patients with stage II and III colorectal cancer: A multicenter prospective cohort study. *J Natl Cancer Inst Monogr* **2017(52):** 19–25.

Glossary

Terms	Acronym	Definition	Reference
95% Confidence Interval	95% CI	A measure of the uncertainty around the main finding of a statistical analysis. Estimates of unknown quantities, such as the odds ratio comparing an experimental intervention with a control, are usually presented as a point estimate and a 95% confidence interval. This means that if someone were to keep repeating a study in other samples from the same population, 95% of the confidence intervals from those studies would contain the true value of the unknown quantity. Alternatives to 95%, such as 90% and 99% confidence intervals, are sometimes used. Wider intervals indicate lower precision; narrow intervals, greater precision.	http://handbook. cochrane.org/ Version 5.1; pt 2, 12.4.1.
Acupressure	—	Application of pressure on acupuncture points.	—
Acupuncture	—	The insertion of needles into humans or animals for remedial purposes.	World Health Organisation. (2007).WHO International Standard Terminologies of Traditional Medicine in the Western Pacific Region.

(Continued)

(*Continued*)

Terms	Acronym	Definition	Reference
Allied and Complementary Medicine Database	AMED	Alternative medicine bibliographic database.	https://www.ebsco.com/products/research-databases/allied-and-complementary-medicine-database-amed
Australian New Zealand Clinical Trial Registry	ANZCTR	Clinical trial registry based in Australia.	http://www.anzctr.org.au/
Chemotherapy-induced peripheral neurotoxicity	CIPN	A condition due to the neurotoxic effects of some anti-cancer drugs. It mainly affects the feet and hands causing sensory, motor and autonomic system dysfunction.	—
Chemotherapy-induced nausea and vomiting	CINV	Nausea and vomiting as side effects of chemotherapy.	—
China National Knowledge Infrastructure	CNKI	Chinese language bibliographic database.	www.cnki.net
Chinese Biomedical Literature Database	CBM	Chinese language bibliographic database.	https://cbmwww.imicams.ac.cn
Chinese Clinical Trial Registry	ChiCTR	Chinese clinical trial registry.	http://www.chictr.org.cn/
Chinese herbal medicine	CHM		—
Chinese medicine	CM		—
Chongqing VIP Information Company	CQVIP	Chinese language bibliographic database.	www.cqvip.com
ClinicalTrials.gov	—	Clinical trial registry based in the United States.	https://clinicaltrials.gov/
Cochrane Central Register of Controlled Trials	CENTRAL	Bibliographic database that provides a highly concentrated source of reports of controlled trials.	https://community.cochrane.org/editorial-and-publishing-policy-resource/overview-cochrane-library-and-related-content/databases-included-cochrane-library/cochrane-central-register-controlled-trials-central

(*Continued*)

(Continued)

Terms	Acronym	Definition	Reference
Combination therapies	—	Two or more Chinese medicines from different therapy groups (e.g. Chinese herbal medicine, acupuncture therapies or other Chinese medicine therapies) administered together.	—
Controlled clinical trial	CCT	A study in which people are allocated to different intervention groups using methods that are not random.	https://training. cochrane.org/ handbook
Convention on International Trade in Endangered Species of Wild Fauna and Flora	CITES	International convention aimed at preventing or regulating trade in threatened and endangered species of plants and animals.	https://www.cites.org/ eng/disc/text.php
Colorectal cancer	CRC	Includes tumours of the right colon (caecum, ascending colon), transverse colon, left colon from the splenic flexure downwards, and rectum to anus.	International Agency for Research on Cancer. (2014) World cancer report 2014. WHO Press, Lyon.
Cumulative Index of Nursing and Allied Health Literature	CINAHL	Bibliographic database.	https://www.ebscohost. com/nursing/ products/cinahl- databases
Dukes stage	—	A system used to classify the stage of the tumour. Stage A indicates invasion of, but not through, the bowel wall; stage B involves penetration of the bowel wall into the muscle layer without lymph node involvement; stage C indicates involvement of lymph nodes; and stage D indicates widespread metastases.	Astler VB, Coller FA. (1954) The prognostic significance of direct extension of carcinoma of the colon and rectum. *Ann Surg* **139(6):** 846–852.
Effect size	—	A generic term for the estimate of the effect of a treatment in a study.	http://handbook. cochrane.org/
Effective rate	—	A measure of the proportion of participants who achieved an improvement, as outlined in Chapter 4.	—

(Continued)

(Continued)

Terms	Acronym	Definition	Reference
Electroacupuncture	—	Electric stimulation of the acupuncture needle following insertion.	World Health Organisation. (2007) WHO International Standard Terminologies of Traditional Medicine in the Western Pacific Region.
European Society for Medical Oncology	ESMO	Society that issues guidelines for CRC and other cancers.	https://www.esmo.org/
European Union Clinical Trials Register	EU-CTR	European clinical trial registry.	https://www.clinicaltrialsregister.eu
Excerpta Medica database	Embase	Bibliographic database.	http://www.elsevier.com/solutions/embase
Fast Track Programme of perioperative care	FTP	A package of techniques which aim to enhance recovery after surgery, reduce morbidity, and hence reduce hospital stay.	Polle SW, Wind J, Fuhring JW, *et al.* (2007) Implementation of a fast-track perioperative care program: What are the difficulties? *Dig Surg* **24(6):** 441–449.
Global Cancer Incidence, Mortality and Prevalence	GLOBOCAN	Surveys by the International Agency for Research on Cancer (IARC) that provide global data on a wide range of cancers.	http://www.iacr.com.fr
Grading of Recommendations Assessment, Development and Evaluation	GRADE	Approach used to grade quality of evidence and strength of recommendations.	http://www.gradeworkinggroup.org/
Hand-foot syndrome	HFS	A chemotherapy-related side effect. Symptoms include redness and tenderness of the palms and soles; there can be peeling of the skin and fissures. Also called palmar-plantar erythrodysesthesia (PPE).	—

(Continued)

(*Continued*)

Terms	Acronym	Definition	Reference
Health-related quality of life	HR-QoL	A conceptual or operational measurement that is commonly used in a health care setting as a means to assess the impact of disease on a person.	Brooker C, ed. (2010) *Mosby's Dictionary of Medicine, Nursing and Health Professions.* Elsevier, United Kingdom;
Heterogeneity	—	Used in a general sense to describe the variation in, or diversity of, participants, interventions and measurement of outcomes across a set of studies, or the variation in the internal validity of those studies. Used specifically, as statistical heterogeneity, to describe the degree of variation in the effect estimates from a set of studies. Also used to indicate the presence of variability among studies beyond the amount expected due solely to the play of chance.	https://training. cochrane.org/ handbook Version 5 1; pt 2, 9.5.1.
Hyperthermic intraperitoneal chemotherapy	HIPEC	The direct delivery of highly concentrated, warmed chemotherapy to the abdominal cavity during surgery.	Van Cutsem E, Cervantes A, Adam R, *et al.* (2016) ESMO consensus guidelines for the management of patients with metastatic colorectal cancer. *Ann Oncol* **27**(**8**): 1386–1422.
I^2	—	A measure of study heterogeneity. Indicates the percentage of variance in a meta-analysis.	https://training. cochrane.org/ handbook Version 5.1; pt 2, 9.5.2.
Integrative medicine	IM	Chinese herbal medicine combined with pharmacotherapy or other conventional therapy.	—

(*Continued*)

(*Continued*)

Terms	Acronym	Definition	Reference
Karnofsky Performance Status	KPS	A descriptive scale used to determine the ability of the patient to tolerate chemotherapy. Relates to ability to carry out activities of daily living.	Yates JW, Chalmer B, Mckegney FP. (1980) Evaluation of patients with advanced cancer using the Karnofsky performance status. *Cancer* **45(8):** 2220–2224.
Mean difference	MD	In meta-analysis, a method used to combine measures on continuous scales, where the mean, standard deviation and sample size in each group are known. The weight given to the difference in means from each study (e.g. how much influence each study has on the overall results of the meta-analysis) is determined by the precision of its estimate of effect; mathematically this is equal to the inverse of the variance. This method assumes that all of the trials have measured the outcome on the same scale.	https://training. cochrane.org/ handbook Version 5.1; pt 2, 9.4.5.1.
Meta-analysis	—	The use of statistical techniques in a systematic review to integrate the results of included studies. Sometimes misused as a synonym for systematic reviews, where the review includes a meta-analysis.	—
Moxibustion	—	A therapeutic procedure involving ignited material (usually moxa) to apply heat to certain points or areas of the body surface for managing disease.	World Health Organisation. (2007) WHO International Standard Terminologies of Traditional Medicine in the Western Pacific Region.
National Comprehensive Cancer Network	NCCN	Alliance of leading cancer centres that issues guidelines for CRC and other cancers.	https://www.nccn.org/

(*Continued*)

(*Continued*)

Terms	Acronym	Definition	Reference
National Cancer Institute-Common Terminology Criteria for Adverse Events	NCI-CTCAE	Series of criteria for evaluating adverse events associated with cancer therapy.	National Institutes of Health and National Cancer Institute. (2008) Common terminology criteria for adverse events (CTCAE), version 4. National Institutes of Health, Bethesda, MD.
Non-controlled studies	—	Observations made on individuals, usually receiving the same intervention, before and after the intervention but with no control group.	https://training. cochrane.org/ handbook
Objective Response Rate	ORR	Response of the tumour to treatment. Sum of complete response (CR) and partial response (PR).	—
Other Chinese medicine therapies	—	Other Chinese medicine therapies include all traditional therapies except Chinese herbal medicine and acupuncture/moxibustion, such as *tai chi, qi gong, tui na* and cupping.	—
Postoperative enteral nutrition	PEN	Provision of liquid nutritional support early in the postoperative period.	McClave SA, Taylor BE, Martindale RG, *et al.* (2016) Guidelines for the provision and assessment of nutrition support therapy in the adult critically ill patient: Society of critical care medicine (SCCM) and American society for parenteral and enteral nutrition (ASPEN). *J Parenter Enteral Nutr* **40(2):** 159–211.
PubMed	PubMed	Bibliographic database.	http://www.ncbi.nlm. nih.gov/pubmed

(*Continued*)

(*Continued*)

Terms	Acronym	Definition	Reference
Qi gong 气功	—	Physical exercises and breathing techniques.	—
Randomised controlled trial	RCT	Clinical trial that uses a random method to allocate participants to treatment and control groups.	—
Response Evaluation Criteria in Solid Tumours	RECIST	System for evaluating response of a tumour to therapy. Originally published in 2000, based on the original World Health Organisation guidelines. In 2009, revisions were made (RECIST 1.1).	Schwartz LH, Litiere S, de Vries E, *et al.* (2016) Recist 1.1-update and clarification: From the Recist committee. *Eur J Cancer* **62:** 132–137.
Risk of bias	—	Assessment of clinical trials to indicate if results may overestimate or underestimate the true effect because of bias in study design or reporting.	https://training. cochrane.org/ handbook Version 5.1; pt 2, Chapter 8.
Risk ratio (Relative risk)	RR	The ratio of risks in two groups. In intervention studies, it is the ratio of the risk in the intervention group to the risk in the control group. A risk ratio of 1 indicates no difference between comparison groups. For undesirable outcomes, a risk ratio that is less than 1 indicates that the intervention was effective in reducing the risk of that outcome.	https://training. cochrane.org/ handbook Version 5.1; pt 2, 9.2.2.2.
Standardised mean difference	SMD	Similar to mean difference (MD). Used when different instruments are used to measure the same construct. The SMD expresses the intervention effect in standard units rather than the original units of measurement. As a rule of thumb, an SMD of 0.2 represents a small effect, 0.5 a moderate effect and 0.8 a large effect.	https://training. cochrane.org/ handbook Version 5.1; pt 2, 9.2.3.2, 12.6.2.
Summary of findings	SoF	Presentation of results and rating the quality of evidence based on the GRADE approach.	http://www. gradeworkinggroup. org/

(*Continued*)

(Continued)

Terms	Acronym	Definition	Reference
Tai chi 太极 (*tai ji* 太极)	—	A Chinese martial art with health benefits.	—
TNM classification system	—	A system developed by the American Joint Cancer Committee (AJCC)/ Union for International Cancer Control (UICC), used to classify the stage of the tumour. 'T' is for tumor and denotes the extent of invasion of the intestinal wall; 'N' is for the number of lymphatic nodes invaded and the amount of lymphatic node involvement; and 'M' is for distant metastasis.	Labianca R, Nordlinger B, Beretta GD, *et al.* (2013) Early colon cancer: ESMO clinical practice guidelines for diagnosis, treatment and follow-up. *Ann Oncol* **24(Suppl 6):** vi64–72.
Transcutaneous electrical nerve stimulation	TENS	Application of transdermal electrical current to acupuncture points via conducting pads.	—
Tui na 推拿	—	Chinese massage: rubbing, kneading or percussion of the soft tissues and joints of the body with the hands, usually performed by one person on another, especially to relieve tension or pain.	World Health Organisation. (2007) WHO International Standard Terminologies of Traditional Medicine in the Western Pacific Region.
Wanfang database	Wanfang	Chinese language bibliographic database.	www.wanfangdata.com
World Health Organisation	WHO	WHO is the directing and coordinating authority for health within the United Nations system. It is responsible for providing leadership on global health matters, shaping the health research agenda, setting norms and standards, articulating evidence-based policy options, providing technical support to countries, and monitoring and assessing health trends. It has issued a range of criteria for assessing outcomes in cancer.	http://www.who.int/about/en/

(Continued)

(*Continued*)

Terms	Acronym	Definition	Reference
Zhong Hua Yi Dian 中华医典	ZHYD	A comprehensive series of electronic books on compact disk. The collection was put together by the Hunan Electronic and Audio-Visual Publishing House. It is the largest collection of Chinese electronic books and includes the major Chinese ancient works, many of which are from rare manuscripts and are the only existing copies. These books cover the period from ancient times up to the period of the Republic of China (1911–1948).	Hu R, ed. (2000) *Zhong Hua Yi Dian* [*Encyclopaedia of Traditional Chinese Medicine*], 4th ed. Hunan Electronic and Audio-Visual Publishing House, Chengsha.
Zhong Yi Fang Ji Da Ci Dian 中医方剂大辞典	ZYFJDCD	Compendium of Chinese herbal formulas with over 96,592 entries derived from classical Chinese books. The Nanjing Chinese Medicine Institute compiled the ZYFJDCD and first published it in 1993.	Peng HR, ed. (1994) *Zhong Yi Fang Ji Da Ci Dian* [*Great Compendium of Chinese Medical Formulae*]. People's Medical Publishing House, Beijing.

Index

Evidence-based Clinical Chinese Medicine

Print ISSN: 2529-7562
Online ISSN: 2529-7554

Series Co Editors-in-Chief

Charlie Changli Xue *(RMIT University, Australia)*
Chuanjian Lu *(Guangdong Provincial Hospital of Chinese Medicine, China)*

Published

More information on this series can also be found at https://www.worldscientific.com/series/ebccm

Forthcoming